T0309104

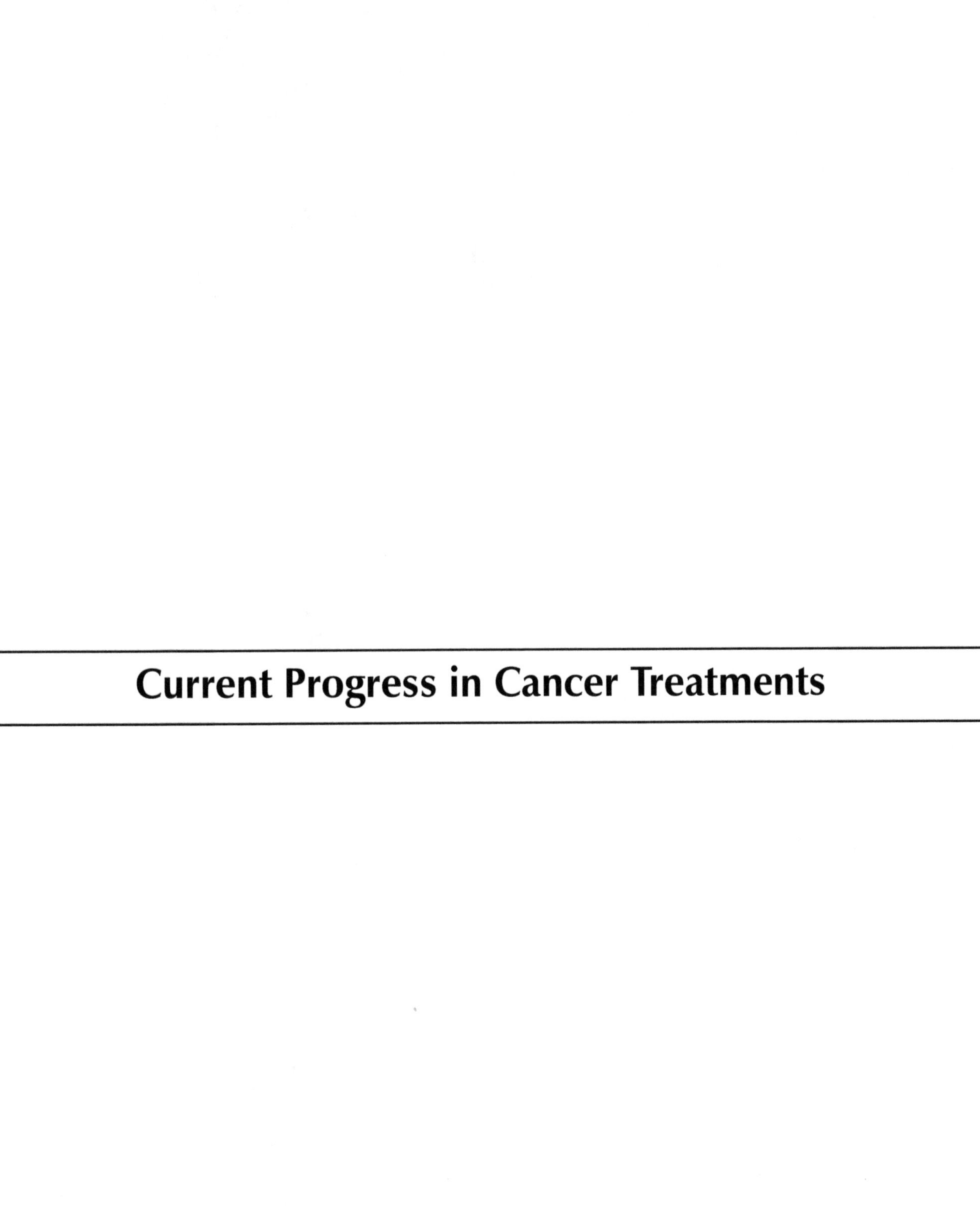

Current Progress in Cancer Treatments

Current Progress in Cancer Treatments

Editor: Judah Horton

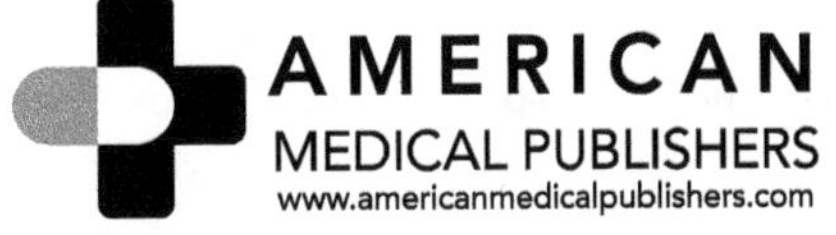

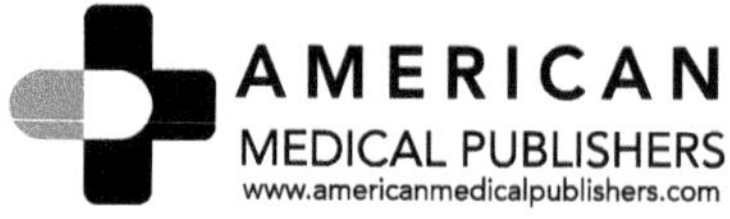

Cataloging-in-Publication Data

Current progress in cancer treatments / edited by Judah Horton.
p. cm.
Includes bibliographical references and index.
ISBN 978-1-63927-647-9
1. Cancer--Treatment. 2. Cancer--Treatment--Technological innovations. 3. Oncology. I. Horton, Judah.
RC270.8 .C87 2023
616.994 06--dc23

American Medical Publishers,
41 Flatbush Avenue,
1st Floor, New York,
NY 11217, USA

ISBN 978-1-63927-647-9 (Hardback)

Contents

Preface

Cancer refers to a type of condition when certain cells in the body grow non-stop and spread to other body parts. It can be treated through a variety of therapeutic approaches, which are selected on the basis of the type and stage of cancer. Radiation therapy, surgery, immunotherapy, chemotherapy, hormone therapy and targeted therapy are some of the traditional therapeutic approaches utilized in the treatment of cancer. Various limitations including multi-drug resistance, lack of selectivity and cytotoxicity act as significant hurdles in effective cancer treatment. The introduction of nanotechnology has transformed the field of cancer diagnosis and therapy. Nanoparticles can be utilized for treating cancer because of their unique benefits, like increased retention and permeability, biocompatibility, improved stability, precise targeting and less toxicity. This book provides comprehensive insights on cancer treatments. It provides significant information to help develop a good understanding of the current progress within this area of study. This book is appropriate for students seeking detailed information on cancer treatments as well as for experts.

This book unites the global concepts and researches in an organized manner for a comprehensive understanding of the subject. It is a ripe text for all researchers, students, scientists or anyone else who is interested in acquiring a better knowledge of this dynamic field.

I extend my sincere thanks to the contributors for such eloquent research chapters. Finally, I thank my family for being a source of support and help.

Editor

1

Repurposing Antibacterial AM404 as a Potential Anticancer Drug for Targeting Colorectal Cancer Stem-Like Cells

Mehreen Ahmed [1], Nicholas Jinks [1], Roya Babaei-Jadidi [1,2], Hossein Kashfi [1], Marcos Castellanos-Uribe [3], Sean T. May [3], Abhik Mukherjee [4] and Abdolrahman S. Nateri [1,*]

1 Cancer Genetics & Stem Cell Group, BioDiscovery Institute, Division of Cancer and Stem Cells, School of Medicine, University of Nottingham, Nottingham NG7 2UH, UK; mehreen.ahmed@nottingham.ac.uk (M.A.); msxnj@exmail.nottingham.ac.uk (N.J.); mszrb3@exmail.nottingham.ac.uk (R.B.-J.); mzxsmk@exmail.nottingham.ac.uk (H.K.)

2 Respiratory Medicine, School of Medicine, University of Nottingham, Nottingham NG7 2UH, UK

3 Nottingham Arabidopsis Stock Centre (NASC), Plant Science Building, School of Biosciences, University of Nottingham, Loughborough LE12 5RD, UK; sbzmc3@exmail.nottingham.ac.uk (M.C.-U.); sbzstm@exmail.nottingham.ac.uk (S.T.M.)

4 Department of Histopathology, Queen's Medical Centre, School of Medicine, University of Nottingham, Nottingham NG7 2UH, UK; mszam2@exmail.nottingham.ac.uk

* Correspondence: a.nateri@nottingham.ac.uk

Abstract: Tumour-promoting inflammation is involved in colorectal cancer (CRC) development and therapeutic resistance. However, the antibiotics and antibacterial drugs and signalling that regulate the potency of anticancer treatment upon forced differentiation of cancer stem-like cell (CSC) are not fully defined yet. We screened an NIH-clinical collection of the small-molecule compound library of antibacterial/anti-inflammatory agents that identified potential candidate drugs targeting CRC-SC for differentiation. Selected compounds were validated in both in vitro organoids and ex vivo colon explant models for their differentiation induction, impediment on neoplastic cell growth, and to elucidate the mechanism of their anticancer activity. We initially focused on AM404, an anandamide uptake inhibitor. AM404 is a metabolite of acetaminophen with antibacterial activity, which showed high potential in preventing CRC-SC features, such as stemness/de-differentiation, migration and drug-resistance. Furthermore, AM404 suppressed the expression of *FBXL5* E3-ligase, where AM404 sensitivity was mimicked by *FBXL5*-knockout. This study uncovers a new molecular mechanism for AM404-altering FBXL5 oncogene which mediates chemo-resistance and CRC invasion, thereby proposes to repurpose antibacterial AM404 as an anticancer agent.

Keywords: AM404; cancer stem cells; colonosphere; CRC; differentiation; drug screening; FBXL5 E3-ligase; patient derived organoids; resistance and metastasis; tissue explants

---

1. Introduction

Colorectal cancer (CRC) is the fourth most common cancer and leads to approximately 500,000 deaths a year worldwide [1]. For patients with CRC, chemotherapy remains the most common treatment but often followed by tumour regrowth due to acquired chemotherapy-resistance. Experimental evidence supports the role of small fraction of cancer stem-like cells (CSCs) in the tumour, including colorectal cancer [2–4]. CSCs exhibit several distinctive features such as enhanced self-renewal and limited differentiation capacity that allow them to be resistant to anti-cancer therapies and tumour-targeted drugs, which in turn, helps them to survive treatment and initiate tumour recurrence [5].

However, selective targeting of CSC is a huge challenge from the therapeutic point of view as strategies not being sufficiently selective for CSCs also increase risks of recurrence among the patients [6]. Therefore, there is an ever-growing need for novel compounds and drugs that target CSCs, preferably in combination with other cytotoxic drugs and tumour-targeted agents to prevent the regrowth of neoplastic cell populations.

Several multidimensional approaches have been utilized to target specific markers or pathways to eliminate CSCs, alter tumour microenvironment, induce differentiation, re-sensitization to chemotherapy, apoptosis, and reversal of epithelial-mesenchymal transition (EMT) [7,8]. Nevertheless, the association of stem cell signatures with disease outcome in several types of cancer is widely established. Due to the characteristic features of cancer and their association with other diseases, it is also important to investigate these cancer traits in order to target them. For example, inflammation is one of the major hallmarks of cancer [9], as evident at the earliest stages of cancer progression and is capable of fostering growth of small tumors into metastatic cancers [10]. In addition, some FDA approved commercially available antibacterial and anti-inflammatory drugs are currently being studied for their potential in targeting CSCs. Such examples include salinomycin, curcumin, metformin, vismodegib, EGCG, imetelstat, heparin, resveratrol, tranilast, amongst others [11–14]. Therefore, investigating the parameters and drugs greatly benefits the study of cancer therapeutics. Based on this hypothesis, we carried out drug screening on a library of 707 FDA (the Food and Drug Administration) approved small molecule compounds with anti-inflammatory, antibacterial activities using 3D colonosphere as a model representing CRC-SC [15,16]. We have validated and used stem cell fluorescent probe (i.e., CDy1) as a reporter for the rapid screening of compounds in their differentiation-inducing potential [17,18]. Our further analysis of patient-derived tumour explant and organoid models and the molecular mechanisms data has identified antibacterial AM404 as a potential candidate for targeting CRC stem-like cells.

AM404 is a metabolite of acetaminophen with antibacterial activity, also known as N-arachidonoylphenolamine with a chemical formula of $C_{26}H_{37}NO_2$ [19]. Acetaminophen (N-acetyl-*para*-aminophenol or paracetamol) is one of the most commonly used over-the-counter drugs for its analgesic and antipyretic properties [20]. Following its administration, AM404 has been reported in human cerebrospinal fluid [21]. Acetaminophen undergoes de-acetylation to p-aminophenol in both liver and nervous system and p-aminophenol is conjugated with arachidonic acid to produce AM404 in the nervous system. It has been suggested that AM404 may be responsible for the analgesic mechanism of paracetamol [19]. Some studies have demonstrated AM404s antibacterial and anti-inflammatory effects in reducing oxidative stress are associated with the presence of the phenolic group in its structure (Figure 1A) [19,22,23]. Currently, there is no established data available for AM404 in colorectal cancer. Our data suggest that ubiquitin-ligase FBXL5 [24–27], might be a key target through which AM404 utilizes its pharmacological effects on CRC cells.

2. Results

2.1. A Screen of the NIH Clinical Collection Small Molecule Library Identifies Potential Anti-Cancer Drug AM404

The 3D colonospheres were obtained from HCT116, DLD-1 and SW480 human CRC cell lines according to their colonosphere forming efficiencies and were employed into a fluorescence-based screening of US National Institute of Health (NIH) clinical library consisting of 707 small molecule inhibitors (Figure S1). One particular advantage of this screening was that it has been carried out on live colonospheres without any fixation step involved. Prior to the compound library screening, we initially carried out a pre-screening study with stem cell dye CDy1 using a HDAC inhibitor and *FBXW7* deleted CRC cells (Figure S1 and Table S1). Vorinostat (SAHA) is a potent HDAC inhibitor that has previously been reported to induce differentiation and has undergone Phase I and II clinical trials [28–30]. On the other hand, our lab and others have reported FBXW7 as one of the most frequently mutated genes in CRC, and have associated its loss with chromosomal instability, cellular proliferation, EMT, and overall tumorigenesis [31–34]. In order to carry out the pilot-screening, we incorporated both vorinostat treatment (to induce differentiation) and HCT116$^{FBXW7(-/-)}$ derived colonospheres (to represent high tumorigenesis), within the CDy1 based screening system.

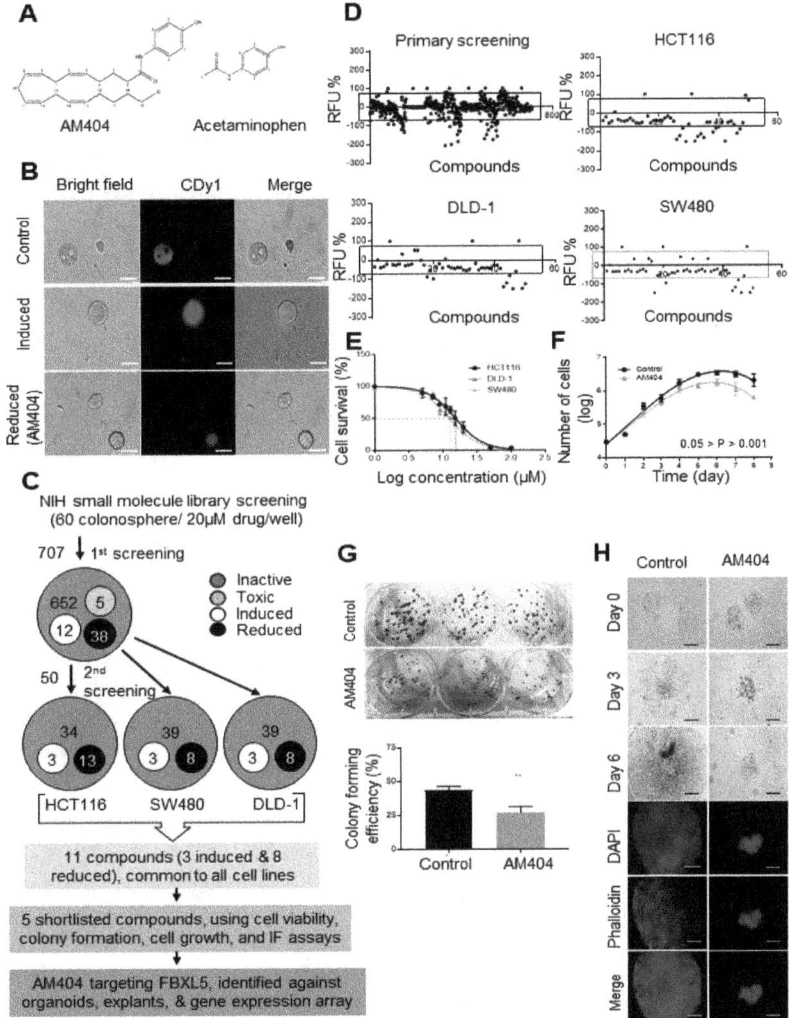

Figure 1. Screening of NIH library containing 707 small-molecule inhibitors, can induce 3D colonosphere differentiation. (**A**) Structural formula of AM404 and acetaminophen. (**B**) Representative images of the fluorescence intensity conferred by CDy1 on compounds and control-treated colonospheres obtained from HCT116 cells. Top row represents untreated colonospheres intensity, whereas middle and bottom row represent induced and reduced intensity as measure of induce and reduced stem-like characteristics upon treatments. Scale bar: 25 μM. (**C**) Summary of screening. (**D**) Primary screening based on fluorescence intensity influenced by small molecules on colonospheres derived from HCT116 cells. Each dot represents one compound ($n = 2$). All compound treated colonosphere intensities were expressed as percentage of the control-treated intensities as an indication of induced or reduced stemness. Compounds outside the square-zone were selected for a rescreening. At the end of rescreening ($n = 3$), 11 common compounds from 3 cell lines were selected based on their potential on CDy1 intensity induction and/or reduction. (**E**) IC_{50} of AM404 in HCT116, DLD-1 and SW480 cell lines. IC_{50} was measured at 15.2, 15.3 and 12.3 μM respectively. (**F**) Growth curve of AM404-treated DLD-1 cells. Student's *t*-test was performed for the statistical analysis. Error bars represent mean ± S.D. ($n = 3$). $0.05 > p > 0.001$. (**G**,**H**) AM404 showing morphological alteration and significant reduction in colony formation assay in DLD-1 cell line. ** $p \leq 0.01$. Scale bar: 75 μm.

Our results showed CDy1 intensities were significantly reduced in vorinostat-treated colonospheres, whereas, it was induced in HCT116$^{FBXW7(-/-)}$ derived colonospheres, further demonstrating successful use of CDy1 as an indicator of stemness/differentiation induction. Based on the pre-screening, well defined colonospheres derived from HCT116 cells were collected carefully with mild agitation and ensured of uniform transfer (~60 colonospheres/well) in 96 well plates. Colonospheres were then treated with 707 compounds (at final concentration of 20 μM) for 72 h before selectively stain the live stem cells, as magnitude of drug-induced stemness and/or differentiation level represented by high and low CDy1 fluorescence intensity respectively. HCT116 cells were primarily chosen for the initial screening based on their highly aggressive, resistant and non-differentiating nature [35]. The concentration of compounds was selected based on previous studies being carried out at 10 μM in monolayer cells, in line with results from our lab showing significantly higher resistance with 3D colonospheres than 2D cells [5,33]. Initial screening identified 50 compounds based on distinct morphology changes, colonosphere sizes and CDy1 intensity (Figure 1B–D and Table S2). Next, we carried out a re-screening using other CRC cell lines (SW480 and DLD-1), in addition to HCT116 cells (Figure 1D) that identified 11 compounds for their ability in inducing and/or reducing stem-like prowess (Table S2). Amongst the compounds that reduced the stem-like characteristics, more recent work showed that the antifungal drug itraconazole targets cell cycle heterogeneity, and epirubicin targets metastasis and DNA-damage induced-drugs resistance in CRC [36,37]. However, the SRB assay was used for over a wide range of doses (1 to 100 μM) to calculate the half-maximal inhibitory concentration (IC50) which defined AM404 as a better candidate with an IC_{50} that is lower than the target threshold (20 μM) for further in-depth evaluations [5]. This result was backed by the previous studies reporting AM404 to be well tolerated on animal models and being less toxic on mammalian cells including human HEK-293, HepG2, and, Panc-1 cells for up to the 4X of the MIC, indicating its relatively safe profile [22,23]. Our results were highly comparable between the DLD-1 and HCT116 cell lines, with IC50 of 15.3 and 15.2 μM respectively, whereas, AM404 shows slightly more sensitivity towards SW480 with an IC_{50} of 12.3 μM (Figure 1E). Next, cells were treated with the IC_{50} of AM404 (Figure 1E) on day 1 and were counted every day for a period of 8 days. AM404-treated DLD-1 cells showed a shift in the population doubling time (PDT) from 21 h to 29 h as shown in control-treated cells. This lag in the doubling time indicates significant impedance on cell growth (Figure 1F). Our results showed a significant reduction in the number of colonies during the treatment along with their morphological alteration upon AM404 treatment (Figure 1G). Reduction in colony size was strongly evident within the first three days of treatment, which was also seen in the growth curve (Figure 1G,H). Phalloidin staining significantly distinguishes the morphological differences conferred by AM404 in DLD-1-treated colonies (Figure 1H). Next, we examined the effect of AM404 on the sensitivity to the drugs 5-fluorouracil (5-FUra) and oxaliplatin (Oxa) that are widely used for cancer treatment, particularly for CRC [38]. Also, we have previously investigated the sensitivity to 5-FUra and Oxa drugs and showed that FBXW7-deficiency-induced chemoresistance [33,39].

Our results indicated that $HCT116^{FBXW7(-/-)}$ cells treated with AM404 were more sensitive to treatment with these drugs, following synergistic effects with CI < 1 (Figure 2A,B, Figure S2) [40,41]. These results further confirmed AM404 as a potential anticancer drug candidate in CRC cells.

2.2. *AM404 Inhibits De-Differentiation and Acquisition of Stem-Like Properties*

The relative changes in colonospheres size/shape were assessed by treating the fully grown colonospheres on day 14. AM404 treatment showed distinct morphological alteration in colonospheres, which could be related to cell polarity, cell-cell attachment, EMT, resulted by differentiation induction; however, the number of colonospheres remained the same after the treatment (Figure 2C). Characterization of the inhibition pathway involved in the mechanism of action of AM404 on CSC-like properties and the sensitivity to chemotherapeutics, as evidenced in the colonospheres, was initially performed by gene expression analysis from mRNA isolated from colonospheres of roughly the same size using qRT-PCR analysis. Notably, a significant reduction in expression level was observed for *CD44*, *NANOG*, *LGR5*, *OCT4* and *BMI-1* stem cell markers, *CXCR4* and *c-JUN* oncogenes, whereas, *KRT20* and *CDX2* differentiation markers and *FBXW7* tumour suppressor genes were significantly increased upon AM404 treatment in the colonospheres (Figure 2D–F). Furthermore, immunofluorescence assay on AM404 treated colonospheres with well-established differentiation marker MUC2 and stemness CD44 also revealed high expression pattern with MUC2 (Figure 2G,H). Thus, several established stem cell markers, CRC prognostic factors, and differentiation markers have also revealed the potential of AM404 in targeting stem-like cells.

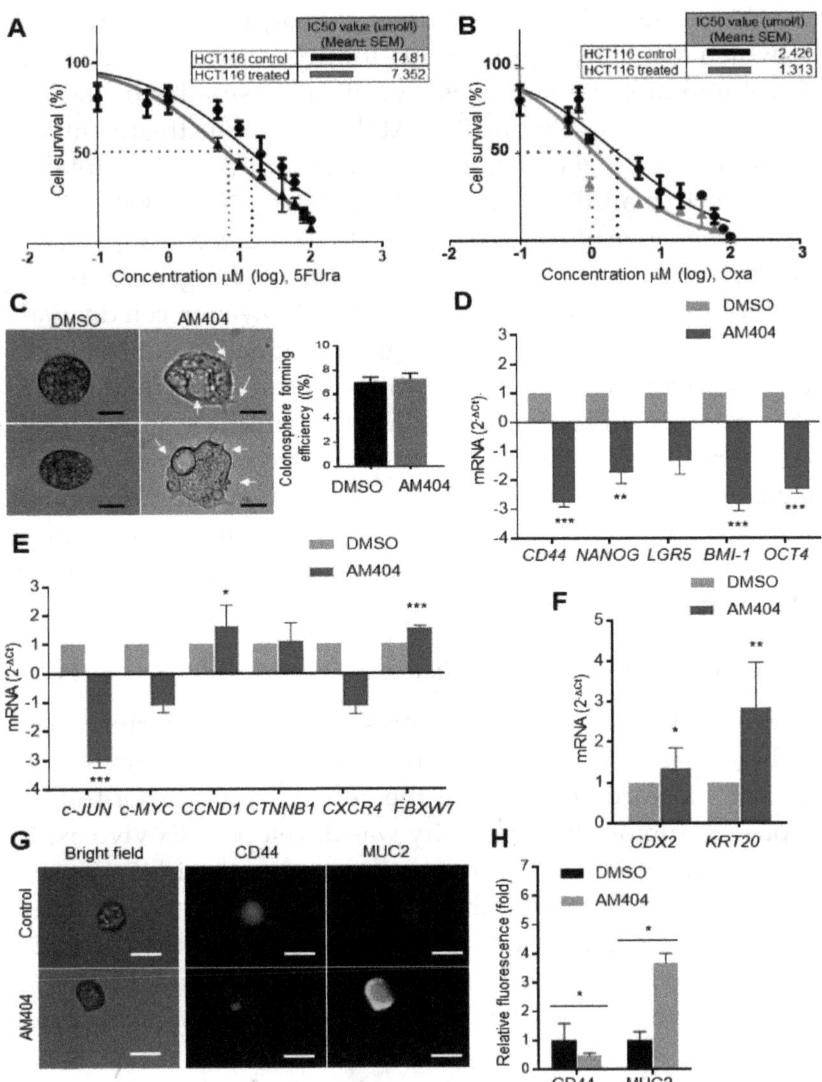

Figure 2. AM404 association with stem-like characterizes and differentiation. (**A**,**B**) Survival of synchronized/ serum-starved FBXW7-deficient HCT116 cell lines (HCT116$^{FBXW7(-/-)}$). Black colour indicates treatment with 10 increasing concentrations of 5-FU (**A**) and Oxaliplatin (**B**), whereas red indicates co-treatment with AM404. SRB colorimetric assay was performed in triplicate for each cell line on three independent occasions. IC_{50} values, calculated by using GraphPad Prism software 7.02, represent the mean of three different experiments ± SEM with $p \leq 0.005$. Cells co-treated with AM404 are found to be more sensitive to 5-FU (**A**) with an IC_{50} of 7.35 vs. 14.8 μM and to Oxaliplatin (**B**) with an IC_{50} of 1.3 vs. 2.4 μM. (**C**) AM404 showing morphological alteration in colonosphere with no change in colonosphere formation efficiency. Scale bar: 25 μM. (**D**–**F**) qRT-PCR analysis of CRC-SC (**D**), stemness (**E**), transcription factor for recurrence, poor survival, metastasis and tumour suppressor, and (**F**) differentiation in DLD-1 derived colonospheres treated with AM404. Student's *t*-test was performed for the statistical analysis. *, $p \leq 0.05$; **, $p \leq 0.01$; ***, $p \leq 0.001$. (**G**) Immunofluorescence assay of AM404 treated colonospheres using stemness and differentiation markers, Scale bars: 25 μm. (**H**) AM404 treatment shows increased MUC2 expression and reduced level of CD44 expression suggesting induction of differentiation upon drug treatment (right panel, $n = 15$, $p \leq 0.05$).

As a first step towards mimicking the patient tumour tissues, we used CRC patients' derived organoids [42,43], to study specific cell-type response to drugs [44]. Organoids were cultured and allowed to start budding for 5–6 days prior to treating them with AM404. The 2 weeks treatment period was chosen based on the majority of control-treated organoids grew >700 μm and covered the limited space within the wells after a total period of 3 weeks. When compared to control-treated tumour organoids, AM404 appeared to induce distinct morphological changes such as branching formation (Figure S3), which may indicate of AM404-induced differentiation (Figure 3A, arrowheads, and Figure S3). The volume of organoids was significantly smaller in the AM404-treated group (197 μm^3 vs. 86 μm^3; $0.05 > p > 0.001$). (Figure 3B). At the end of the treatment, only 10% of organoids were measured to be as more than 700 μM, as compared to the 30% of total organoids in control group. Similarly, in reference to all the organoids being larger than 300 μM in control group, 20% organoids were still within the range of 100–300 μM in AM404 treated group, on day 14 of the treatment (Figure 3C). This result shows a high population of AM404-treated organoids being in smaller diameter range, suggesting its inhibitory effect on organoid growth. However, cell dead/alive status identified by PI/Hoechst staining. AM404 treatment showed slight/no reduction in PI staining followed by 6 days treatment period in tumour organoids (Figure 3D), while differentiation markers *CDX2* expression were significantly increased (Figure 3E). In addition, after AM404 withdraw on day 14 of the treatment, signs and symptoms of the differentiation, only some of the treated organoids were reversed. This result suggests minimal/no changes in cell death caused by AM404 on tumour organoids. Our results are consistent with previously reported evidence that AM404 is well tolerated on mammalian cells and in animal models [22,23]. Taken together, these results may indicate that AM404 induces differentiation and thereby affects CRC-SCs.

2.3. *Ex Vivo Treatment of CRC Patient Biopsies Evaluates AM404 Response As an Anticancer Drug*

Our results from monolayer cells, colonospheres, and patient-derived organoids have shown that AM404 impedes the growth and can induce morphology change while reducing the stem-like properties. Further studies towards mimicking the clinical response of the tumour environment, an ex vivo platform capturing tumour heterogeneity was developed. Ex vivo explants have previously been reported to be more viable in the short-term culture method [45,46]. Fresh tumour tissues were obtained from CRC patients following their surgery and processed immediately for culturing explants. To validate AM404's response on stemness, differentiation and proliferation deliberated in tumour tissues, we have selected 15–17 h for the explants to recover after initial generation, based on published data [45,46]. Following analyses of AM404 responses were also performed for 24 h, at its IC_{50} (Figure 1E).

IHC analysis of AM404 treated explants showed a trend of decreasing cell proliferation and stemness with increasing differentiation marker (Figure 4). This was found to be consistent for tumour explants generated from all the CRC patients, with 5–6 images analysed per tumour sample. Overall, 24-h treatment with AM404 significantly reduced Ki-67 staining and the proliferation level in tumour explants by 20% (Figure 4A, right panel). However, Caspase-3 staining showed, not a significant number of cells will necessarily die in response to AM404 (Figure 4B). Therefore, to associate AM404 with cellular differentiation and stem-like activity, we utilized CDX2 and CD44v6 as markers for differentiation and 'stemness' in tumour explants (Figure 4C,D).

Overexpression of CDX2 has been shown previously to induce differentiation as well as to inhibit proliferation and is therefore, frequently downregulated during tumorigenesis [47]. We used the H-score system to quantify CDX2 expression in both control-treated and AM404 treated groups (Figure 4C, left panel). Our result showed a significant increase in CDX2 expression in tumour explants treated with AM404 (Figure 4C, right panel). CD44v6 is a multifunctional transmembrane glycoprotein and it has long been used as a marker of colorectal cancer stem cells, and is associated with cell adhesion, growth, differentiation, migration and tumour progression. CD44v6 positive cells have been reported to have the characteristics of stem cells and have a higher level of proliferation and invasion than CD44v6 negative cells [48,49].

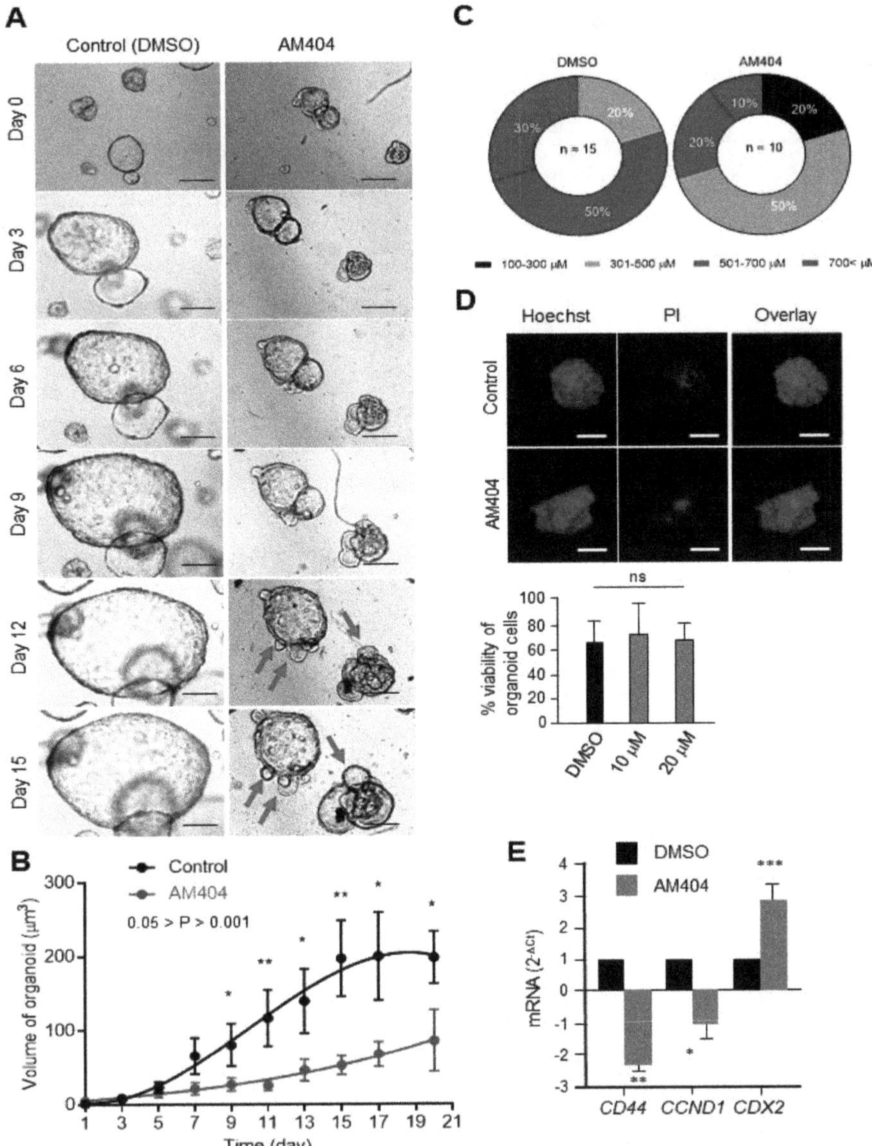

Figure 3. AM404 treatment altered CRC patients-derived organoids growth and morphology patterns. (**A**) Representative images of tumour organoids treated with AM404 for a period of 2 weeks. Tumour organoids were cultured and allowed to grow for 5-6 days prior to the treatment. AM404 was added to its IC_{50}. Both AM404 and control-treated groups were maintained with changing of medium every other day. Morphological alteration and variation in growth were observed throughout the treatment period. Images were taken using Leica microscope. Scale bar: 75 µm. (**B**) AM404 treatment causes growth impairment in tumour organoid. Volumes of organoids were measured every 2 days. AM404 treatment shows significant inhibition to the tumour growth as compared to control-treated group. Error bars represent mean ± SEM. ($n = 15$; control, $n = 10$, AM404). $0.05 > p > 0.001$. (**C**) Number of organoids in different size groups at the end of the treatment. Numbers in each size group are expressed as percentage of the total. In treated group, only 10% of organoids were measured as more than 700 µM, as compared to the 30% of total organoids in control group. (**D**) Hoechst/PI staining on AM404 treated organoids. The similar pattern in PI staining in both AM404 and control-treated group indicates no changes in cell death upon AM404 treatment. Scale bar: 25 µM. (**E**) qRT-PCR analysis of AM404 treated compared with control untreated patients derived organoids for CD44, cyclin-D1 and CDX2. Student's *t*-test was performed for the statistical analysis. *, $p \leq 0.05$; **, $p \leq 0.01$; ***, $p \leq 0.001$.

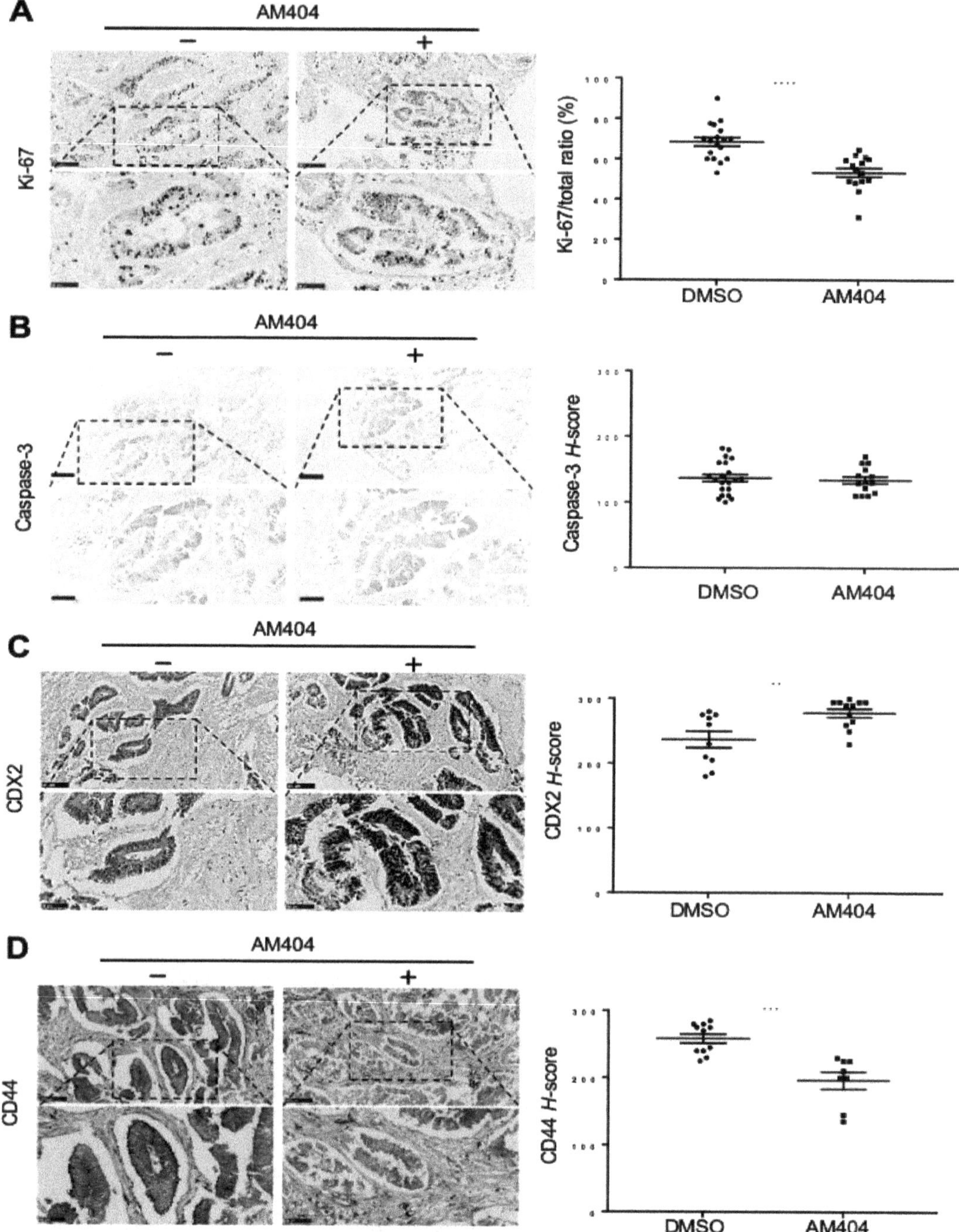

Figure 4. AM404 treatment impacts on cancer cell proliferation, stemness and differentiation in the patients-derived CRC tissues explants (7 patients). (**A**–**D**) Proliferation was assessed by quantitating Ki-67 (A) IHC staining, cell survival by caspase-3 (**B**), whereas differentiation and stemness levels were assessed by CDX2 (**C**) and CD44 (**D**) staining quantification respectively. IHC stains were counterstained with hematoxylin and eosin. Representative images (top panel) shows the images at 20× magnification with a scale bar of 100 µm. Bottom panel shows the selected parts in higher 40× magnification with scale bar 50 µm in control (DMSO) and AM404-treated groups. Each dot (Right panels) represents an image used for quantification. Student's *t*-test was performed for the statistical analysis. Control treated groups represents the level of intrinsic proliferation, stemness and differentiation level in tumours. For the Ki-67 staining, Ki-67 + ve cells were counted and expressed as a percentage of the total cells. In case of CD44 and CDX2 and Caspase-3, H-scores were counted as a measure for the quantification. AM404 treatment showed significant reduction in proliferation and stemness levels, and significant increase in the differentiation level in tumour explants.

In line with the proliferation pattern, CD44v6 expression was also reduced by AM404 treatment on the tissue explants (Figure 4D, right panel). Thus, treating these tumour explants with AM404 showed a reduction in proliferation and stemness while also increasing the level of differentiation characteristics.

2.4. FBXL5 Attenuates AM404-Induced Anticancer Activity

To identify the targets associated with AM404's mechanism on CRC, the transcriptome of DLD-1-colonospheres treated with AM404 and controls was compared. Microarray analysis emphasizing on 2 or more-fold changes ($p < 0.001$) revealed 323 differentially expressed genes (Figure 5A, Figure S4 and Table S3). As predicted by the status of colonospheres, the gene ontology (GO) pathways for 75 genes with 2.5 or more-fold changed were mainly associated with cell cycle, DNA damage, and protein ubiquitination/ degradation signalling (Figure S5A,B). Among these top biological processes, and 16 genes with changes of 3-fold or greater (Figure 5B,C), protein ubiquitination was one of the major gene expression regulatory groups. In general, the specificity of proteolysis for any particular substrate is determined by its association with a specific E3-receptor subunit. F-box proteins are the substrate-recognition components of the Skp1-Cul1-F-box-protein (SCF) E3-ubiquitin ligases. Accordingly, F-box proteins can function as oncoproteins when overexpressed (if their substrates are tumour suppressors) or as tumour suppressors (if their substrates are oncoproteins). For example, we have extensively studied FBXW7, a commonly mutated tumour suppressor gene in human tumours including 10–15% of CRC, which, we found to be significantly increased upon AM404 treatment (Figure 2D) [34,39,50]. However, characterization of many other F-box proteins is required for their roles in cancer, which could be a key breakthrough for cancer therapy and offer a potential new biomarker(s) for early detection of epithelial tumour progression including CRC. Therefore, we have selected *FBXL5* gene, which showed over three folds decrease upon AM404 treatment (Figure 5B–F), functioned as an oncogene in the progression of colon cancer through regulating PTEN/PI3K/AKT signalling [24] and HIF-1α transcriptional activity [26].

FBXL5 (F-box and leucine-rich repeat protein 5), also known as FBL4 and FBL5, is a member of the F-box protein family, characterized by an F-box motif consisting of 40 amino acids [24,26,51]. It is predominantly an iron and oxygen-regulated SCF-type E3 ubiquitin ligase containing an N-terminal hemerythrin-like domain, α-helix-rich structure [51,52]. Therefore, we initially sought to examine whether the expression of *FBXL5* was altered in patients' colorectal cancers.

These results indicated a lower expression of *FBXL5* mRNA in normal/healthy tissues adjacent to the tumours (Figure 6A). Notably, Yao et al., showed post-surgical patients with high expression of *FBXL5* had shorter overall survival than patients with low FBXL5 expression [24]. Based on our data suggesting AM404's effect in CSC-like activity (Figure 2), and recent studies indicating FBXL5 regulating CRC metastasis [23,25,26], we then wanted to elucidate whether AM404 exerted its noted effects via FBXL5 in CRC cells [24,26,27]. We have therefore generated CRISPR-Cas9 mediated *FBXL5*-knockout in DLD-1 cell line (Figure 6B and Figure S6). The cytotoxicity assay of the *FBXL5*-knockout cell line further confirmed that loss of FBXL5 induced sensitivity of cells (11.5 μM vs. 15.3 μM; $0.05 > p > 0.001$) to AM404 than that of the control-treated cells (Figure 6C). In addition, knockout of *FBXL5* caused an inhibition of colony formation efficiency in DLD-1 cells (KO1 & KO2) (Figure S6A). Our microscopic study for Phalloidin stained DLD cells showed that *FBXL5*-knockout cells (KO) displayed branched, flat, and elongated shape with prominent actin fibers (Figure 6D). Furthermore, we synchronised cells by serum starvation, and performed scratch wound healing assays [53]. The result showed that AM404 significantly reduces the migration of DLD-1 cells (Figure S6B and Figure 6E, Black vs. Red columns). Consistent with the cell morphology observation, the wound-closure of *FBXL5*-knockout cells versus control cells expressing Cas9 is significantly reduced (Figure S6B and Figure 6E, Black vs. Gray columns). AM404, being sensitive to *FBXL5*-knockout cells, showed to mimic this effect and caused further additive effect in inhibiting cell migration (Figure S6B and Figure 6E, Red vs. Blue columns). Furthermore, in between two treatment groups, AM404 treatment caused significant reduction in cell migration in *FBXL5*-knockout cells than that of WT DLD-1 cells (Figure 6E). This finding postulates FBXL5 as a potential target via which AM404 exerts its effects on CRC cells migration.

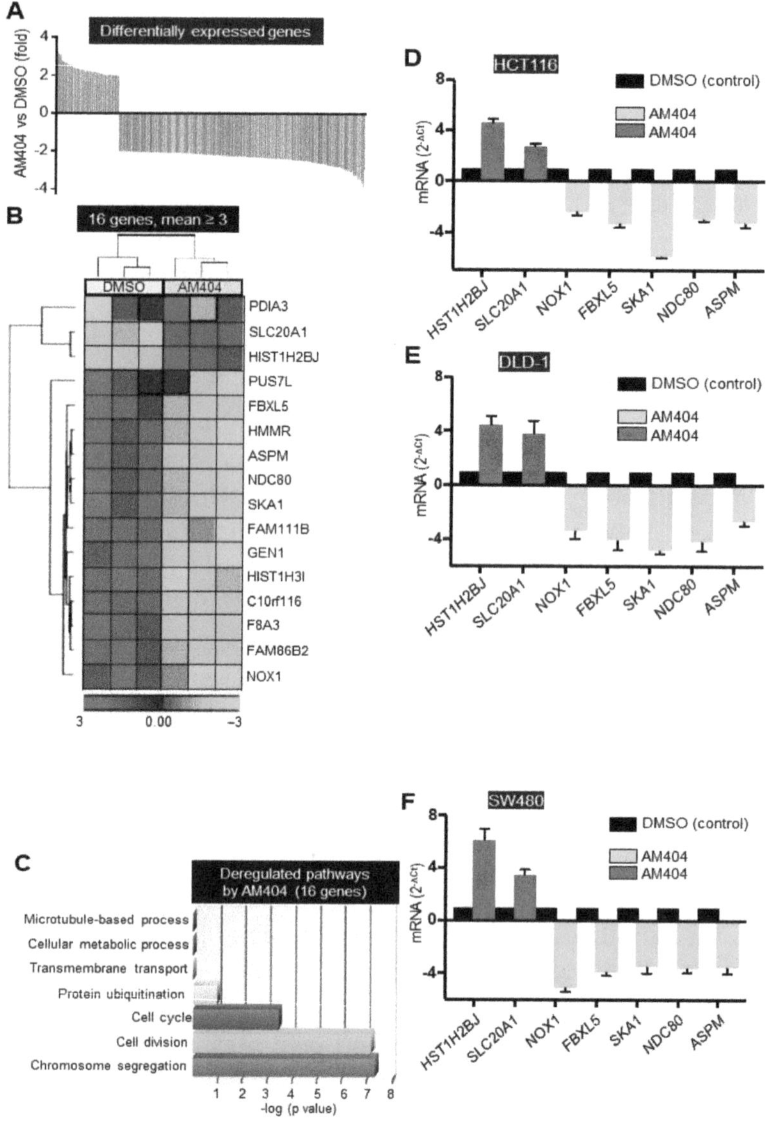

Figure 5. AM404 treatment altered genes expression profile of DLD-1 colonospheres. (**A**) Differentially expressed genes on colonospheres treated with AM404. Each bar represents one gene that has a *p*-value of 0.001 or less and is 2 or higher fold increased or decreased on colonospheres following the drug treatments. (**B**) Heat-map representation of unsupervised clustering of the 16 differentially expressed genes (mean ≥3-fold change) by AM404 in colonospheres. Each row represents a gene. Each column represents a sample: yellow, control (DMSO treated) and blue, AM404 treated colonospheres. Colour code within the graph represents log2 of the fold change of expression: green, downregulated; red, upregulated. Horizontal and vertical clusters were created based in Euclidean distance. (**C**) Gene ontology biological processes revealing the top biological processes affected by the sixteen genes represented in B. Functional annotation clustering with default settings was used; medium stringency and Benjamini–Hochberg correction was applied. Only the enriched GO terms with FDR < 0.05 were selected and displayed in the bar chart. The full list of differentially expressed genes can be found in Tables S2 and S3 and their GO biological processes enrichment in Figures S3 and S4. (**D**–**F**) mRNA expression levels of seven genes with differential expression including *FBXL5* by AM404 obtained from the microarray analysis were confirmed by RT-qPCR analysis in colonospheres derived from HCT116 (**D**), DLD-1 (**E**) and SW480 (**F**) cells. Student's *t*-test was performed for the statistical analysis. Error bars represent SEM.

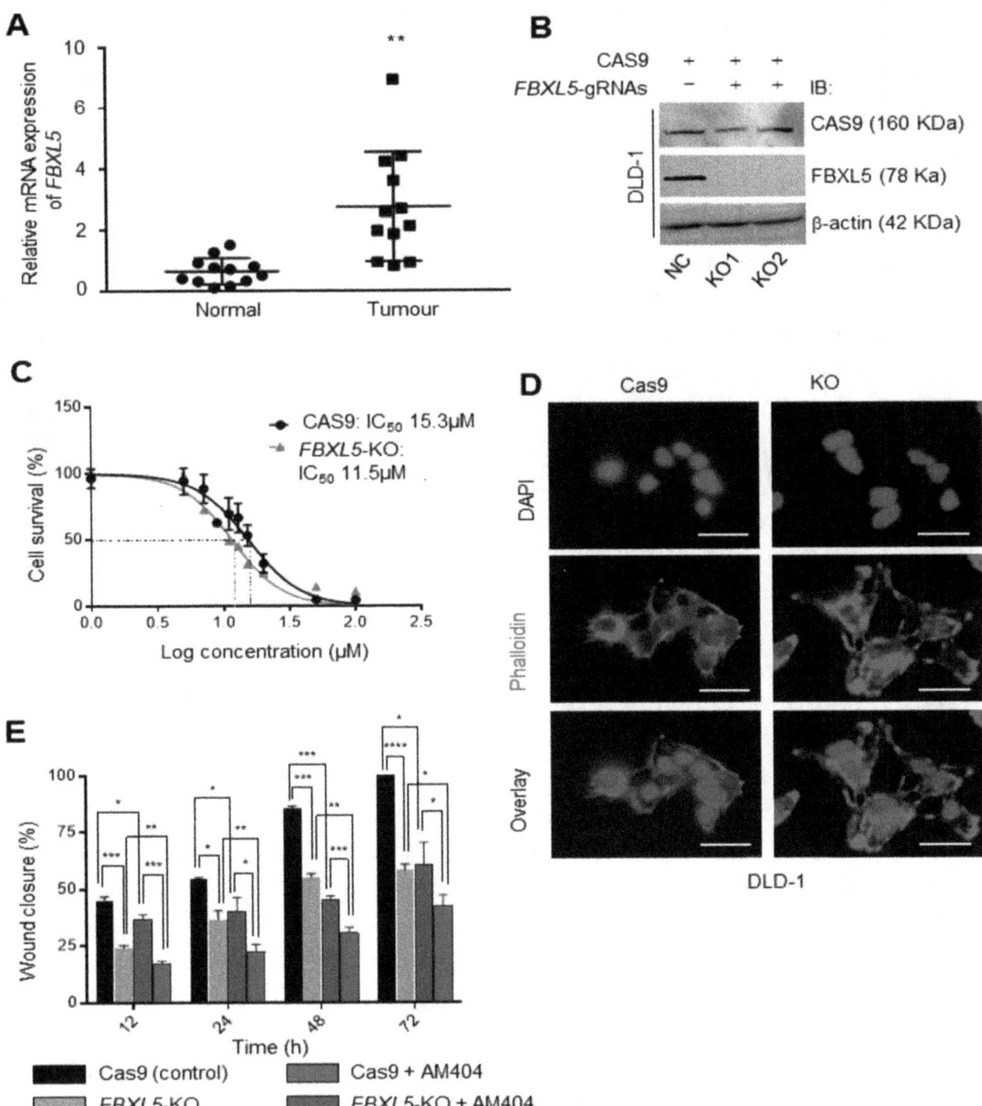

Figure 6. AM404 association with FBXL5 in CRC. (**A**) qRT-PCR analysis of *FBXL5* mRNA expression in a cohort of twenty-two; normal adjacent and tumour tissues from patients with CRC in Nottingham, UK, normalized to Hypoxanthine-guanine phosphoribosyltransferase (HPRT). Student's *t*-test was performed for the statistical analysis. Data are mean ± SEM ($n = 3$; **, $p \leq 0.01$). Experiments were performed in triplicate for each sample and repeated on two independent occasions. (**B**) Western blot analysis of FBXL5 expression in DLD-Cas9 (control) and DLD-Cas9:FBXL5-gRNAs (CRISPR-knockout) cell lines (KO1 and KO2). β-actin was used as loading control (Figure S7). (**C**) IC_{50} of AM404 on *FBXL5*-KO cell lines. FBXL5-KO cells are found to be more sensitive to AM404 with an IC_{50} of 11.5 μM. (**D**) FBXL5 modulates cell adhesion and morphology. These cells were stained with Phalloidin and visualized under fluorescent microscope. Scale bars, 50 μm. (**E**) AM404 significantly inhibited migration in DLD-1 and FBOXL5-KO-DLD-1 cells in vitro. Migration of DLD-1 and FBOXL5-KO-DLD-1 cells was performed with scratch wound healing assay. Starved cells were scratch-wounded and wound width was measured to determine the healed distance (please see Figure S6B). Significant reduction in cell migration was observed for both cell lines. Bars are expressed as mean ± SEM. ($n = 3$). *, $p < 0.05$; **, $p < 0.01$; ***, $p < 0.001$; ****, $p < 0.0001$.

3. Discussion

In summary, the 3D models used throughout the study provides means of reproducible, rapid, low cost and patient relevant platform not only for drug screening, but also for the preclinical evaluation of novel anticancer agents. Based on this platform, we have identified the anti-bacterial AM404 as a potential candidate to target CRC cells via supressing the oncogenic E3 ligase FBXL5. We speculate that AM404 modulated FBXL5 expression might reduce polarized epithelial cells to inhibit migration to distant sites.

Infection and chronic inflammation are major causes of cancer. Our understanding of the molecular pathways and links between inflammation and cancer is continuously improving. AM404 is currently being studied for its antibacterial and anti-inflammatory effects notably for reducing the production of IL-1β, IL-6 as well as decreasing oxidative stress and for their association with circulating tumour necrosis factor (TNF)-α [19]. Previously, AM0404 has been reported to inhibit NF-κB and NFAT activation on neuroblastoma and glioma cells. NF-κB is one of the key transcription factors in cancer associated inflammation transition process, regulated via TNF and various cytokines including IL-6 [54,55]. In neuroblastoma cells, AM404 inhibited the NF-κB activation by targeting IKKβ phosphorylation and activation 57 In addition, AM404 also impaired COX-2 expression, PGE2 release, migration and invasion in a cell specific manner [56,57]. Inhibition of COX-2 has an anti-tumorigenic effect in cancers that occurs due to prolonged chronic inflammation. Several pathways including Wnt–β catenin, PIK3CA/AKT/PTEN, and NF-κB, have been postulated as targets for NSAIDs [54]. FBXL5 has previously been interpreted as oncogene whilst its association in iron regulation is required for HSC self-renewal [52]. In CRC progression, FBXL5 has shown to induce cell proliferation, growth, tumorigenesis and inhibit cell apoptosis by modulating PTEN/PI3K/AKT signalling and its overexpression resulted in high tumour formation ability [24,27]. Furthermore, they have also been reported to negatively regulate several EMT inducers, such as Notch, c-Myc and mTOR, particularly in gastric and cervical cancer [24,51]. We showed that AM404 associated cell homeostasis caused reduction of CRC 'stemness' features, including cell proliferation, migration, tumour growth, morphology, and induction of CRC differentiation. It has been markedly reported that, silencing FBXL5 showed decrease in metastasis with significant increase in expression of E-cadherin at posttranscriptional level [27]. In line with this, we showed that AM404 significantly reduced the expression level of N-cadherin and Vimentin (Figure 2E), and by mimicking the effect of *FBXL5* deletion, it also significantly prevented the invasion in CRC cells (Figure S5B and Figure 6E). When used in FBXL5-KO-cells, AM404 showed sensitivity and further additive effect in preventing cells invasion suggesting AM404 as a new compound to target FBXL5 in blocking CRC cell migration. We currently do not have an in vivo intestinal/colon model that implicit FBXL5 as a potential therapeutic target for cancer stem cells, although an essential role of FBXL5-mediated cellular iron homeostasis in the maintenance of hematopoietic stem cells has already been reported [52].

This study demonstrates the application of colonospheres, organoids and explant models to screen new compounds and helps improving our understanding of the inflammatory mediators involved in CRC. This study thereby also helps reducing, and potentially replacing animal models and may provide novel preventive, diagnostic and therapeutic strategies.

One of the major hallmarks of cancer highly focuses on inflammation specifically for cancer progression, development and proliferation. Due to this correlation, preclinical focuses highlighted several antibacterial, anti-inflammatory drugs for repurposing in cancer treatment. In the study of Sharma et al., [19] AM404 was detectable in plasma of only eight of the 26 plasma samples, with three being above 5 nmol/L, which warranted an unidentified mechanism in some individuals through which AM404 leaks out of the brain and into the blood. In most cases, otherwise, the plasma concentration was below the detectable range. However, when we used the measured IC_{50} in colonospheres, organoids or tissue explants systems that recapitulate patient response, this concentration showed induction of differentiation rather than cell toxicity or cell death as evident in Figures 3 and 4. The heterogeneous cell population could explain why the cells may respond differently to treatment in these systems [58]. In addition, the concentration at which different drugs exert their pharmacological effects varies largely on the dynamics of the drugs and different cell types. Many drugs are used at concentrations of nM–mM range, with concentrations >10 μM. For example, BBI608 with 30 μM, 20 μM ECGC, 10 mM metformin, or vismodegib 10 μM [59–62]. Therefore, we presume this concentration may not be too toxic for future clinical use.

Based on our results, we conclude that AM404 as a new compound and FBXL5 as an associated key target gene with high therapeutic pharmacological potential could be used against human colorectal cancer and other infectious diseases.

4. Materials and Methods

4.1. Human Tissues

Tumour and adjacent healthy tissue samples of 17 CRC patients were collected [43] from Nottingham Health Sciences Biobank (NHSB), Queens Medical Centre, University of Nottingham. Ethical approval and research and development approval including written informed consent were obtained by Nottingham Health Science Biobank (NHSB), Histopathology Department, School of Medicine, University of Nottingham, Nottingham NG7 2UH. We collected samples from Biobank via access committee of NHSB approval number: ACP000098 A Nateri CRC. Tissue samples were used for culturing patient-relevant 3D organoid and ex vivo tissue explant models [45,46]. All procedures were conducted following the Declaration of Helsinki and local ethics committee approval. Tissue samples were collected only from patients who provided written informed consent.

4.2. Ex Vivo Explant Culture of CRC Tissues

Explant tumour models [45,46] were cultured from patients' tissues obtained as outlined above. Primary tumour tissue samples were cut in 2–4 mm segments and were maintained in complete organoid medium supplemented with Noggin 12–15 h or overnight. Explant samples were treated with the drug for 24 h. Tissues were fixed overnight in 10% neutral-buffered formalin (NBF), paraffin embedded, and sectioned at 4-mm thickness for hemotoxylin and eosin (H&E) staining or immunohistochemistry (IHC).

4.3. Organoid Culture

CRC patient-derived organoids were cultured as previously established and characterized in our lab [42,43]. Colonic crypts were made to release from intestinal epithelium and were re-suspended in Matrigel in the presence of complete organoid medium [43]. Once the organoids started to grow (usually day 4–5), they were treated with drug and/or complete organoid medium as vehicle control for their morphology, growth evaluation and live/dead staining. Considering the 3D enteroid structures with crypt like projections, volume of organoids was measured by taking 3–4 separate diameters for each organoid. Half of the average of this diameter was considered as radius (r), organoid volume was measured using the following formula: $V = 4/3\pi r^3$. Re-treatment and/or organoid medium replacement was carried out every two days, for the whole experimental period. Microscopy was performed using a DMI3000 B fluorescence microscope (Leica Biosystem, Milton Keynes, UK) at ×10 and ×40 magnification for recording organoid growth and/or live/dead staining.

4.4. Organoids Live/Dead Staining

Live organoids were stained with Hoechst 33342, a blue-fluorescence dye to stain all cells and propidium iodide (PI, Sigma Aldrich, Dorset, UK), a red-fluorescence dye to stain dead cells, according to double Hoechst 33342/PI stain apoptosis detection kit (GenScript, Leiden, Netherlands). Stained organoids were carefully collected and fixed, in order to distinguish live/dead staining with the Leica DMI3000 B fluorescence microscope.

4.5. Immunohistochemistry (IHC)

Fixed tissues were processed by a Leica TP1020 semi-enclosed benchtop tissue processor via automatic passages from ethanol (70%, 90% and 100%) to methanol, xylene and, lastly, paraffin. Samples were embedded in paraffin blocks to be cut in 4 μm-thick sections with a microtome and placed onto the glass slides for IHC analysis. Immunohistochemical analysis was carried out with and without (antibody control) Ki-67 (Dako, Stockport, UK), active caspase-3, CDX2, CD44 (Cell Signaling, London, UK), and FBXL5 (Abcam, Cambridge, UK) antibodies followed by incubation with secondary antibodies and detection reagents. A section from a CRC tissue known to express the protein of interest was also used as positive control [33]. Slides were scanned at 20× magnification. Images were analysed using NanoZoomer Digital Pathology software (Hamamatsu Ltd., Welwyn Garden City, UK). Immunostaining was evaluated by H-score method to calculate the sum and intensity of positively stained tumour cells. The H-score is ranged from 0 to 300, using the formula: (1 × % weakly stained nuclei) + (2 × % moderately stained nuclei) + (3 × % strongly stained nuclei) [63].

4.6. Cell Culture and Colonosphere Formation Assay

Human colorectal carcinoma HCT116, DLD-1, and SW480 cell lines were used throughout the study. These were purchased from ATCC and were further characterised in our laboratory [33,34,64]. Cells were routinely tested and approved mycoplasma-free. All cells were propagated in complete medium and used for experiments within 5 passages from thawing. 3D colonospheres were cultured for 13–14 days as previously established [15,16]. Well-defined colonospheres were then treated with drug compound for 72 h for further employment into NIH clinical collection screening, colonosphere formation and morphology evaluation, immunofluorescence assay, RNA extraction for qRT-PCR and gene array.

4.7. Screening of NIH Clinical Collection Using 3D Colonosphere

As a representation of CRC-SC [16], colonospheres obtained from the above CRC cell lines were employed into a fluorescence-based screening of US National Institute of Health (NIH, Evotec, South San Francisco, CA, US) clinical library consisting of 707 small molecule inhibitors. The fluorescent Rosamine dye CDy1- (Active Motif, La Hulpe, Belgium) based screening in 96 well-plates was used to examine the effect drugs in the differentiation/stemness activities of colonospheres [17,18]. Fluorescence intensities were measured using a CLARIOstar microplate reader (BMG LABTECH, Aylesbury, UK) with optic setting for excitation and emission as 544–10 and 577–10 nm respectively. Based on this platform, throughout the screening, fluorescence intensity of vehicle (DMSO) treated colonospheres was used as control. All treated colonosphere intensities were expressed as a percentage of the control as an indication of induced or reduced stem-like activity.

4.8. Cytotoxicity Assay

Same passage number of HCT116, DLD-1 and SW480 cells were seeded in 96-well plate and were allowed to grow. Subsequently, cells were serum-starved for 18 h and then were treated with a drug by itself or with 5-FU and Oxaliplatin (Tocris, Abingdon, UK) for 72 h. Sulforhodamine-B colorimetric assay (230162, Sigma Aldrich, Gillingham, UK) was performed as previously described [33].

4.9. Clonogenic Assay

DLD-1 cells were seeded in 6-well plates (200 cells per well). Cells were allowed to form into colonies and were treated with AM404 on day 7. Colonies were re-treated or replaced with fresh medium every three days throughout day 14. They were then fixed with 4% paraformaldehyde and stained with 0.01% crystal violet (Sigma Aldrich, Gillingham, UK), before the manual counting and colony size measurement.

4.10. Cell Migration and Wound Healing Assays

Wound healing assay was conducted on DLD-1 cells to investigate AM404's effect on migration [53]. Cells were cultured in a monolayer confluent manner. In order to suppress cell proliferation and avoid interference with the migration measurement, they were serum starved for 18 h. A wound was stimulated using pipette tip, creating gap in the confluent monolayer cells and removed of any mechanical debris by subsequent washes. Images were taken for the time point of 0 h, using a phase-contrast microscope. Cells were treated with the drug and/or medium immediately and returned to the incubator. Image acquisition integrity was assured by several reference points close to scratch. Images were taken periodically at time points of 12 h, 24 h, 48 h and 72 h following the abovementioned approach. The distances between the scratch sides (μm) were measured and compared between 0 h and 72 h.

4.11. *Immunofluorescence and Western Blotting*

Immunofluorescence and Western blotting analyses were conducted to study the expression pattern and distribution of a protein within cells as previously described [15].

4.12. *Knockout of FBXL5 Using the CRISPR/Cas9 System*

Two copies of 19- and 20-bp guide sequence targeting DNA within the first and eleventh exon of FBXL5, with high-specificity protospacer adjacent motif (PAM, Sanger, Cambridge, UK) target sites was cloned in LV04 Sanger Lentiviral CRISPR vector (Sigma) respectively. DLD-1 and SW480 stably expressing Cas9 cells were transduced with LV40-FBXL5 gRNAs. Single transduced cells were isolated by puromycin selection and individual clones extended and screened by immunoblotting with anti-FBXL5 antibody (Abcam). Genomic DNA was isolated from individual edited clones, and PCR amplified exons products were sequenced to confirm homogeneous representation in the edited cells.

4.13. *RNA, Transcriptomic, qRT-PCR Assay*

Total RNA was isolated from CRC cells, colonospheres and tissues with TRIzol reagent (Sigma Aldrich) and RNeasy Mini Kit (QIAGEN) following the manufacturer's protocol. The quality and integrity of the total RNA were evaluated on the Agilent-2100 Bioanalyzer system (Agilent, Stockport, UK). Only samples surpassing the minimal quality threshold (RIN > 8.0) were used in the subsequent transcriptomic assessment. cDNA was prepared from 200 ng of RNA as per the GeneChipTM WT-PLUS Reagents (Thermo Fisher Scientific/Affymetrix, Winsford, UK), and followed by in vitro transcription to produce cRNA, end-labelled and hybridized for 16 h at 45 C to GeneChip™ Human Gene 2.1 ST Arrays (Thermo Fisher Scientific/ Affymetrix, Winsford, UK). All steps were performed by a GeneAtlas™ Personal Microarray system (Thermo Fisher Scientific/ Affymetrix, Winsford, UK) according to manufacturer's instructions at the Nottingham Arabidopsis Stock Centre (NASC, School of Biosciences, and University of Nottingham). Differentially expressed genes were considered significant if p-value with FDR ≤ 0.05 and fold-change of >2 or <-2.

Transcriptomic data were then processed by a standardized sequence of analyses (gene ontology (GO) enrichment) using Ingenuity Pathway Analysis. For qPCR assays, cDNAs were generated by using PrimeScript RT Reagent Kit (Perfect Real Time) (Takara-Clontech Laboratories, Saint-Germain-en-Laye, France) and cDNA samples were then amplified using LightCycler 480 SYBR Green I Master Mix (Roche, Welwyn Garden City, UK) and LightCycler 480 II instrument (Roche). Results were normalized to those obtained with β-actin, and all assays were performed in triplicate. Details of primers used are shown in Table S1.

4.14. *Data Analysis and Statistics*

GraphPad Prism 7 (GraphPad Software, San Diego, CA, USA) and Microsoft Office Excel (Microsoft, Redmond, WA, USA) were used to generate graphs and carry out statistical analysis. Fiji (ImageJ) software (ImageJ 1.51j8, NIH, Bethesda, MD, USA) was used to analyse images. Gene expression data were analysed using Partek Genomics Suite 7.0 (Partek Incorporated, St. Louis, MO, USA). Data are reported as means ± SEM using the Student t test and the Mann–Whitney U test, as appropriate and for all analyses, $p < 0.05$ was considered statistically significant. * $p < 0.05$; ** $p < 0.01$; *** $p < 0.001$ values are shown.

5. Conclusions

Our data demonstrate a new molecular mechanism, by which an uncharacterised antibacterial AM404 drug altering the oncogenic activity of FBXL5 receptor subunit of E3-ligase, to alter differentiation, migration and drug-resistant of CRC cells. Needless to say, that, the connection between inflammation and tumorigenesis involved at different stages during pathogenesis in all malignancies, and therefore these cancer-related cellular processes alterations through AM404 may offer possibilities for the anticancer potential of AM404 targeting the FBXL5-E3 ligase signalling in different types of cancers.

Supplementary Materials:
Table S1: List of primers and their sequences used for qRT-PCR assay, Table S2: List of drugs selected during different stages of the screening, Table S3: List of differentially expressed genes upon AM404 treatment, Figure S1: Optimisation of screening methodology using CDy1, Figure S2: Isobologram analysis shows the combined effect, Figure S3: AM404 treatment presents enteroid-like structures and induces differentiation in organoids. Percentage of enterosphere, cyst, enteroids and dead cells at day 3, 7 and 15 days of treatment, Figure S4: Principal components analysis (PCA) of microarray data between DMSO (control, red) and AM404 treated (blue) cells transcriptomes, Figure S5: Gene ontology (GO) pathway for 75 differentially expressed genes (2.5 or more-fold change), Figure S6: Clonogenic assay of AM404 on *FBXL5* KO DLD-1 cells, Figure S7: Whole Western Blot image and intensity ratio.

Author Contributions: Conceptualization, M.A., R.B.-J. and A.S.N.; methodology, M.A., N.J., H.K., R.B.-J., M.C.-U. and A.S.N; software, M.C.-U., M.A., and R.B.-J.; validation, M.A., N.J., H.K., R.B.-J. and A.M.; investigation, M.A., N.J., H.K., R.B.-J. and M.C.-U.; resources, S.T.M. and A.S.N.; data curation, M.A., N.J., H.K., R.B.-J., M.C.-U.; writing—original draft preparation, M.A., R.B.-J. and A.S.N.; writing—review and editing, M.A., N.J., H.K., R.B.-J., M.C.-U., S.T.M., M.A. and A.S.N.; visualization, M.A., N.J., H.K., R.B.-J., M.C.-U., M.A.; supervision, R.B.-J., M.A. and A.S.N.; project administration, A.S.N.; funding acquisition, A.S.N. All authors have read and agreed to the published version of the manuscript.

Acknowledgments: We thank D. Bates and L.V. Dekker for useful comments on the manuscript. We also appreciate the fantastic fundraising efforts of Alison Sims and her family in memory of Daz Sims to support the work in our laboratory.

References

1. Arnold, M.; Sierra, M.S.; Laversanne, M.; Soerjomataram, I.; Jemal, A.; Bray, F. Global patterns and trends in colorectal cancer incidence and mortality. *Gut* **2017**, *66*, 683–691. [CrossRef] [PubMed]
2. O'Brien, C.A.; Pollett, A.; Gallinger, S.; Dick, J.E. A human colon cancer cell capable of initiating tumour growth in immunodeficient mice. *Nature* **2007**, *445*, 106–110. [CrossRef] [PubMed]
3. Ricci-Vitiani, L.; Lombardi, D.G.; Pilozzi, E.; Biffoni, M.; Todaro, M.; Peschle, C.; De Maria, R. Identification and expansion of human colon-cancer-initiating cells. *Nature* **2007**, *445*, 111–115. [CrossRef] [PubMed]
4. Singh, A.; Settleman, J. EMT, cancer stem cells and drug resistance: An emerging axis of evil in the war on cancer. *Oncogene* **2010**, *29*, 4741–4751. [CrossRef] [PubMed]
5. Sachlos, E.; Risueño, R.M.; Laronde, S.; Shapovalova, Z.; Lee, J.H.; Russell, J.; Malig, M.; McNicol, J.D.; Fiebig-Comyn, A.; Graham, M.; et al. Identification of Drugs Including a Dopamine Receptor Antagonist that Selectively Target Cancer Stem Cells. *Cell* **2012**, *149*, 1284–1297. [CrossRef] [PubMed]
6. Dashzeveg, N.K.; Taftaf, R.; Ramos, E.K.; Torre-Healy, L.; Chumakova, A.; Silver, D.J.; Alban, T.J.; Sinyuk, M.; Thiagarajan, P.S.; Jarrar, A.M.; et al. New Advances and Challenges of Targeting Cancer Stem Cells. *Cancer Res.* **2017**, *77*, 5222–5227. [CrossRef] [PubMed]
7. Marquardt, S.; Solanki, M.; Spitschak, A.; Vera, J.; Pützer, B.M. Emerging functional markers for cancer stem cell-based therapies: Understanding signaling networks for targeting metastasis. *Semin. Cancer Biol.* **2018**, *53*, 90–109. [CrossRef]
8. Batlle, E.; Clevers, H. Cancer stem cells revisited. *Nat. Med.* **2017**, *23*, 1124–1134. [CrossRef]
9. Hanahan, D.; Weinberg, R. Hallmarks of cancer: The next generation. *Cell* **2011**, *144*, 646–674. [CrossRef]

10. Elinav, E.; Nowarski, R.; Thaiss, C.A.; Hu, B.; Jin, C.; Flavell, R.A. Inflammation-induced cancer: Crosstalk between tumours, immune cells and microorganisms. *Nat. Rev. Cancer* **2013**, *13*, 759–771. [CrossRef]
11. Ahmed, M.; Chaudhari, K.; Babaei-Jadidi, R.; Dekker, L.V.; Shams Nateri, A. Concise Review: Emerging Drugs Targeting Epithelial Cancer Stem-Like Cells. *Stem Cells* **2017**, *35*, 839–850. [CrossRef] [PubMed]
12. Gupta, P.B.; Onder, T.T.; Jiang, G.; Tao, K.; Kuperwasser, C.; Weinberg, R.A.; Lander, E.S. Identification of selective inhibitors of cancer stem cells by high-throughput screening. *Cell* **2009**, *138*, 645–659. [CrossRef] [PubMed]
13. Shibata, H.; Yamakoshi, H.; Sato, A.; Ohori, H.; Kakudo, Y.; Kudo, C.; Takahashi, Y.; Watanabe, M.; Takano, H.; Ishioka, C.; et al. Newly synthesized curcumin analog has improved potential to prevent colorectal carcinogenesis in vivo. *Cancer Sci.* **2009**, *100*, 956–960. [CrossRef] [PubMed]
14. Naujokat, C.; Laufer, S.J.J. Targeting cancer stem cells with defined compounds and drugs. *J. Cancer Res. Update* **2013**, *2*, 36–67. [CrossRef]
15. Shaheen, S.; Ahmed, M.; Lorenzi, F.; Nateri, A.S. Reports Spheroid-Formation (Colonosphere) Assay for in vitro Assessment and Expansion of Stem Cells in Colon Cancer. *Stem Cell Rev. Rep.* **2016**, *12*, 492–499. [CrossRef]
16. Hwang, W.L.; Jiang, J.K.; Yang, S.H.; Huang, T.S.; Lan, H.Y.; Teng, H.W.; Yang, C.Y.; Tsai, Y.P.; Lin, C.H.; Wang, H.W.; et al. MicroRNA-146a directs the symmetric division of Snail-dominant colorectal cancer stem cells. *Nat. Cell Biol.* **2014**, *16*, 268–280. [CrossRef]
17. Kang, N.Y.; Yun, S.W.; Ha, H.H.; Park, S.J.; Chang, Y.T. Embryonic and induced pluripotent stem cell staining and sorting with the live-cell fluorescence imaging probe CDy1. *Nat. Protoc.* **2011**, *6*, 1044–1052. [CrossRef]
18. Vendrell, M.; Park, S.J.; Chandran, Y.; Lee, C.L.; Ha, H.H.; Kang, N.Y.; Yun, S.W.; Chang, Y.T. A fluorescent screening platform for the rapid evaluation of chemicals in cellular reprogramming. *Stem Cell Res.* **2012**, *9*, 185–191. [CrossRef]
19. Saliba, S.W.; Marcotegui, A.R.; Fortwängler, E.; Ditrich, J.; Perazzo, J.C.; Muñoz, E.; de Oliveira, A.C.P.; Fiebich, B.L. AM404, paracetamol metabolite, prevents prostaglandin synthesis in activated microglia by inhibiting COX activity. *J. Neuroinflamm.* **2017**, *14*, 246. [CrossRef]
20. Mazaleuskaya, L.L.; Sangkuhl, K.; Thorn, C.F.; FitzGerald, G.A.; Altman, R.B.; Klein, T.E. PharmGKB summary: Pathways of acetaminophen metabolism at the therapeutic versus toxic doses. *Pharm. Genom.* **2015**, *25*, 416–426. [CrossRef]
21. Sharma, C.V.; Long, J.H.; Shah, S.; Rahman, J.; Perrett, D.; Ayoub, S.S.; Mehta, V. First evidence of the conversion of paracetamol to AM404 in human cerebrospinal fluid. *J. Pain Res.* **2017**, *10*, 2703–2709. [CrossRef] [PubMed]
22. Costa, B.; Siniscalco, D.; Trovato, A.E.; Comelli, F.; Sotgiu, M.L.; Colleoni, M.; Maione, S.; Rossi, F.; Giagnoni, G. AM404, an inhibitor of anandamide uptake, prevents pain behaviour and modulates cytokine and apoptotic pathways in a rat model of neuropathic pain. *Br. J. Pharmacol.* **2006**, *148*, 1022–1032. [CrossRef] [PubMed]
23. Gerits, E.; Spincemaille, P.; De Cremer, K.; De Brucker, K.; Beullens, S.; Thevissen, K.; Cammue, B.P.A.; Vandamme, K.; Fauvart, M.; Verstraeten, N.; et al. Repurposing AM404 for the treatment of oral infections by Porphyromonas gingivalis. *Clin. Exp. Dent. Res.* **2017**, *3*, 69–76. [CrossRef] [PubMed]
24. Yao, H.; Su, S.; Xia, D.; Wang, M.; Li, Z.; Chen, W.; Ren, L.; Xu, L. F-box and leucine-rich repeat protein 5 promotes colon cancer progression by modulating PTEN/PI3K/AKT signaling pathway. *Biomed. Pharm.* **2018**, *107*, 1712–1719. [CrossRef] [PubMed]
25. Xiong, Y.; Sun, F.; Dong, P.; Watari, H.; Yue, J.; Yu, M.F.; Lan, C.Y.; Wang, Y.; Ma, Z.B. iASPP induces EMT and cisplatin resistance in human cervical cancer through miR-20a-FBXL5/BTG3 signaling. *J. Exp. Clin. Cancer Res.* **2017**, *36*, 48. [CrossRef]
26. Machado-Oliveira, G.; Guerreiro, E.; Matias, A.C.; Facucho-Oliveira, J.; Pacheco-Leyva, I.; Bragança, J. FBXL5 modulates HIF-1alpha transcriptional activity by degradation of CITED2. *Arch. Biochem. Biophys.* **2015**, *576*, 61–72. [CrossRef]
27. Dragoi, A.M.; Swiss, R.; Gao, B.; Agaisse, H. Novel strategies to enforce an epithelial phenotype in mesenchymal cells. *Cancer Res.* **2014**, *74*, 3659–3672. [CrossRef]
28. Richon, V.M. Cancer biology: Mechanism of antitumour action of vorinostat (suberoylanilide hydroxamic acid), a novel histone deacetylase inhibitor. *Br. J. Cancer.* **2006**, *95*, S2. [CrossRef]

29. Finnin, M.S.; Donigian, J.R.; Cohen, A.; Richon, V.M.; Rifkind, R.A.; Marks, P.A.; Breslow, R.; Pavletich, N.P. Structures of a histone deacetylase homologue bound to the TSA and SAHA inhibitors. *Nature* **1999**, *401*, 188–193. [CrossRef]
30. Richon, V.M.; Emiliani, S.; Verdin, E.; Webb, Y.; Breslow, R.; Rifkind, R.A.; Marks, P.A. A class of hybrid polar inducers of transformed cell differentiation inhibits histone deacetylases. *Proc. Natl. Acad. Sci. USA* **1998**, *95*, 3003–3007. [CrossRef]
31. Sancho, R.; Jandke, A.; Davis, H.; Diefenbacher, M.E.; Tomlinson, I.; Behrens, A. F-box and WD repeat domain-containing 7 regulates intestinal cell lineage commitment and is a haploinsufficient tumor suppressor. *Gastroenterology* **2010**, *139*, 929–941. [CrossRef] [PubMed]
32. Welcker, M.; Clurman, B.E. FBW7 ubiquitin ligase: A tumour suppressor at the crossroads of cell division, growth and differentiation. Nature reviews. *Cancer* **2008**, *8*, 83–93. [CrossRef] [PubMed]
33. Li, N.; Babaei-Jadidi, R.; Lorenzi, F.; Spencer-Dene, B.; Clarke, P.; Domingo, E.; Tulchinsky, E.; Vries, R.G.J.; Kerr, D.; Pan, Y.; et al. An FBXW7-ZEB2 axis links EMT and tumour microenvironment to promote colorectal cancer stem cells and chemoresistance. *Oncogenesis* **2019**, *8*, 13. [CrossRef] [PubMed]
34. Babaei-Jadidi, R.; Li, N.; Saadeddin, A.; Spencer-Dene, B.; Jandke, A.; Muhammad, B.; Ibrahim, E.E.; Muraleedharan, R.; Abuzinadah, M.; Davis, H.; et al. FBXW7 influences murine intestinal homeostasis and cancer, targeting Notch, Jun, and DEK for degradation. *J. Exp. Med.* **2011**, *208*, 295–312. [CrossRef]
35. Yeung, T.M.; Gandhi, S.C.; Wilding, J.L.; Muschel, R.; Bodmer, W.F. Cancer stem cells from colorectal cancer-derived cell lines. *Proc. Natl. Acad. Sci. USA* **2010**, *107*, 3722–3727. [CrossRef]
36. Buczacki, S.J.A.; Popova, S.; Biggs, E.; Koukorava, C.; Buzzelli, J.; Vermeulen, L.; Hazelwood, L.; Francies, H.; Garnett, M.J.; Winton, D.J. Itraconazole targets cell cycle heterogeneity in colorectal cancer. *J. Exp. Med.* **2018**, *215*, 1891–1912. [CrossRef]
37. Tarpgaard, L.S.; Qvortrup, C.; Nygård, S.B.; Nielsen, S.L.; Andersen, D.R.; Jensen, N.F.; Stenvang, J.; Detlefsen, S.; Brünner, N.; Pfeiffer, P.; et al. A phase II study of Epirubicin in oxaliplatin-resistant patients with metastatic colorectal cancer and TOP2A gene amplification. *BMC Cancer* **2016**, *16*, 91. [CrossRef]
38. Longley, D.B.; Harkin, D.P.; Johnston, P.G. 5-fluorouracil: Mechanisms of action and clinical strategies. *Nat. Rev. Cancer* **2003**, *3*, 330–338. [CrossRef]
39. Lorenzi, F.; Babaei-Jadidi, R.; Sheard, J.; Spencer-Dene, B.; Nateri, A.S. Fbxw7-associated drug resistance is reversed by induction of terminal differentiation in murine intestinal organoid culture. *Mol. Ther. Methods Clin. Dev.* **2016**, *3*, 16024. [CrossRef]
40. Chou, T.C.; Talalay, P. Quantitative analysis of dose-effect relationships: The combined effects of multiple drugs or enzyme inhibitors. *Adv. Enzym. Regul.* **1984**, *22*, 27–55. [CrossRef]
41. Foucquier, J.; Guedj, M. Analysis of drug combinations: Current methodological landscape. *Pharmacol. Res. Perspect.* **2015**, *3*, e00149. [CrossRef]
42. Sato, T.; Vries, R.G.; Snippert, H.J.; van de Wetering, M.; Barker, N.; Stange, D.E.; van Es, J.H.; Abo, A.; Kujala, P.; Peters, P.J.; et al. Single Lgr5 stem cells build crypt-villus structures in vitro without a mesenchymal niche. *Nature* **2009**, *459*, 262–265. [CrossRef]
43. Kashfi, S.M.H.; Almozyan, S.; Jinks, N.; Koo, B.K.; Nateri, A.S. Morphological alterations of cultured human colorectal matched tumour and healthy organoids. *Oncotarget* **2018**, *9*, 10572–10584. [CrossRef]
44. Xu, H.; Jiao, Y.; Qin, S.; Zhao, W.; Chu, Q.; Wu, K. Organoid technology in disease modelling, drug development, personalized treatment and regeneration medicine. *Exp. Hematol. Oncol.* **2018**, *7*, 30. [CrossRef] [PubMed]
45. Karekla, E.; Liao, W.J.; Sharp, B.; Pugh, J.; Reid, H.; Quesne, J.L.; Moore, D.; Pritchard, C.; MacFarlane, M.; Pringle, J.H. Ex Vivo Explant Cultures of Non-Small Cell Lung Carcinoma Enable Evaluation of Primary Tumor Responses to Anticancer Therapy. *Cancer Res.* **2017**, *77*, 2029–2039. [CrossRef] [PubMed]
46. Majumder, B.; Baraneedharan, U.; Thiyagarajan, S.; Radhakrishnan, P.; Narasimhan, H.; Dhandapani, M.; Brijwani, N.; Pinto, D.D.; Prasath, A.; Shanthappa, B.U.; et al. Predicting clinical response to anticancer drugs using an ex vivo platform that captures tumour heterogeneity. *Nat. Commun* **2015**, *6*, 6169. [CrossRef] [PubMed]
47. Qualtrough, D.; Hinoi, T.; Fearon, E.; Paraskeva, C. Expression of CDX2 in normal and neoplastic human colon tissue and during differentiation of an in vitro model system. *Gut* **2002**, *51*, 184–190. [CrossRef]

48. Merlos-Suárez, A.; Barriga, F.M.; Jung, P.; Iglesias, M.; Céspedes, M.V.; Rossell, D.; Sevillano, M.; Hernando-Momblona, X.; da Silva-Diz, V.; Muñoz, P.; et al. The Intestinal Stem Cell Signature Identifies Colorectal Cancer Stem Cells and Predicts Disease Relapse. *Cell Stem Cell* **2011**, *8*, 511–524. [CrossRef]
49. Todaro, M.; Gaggianesi, M.; Catalano, V.; Benfante, A.; Iovino, F.; Biffoni, M.; Apuzzo, T.; Sperduti, I.; Volpe, S.; Cocorullo, G.; et al. CD44v6 is a marker of constitutive and reprogrammed cancer stem cells driving colon cancer metastasis. *Cell Stem Cell* **2014**, *14*, 342–356. [CrossRef]
50. Nateri, A.S.; Riera-Sans, L.; Da Costa, C.; Behrens, A. The ubiquitin ligase SCFFbw7 antagonizes apoptotic JNK signaling. *Science* **2004**, *303*, 1374–1378. [CrossRef]
51. Diaz, V.M.; de Herreros, A.G. F-box proteins: Keeping the epithelial-to-mesenchymal transition (EMT) in check. *Semin. Cancer Biol.* **2016**, *36*, 71–79. [CrossRef] [PubMed]
52. Muto, Y.; Nishiyama, M.; Nita, A.; Moroishi, T.; Nakayama, K.I. Essential role of FBXL5-mediated cellular iron homeostasis in maintenance of hematopoietic stem cells. *Nat. Commun.* **2017**, *8*, 16114. [CrossRef] [PubMed]
53. Liang, C.C.; Park, A.Y.; Guan, J.L. In vitro scratch assay: A convenient and inexpensive method for analysis of cell migration in vitro. *Nat. Protoc.* **2007**, *2*, 329. [CrossRef] [PubMed]
54. Diakos, C.I.; Charles, K.A.; McMillan, D.C.; Clarke, S.J. Cancer-related inflammation and treatment effectiveness. *Lancet Oncol.* **2014**, *15*, e493–e503. [CrossRef]
55. Lasry, A.; Zinger, A.; Ben-Neriah, Y. Inflammatory networks underlying colorectal cancer. *Nat. Immunol.* **2016**, *17*, 230. [CrossRef]
56. Caballero, F.J.; Soler-Torronteras, R.; Lara-Chica, M.; García, V.; Fiebich, B.L.; Muñoz, E.; Calzado, M.A. AM404 inhibits NFAT and NF-κB signaling pathways and impairs migration and invasiveness of neuroblastoma cells. *Eur. J. Pharmacol.* **2015**, *746*, 221–232. [CrossRef]
57. De Lago, E.; Gustafsson, S.B.; Fernández-Ruiz, J.; Nilsson, J.; Jacobsson, S.O.; Fowler, C.J. Acyl-based anandamide uptake inhibitors cause rapid toxicity to C6 glioma cells at pharmacologically relevant concentrations. *J. Neurochem.* **2006**, *99*, 677–688. [CrossRef]
58. Kleppe, M.; Levine, R.L. Tumor heterogeneity confounds and illuminates: Assessing the implications. *Nat. Med.* **2014**, *20*, 342–344. [CrossRef]
59. Li, Y.; Rogoff, H.A.; Keates, S.; Gao, Y.; Murikipudi, S.; Mikule, K.; Leggett, D.; Li, W.; Pardee, A.B.; Li, C.J. Suppression of cancer relapse and metastasis by inhibiting cancer stemness. *Proc. Natl. Acad. Sci. USA* **2015**, *112*, 1839–1844. [CrossRef]
60. Chen, D.; Pamu, S.; Cui, Q.; Chan, T.H.; Dou, Q.P. Novel epigallocatechin gallate (EGCG) analogs activate AMP-activated protein kinase pathway and target cancer stem cells. *Bioorg. Med. Chem.* **2012**, *20*, 3031–3037. [CrossRef]
61. Jung, J.W.; Park, S.B.; Lee, S.J.; Seo, M.S.; Trosko, J.E.; Kang, K.S. Metformin represses self-renewal of the human breast carcinoma stem cells via inhibition of estrogen receptor-mediated OCT4 expression. *PLoS ONE* **2011**, *6*, e28068. [CrossRef] [PubMed]
62. Singh, B.N.; Fu, J.; Srivastava, R.K.; Shankar, S. Hedgehog signaling antagonist GDC-0449 (Vismodegib) inhibits pancreatic cancer stem cell characteristics: Molecular mechanisms. *PLoS ONE* **2011**, *6*, e27306. [CrossRef] [PubMed]
63. Detre, S.; Saclani Jotti, G.; Dowsett, M. A "quickscore" method for immunohistochemical semiquantitation: Validation for oestrogen receptor in breast carcinomas. *J. Clin. Pathol.* **1995**, *48*, 876–878. [CrossRef] [PubMed]
64. Muhammad, B.A.; Almozyan, S.; Babaei-Jadidi, R.; Onyido, E.K.; Saadeddin, A.; Kashfi, S.H.; Spencer-Dene, B.; Ilyas, M.; Lourdusamy, A.; Behrens, A.; et al. FLYWCH1, a Novel Suppressor of Nuclear Beta-Catenin, Regulates Migration and Morphology in Colorectal Cancer. *Mol. Cancer Res.* **2018**, *16*, 1977–1990. [CrossRef]

2

Cell Surface GRP78 as a Death Receptor and an Anticancer Drug Target

Ruowen Ge * and Chieh Kao

Department of Biological Sciences, National University of Singapore, Singapore 117558, Singapore; ekingo@gmail.com

* Correspondence: dbsgerw@nus.edu.sg

Abstract: Cell surface GRP78 (csGRP78, glucose-regulated protein 78 kDa) is preferentially overexpressed in aggressive, metastatic, and chemo-resistant cancers. GRP78 is best studied as a chaperone protein in the lumen of endoplasmic reticulum (ER), facilitating folding and secretion of the newly synthesized proteins and regulating protein degradation as an ER stress sensor in the unfolded protein pathway. As a cell surface signal receptor, multiple csGRP78 ligands have been discovered to date, and they trigger various downstream cell signaling pathways including pro-proliferative, pro-survival, and pro-apoptotic pathways. In this perspective, we evaluate csGRP78 as a cell surface death receptor and its prospect as an anticancer drug target. The pro-apoptotic ligands of csGRP78 discovered so far include natural proteins, monoclonal antibodies, and synthetic peptides. Even the secreted GRP78 itself was recently found to function as a pro-apoptotic ligand for csGRP78, mediating pancreatic β-cell death. As csGRP78 is found to mainly configur as an external peripheral protein on cancer cell surface, how it can transmit death signals to the cytoplasmic environment remains enigmatic. With the recent encouraging results from the natural csGRP78 targeting pro-apoptotic monoclonal antibody PAT-SM6 in early-stage cancer clinical trials, the potential to develop a novel class of anticancer therapeutics targeting csGRP78 is becoming more compelling.

Keywords: cell surface GRP78 (csGRP78); death receptor; apoptosis; anticancer drug

---

1. Introduction

Glucose-regulated protein 78 kDa (GRP78), also referred to as HSPA5 (heat shock 70 kDa protein 5) and BiP (immunoglobulin heavy-chain binding protein), was first discovered and characterized as an endoplasmic reticulum (ER) resident protein [1,2]. The traditional function of GRP78 is a molecular chaperone in the ER lumen, helping to regulate protein quality control, facilitating protein folding, assembly, and misfolded protein degradation in the unfolded protein response (UPR) pathway [3]. GRP78 serves as a major ER stress sensor and is upregulated under ER stress, helping to maintain ER homeostasis and cell survival. In cancer, GRP78 is significantly upregulated due to the highly stressful microenvironment of cancer, serving as a pro-survival and anti-apoptotic protein for cancer cells [4].

In addition to function as an ER chaperon and stress sensor, GRP78 is also found in other sub-cellular locations such as on the cell surface or secreted into the extracellular environment. Cell surface GRP78 (csGRP78) functions as an important signal receptor, transmitting signals from the extracellular environment into cells [5]. To date, several ligands have been discovered to interact with csGRP78, including secreted proteins and plasma membrane-anchored proteins. Through interactions with these ligands, csGRP78 activates multiple intracellular cell signaling pathways, impacting cell proliferation, survival, migration, or apoptosis. Various pro-proliferative, pro-survival ligands, and pro-apoptotic ligands have been discovered, including natural proteins, monoclonal antibodies (Mabs), and synthetic peptides, even the secreted extracellular GRP78 itself [6]. In addition to extracellular ligands, several plasma membrane-bound proteins have also been demonstrated to interact with csGRP78, such as the glycosylphosphatidylinositol-anchored (GPI-anchored) proteins Cripto, T-cadherin, and CD109 [7–9].

Due to its preferential presence on the cell surface of cancer cells, csGRP78 has emerged as an attractive target for anticancer drugs [4]. Many excellent previous reviews have presented the diverse roles of GRP78 in multiple subcellular locations, and the different functions that GRP78 plays in cancer as well as other diseases [5,10–18]. However, the role of csGRP78 as a cell surface death receptor has not been comprehensively evaluated. In this perspective, we focus on csGRP78 as a death receptor and discuss its significance as a target for proapoptotic ligand-mediated anticancer drug development.

2. csGRP78 as a Death Receptor

The classical death receptors are members of the tumor necrosis receptor superfamily characterized by the presence of a cytoplasmic death domain, which is critical for the death receptor to initiate downstream cytotoxic signaling pathways involving caspases [19]. However, csGRP78 has been shown to be a predominantly external peripheral protein on the plasma membrane in several cultured cancer cell lines, with no transmembrane and cytosolic domain present [20]. A substantial level of csGRP78 achieved plasma membrane localization by interacting with GPI-anchored proteins. A membrane embedded form of csGRP78 was shown to be present only under ER stress conditions in these cancer cells, and at a very low level. Hence, how csGRP78 functions as a death receptor to transmit extracellular death signals to intracellular cytotoxic signaling pathways is intriguing and remains largely unknown. The known pro-apoptotic ligands of csGRP78, including natural proteins, monoclonal antibodies, and synthetic peptides, are summarized in Figure 1.

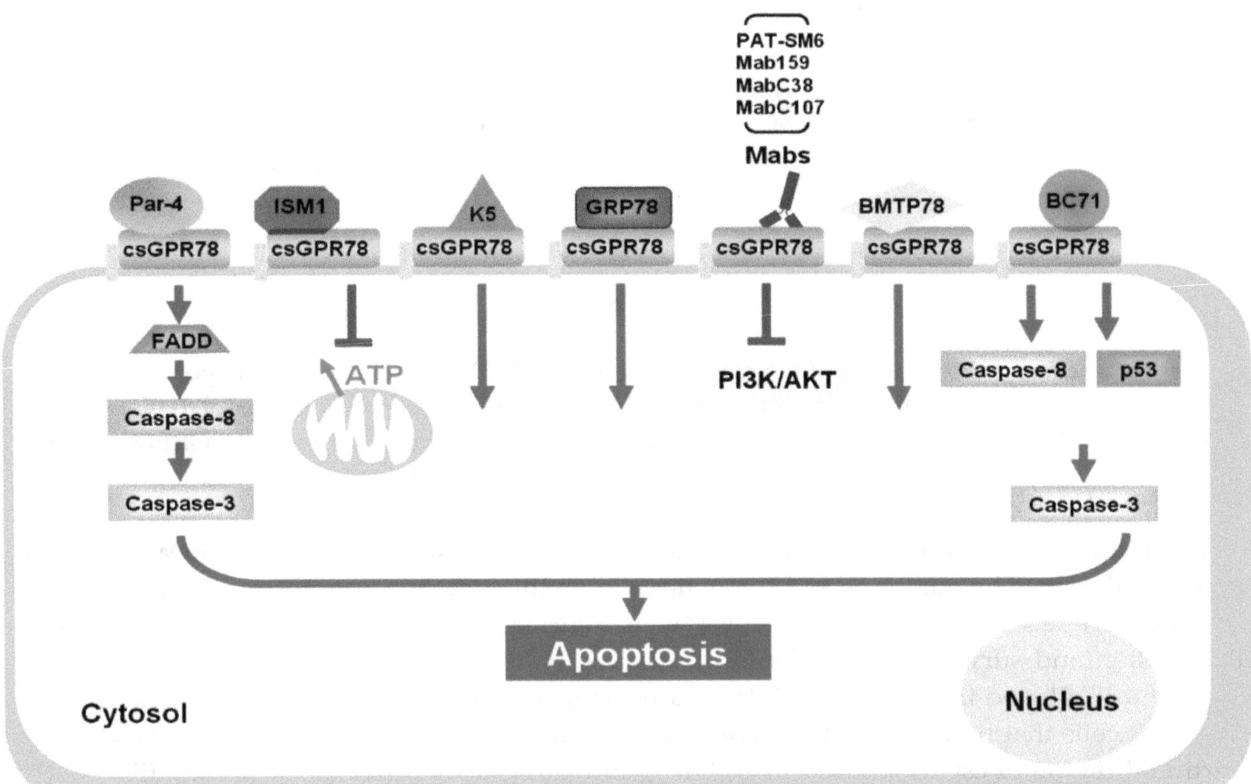

Figure 1. Summary of the pro-apoptotic ligands of csGRP78 and their mechanism of action. Par-4 (Prostate Apoptosis Response-4, ISM1 (Isthmin 1), K5 (plasminogen Kringle 5), Mabs (monoclonal antibodies), FADD (Fas associated protein with death domain), PI3K (PI3 kinase).

3. Natural Proapoptotic Protein Ligands of csGRP78

To date, at least four naturally secreted proteins have been shown to function as proapoptotic ligands of csGRP78, triggering cell death signaling (Figure 1).

3.1. Prostate Apoptosis Response-4 (Par-4)

A well-studied proapoptotic ligand of csGRP78 is the secreted prostate apoptosis response-4 (Par-4) protein [21]. Par-4 is expressed in various tissues and was first identified as a tumor suppressor localized in the cytosol and nucleus. It promotes apoptosis through the mitochondrial mediated intrinsic apoptotic pathway [22]. Subsequently, Par-4 is found to be secreted into the extracellular environment by both cancer cells and normal cells. Extracellular Par-4 functions as a proapoptotic protein, selectively targeting csGRP78 on cancer cells to trigger cancer-specific apoptosis via its SAC (selective for apoptosis induction in cancer cells) domain. Par-4 induces apoptosis by recruiting and activating the adaptor protein, Fas-associated protein with death domain (FADD), leading to downstream caspase-8 activation [21,23]. Moreover, apoptosis induced by the death ligand TRAIL (TNF-related apoptosis-inducing ligand) is dependent on extracellular Par-4 signaling via csGRP78. Notably, Par-4 interacts with the N-terminal region of csGRP78 (Figure 2). Systemic application of recombinant Par-4 or its proapoptotic domain SAC potently inhibited tumor growth in mice [21,24].

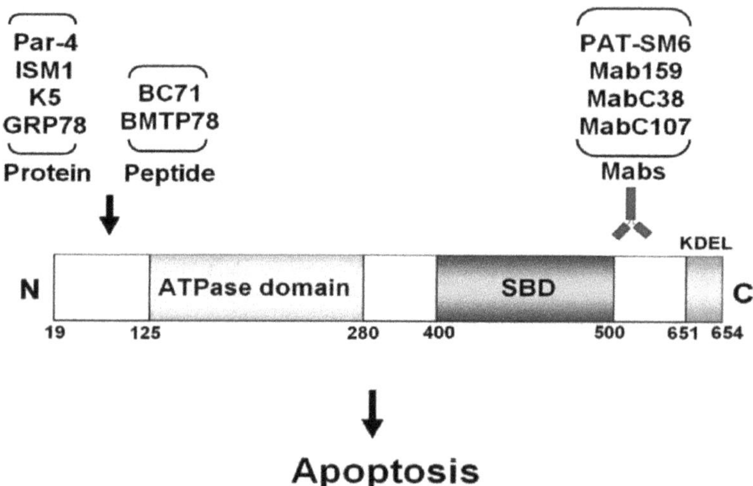

Figure 2. Schematic illustration of the region of human GRP78 that the various proapoptotic ligands interact with. SBD: substrate binding domain, KDEL: the 4 residue ER retention signal at the C-terminus of GRP78. The amino acid boundary of the domains are labelled at the bottom of the GRP78 protein.

3.2. Isthmin 1 (ISM1)

Isthmin 1 (ISM1) is a secreted 70 kDa protein (theoretical molecular weight 50 kDa) in vertebrates. It was first identified by our lab as an angiogenesis inhibitor, inducing apoptosis in endothelial cells via $\alpha v\beta 5$ integrin as a soluble protein [25]. However, in a surface-anchored form, ISM1 support endothelial cell adhesion and survival instead [26]. Subsequently, csGRP78 was identified as a high-affinity receptor for ISM1, and ISM1/csGRP78 interaction triggers apoptosis in both activated endothelial cells and cancer cells that harbor high levels of csGRP78 [27]. Interestingly, ISM1 also interacts with the N-terminal region of csGRP78, similar to Par-4 (our unpublished result, Figure 2). ISM1/csGRP78 interaction lead to the internalization of ISM1 via clathrin-mediated endocytosis and the trafficking of ISM1 to mitochondria, resulting in mitochondria dysfunction by blocking ATP/ADP exchange on the mitochondrial membrane [28]. The decline of cytosolic ATP concentration eventually caused apoptosis. Systemic infusion of recombinant ISM1 via intravenous route potently suppressed xenograft tumor growth in mice [27].

3.3. *Plasminogen Kringle 5 (K5)*

Plasminogen kringle 5 (K5) is a natural proteolytic fragment of the blood protein plasminogen, containing its fifth kringle domain. It functions as an angiogenesis inhibitor, inducing apoptosis of endothelial cells [29]. K5 was identified as a ligand for csGRP78, binding to the N-terminal domain of GRP78 [30,31] (Figure 2). It abrogates cell migration and trigger apoptosis via csGRP78 on endothelial cells and cancer cells. Anti-GRP78 antibody targeting the N-terminal region of GRP78 attenuated K5-induced inhibition of endothelial cell migration. Vaspin (visceral adipose tissue-derived serine proteinase inhibitor), an adipokine, was identified as a novel high-affinity ligand of csGRP78 that competes with K5 for csGRP78 binding and antagonize K5 function. Vaspin dose-dependently suppressed K5-induced intracellular Ca^{2+} influx and subsequent apoptosis in endothelial cells [32]. Recently, K5 was shown to dose-dependently downregulate GRP78 expression in gastric cancer cells. Downregulation of GRP78 contributes to K5-induced apoptosis in gastric cancer cells [33].

3.4. *Secreted GRP78*

GRP78 is known to also exist as a secreted soluble protein in the extracellular environment and in the serum [5]. Recently, extracellular GRP78 itself was identified as a proapoptotic ligand of csGRP78, triggering caspase-mediated apoptosis in stressed pancreatic beta cells [6]. Pro-inflammatory cytokines induce ER stress in beta cells, leading to the secretion and plasma membrane translocation of GRP78 [34]. csGRP78 was shown to serve as a death receptor for the secreted extracellular GRP78 which serves as a self-ligand to activate a proapoptotic pathway in these cells, leading to cell death. In addition, recombinant GRP78 induced apoptosis in cytokine-treated beta cells, but not in untreated control cells. Anti-GRP78 antibody targeting both N- and C-terminal regions of GRP78 blocked extracellular GRP78-induced apoptosis. These results suggest a possible pathway of active self-destruction in cytokine-exposed pancreatic beta cells mediated through GRP78, with soluble extracellular GRP78 activating csGRP78 for this self-destruction. csGRP78 may be an important modulator of beta cell death upon inflammatory stress responses and a therapeutic target for type I diabetes.

4. Monoclonal Antibodies as Proapoptotic Ligands of csGRP78

Different anti-GRP78 Mabs generate different biological consequences in the target cells depending on the Mab and the particular region of GRP78 it targets. The consequences of a Mab binding to csGRP78 include stimulation of cell proliferation, suppression of cell proliferation, triggering apoptosis, or no effect at all. It remains unclear why different anti-GRP78 Mabs generate different biological effects in cells. Previously, it has been postulated that an antibody targeting the C-terminal region of GRP78 may be a pan suppressor of proliferative/survival signaling of csGRP78 in cancer cells. However, not all antibodies against the C-terminal region of GRP78 present suppressive activity in cancer [35,36]. The GRP78 C-terminal targeting Mabs C38 and C107 both significantly suppressed tumor growth in prostate and melanoma models by activating caspase-mediated apoptosis [37,38]. A mouse Mab targeting the KDEL ER retention sequence at the C-terminus of GRP78 also inhibited cell proliferation and induced apoptosis [39]. However, a human Mab targeting the C-terminal 20 residues affected neither cell proliferation nor apoptosis [40]. Mab159, a GRP78-specific mouse monoclonal IgG, suppressed multiple types of cancer growth and metastasis in mice by inducing cancer cell apoptosis and suppressing PI3K/AKT signaling [41]. The GRP78 region targeted by Mab159 is also towards the C-terminal region [42] (Figure 2). PAT-SM6, a human monoclonal IgM isolated from a gastric cancer patient, induced apoptosis of multiple myeloma and melanoma cells in vitro and suppressed cancer growth in xenograft models [43,44]. PAT-SM6 recognized an O-linked carbohydrate moiety of csGRP78 with a molecular weight of 82 kDa, specifically present in cancer cells [45]. Nevertheless, to date, no report has demonstrated that csGRP78 is of a different protein composition, comparing to the ER lumen GRP78. csGRP78 expression is known to increase with the progression of multiple myeloma and is highly elevated in multiple myeloma patients presenting drug-resistant and extramedullary disease phenotypes. About one-third of multiple myeloma patients with relapsed or refractory disease showed stability after two weeks of PAT-SM6 treatment in a phase I clinical trial [46]. PAT-SM6 in combination with bortezomib and lenalidomide leads to partial remission of both intra- and extramedullary lesions in a patient with drug-resistant multiple myeloma [47].

5. Synthetic Peptides as Proapoptotic Ligands of csGRP78

Several synthetic peptides able to induce apoptosis by targeting the N-terminal region of GRP78 have been developed (Figure 2). Peptides WIFPWIQL and WDLAWMFRLPVG were selected by phage-binding assays for their ability to bind GRP78 specifically [48]. When these two GRP78-binding peptides were fused with a proapoptotic peptidomimetic, the two resulting peptides, WIFPWIQL-GG-$_{D}$(KLAKLAK)$_2$ (later called BMTP78) and WDLAWMFRLPVG-GG-$_{D}$(KLAKLAK)$_2$, both selectively targeted tumors and suppressed tumor growth in vivo by inducing cancer cell apoptosis. BMTP78 selectively killed breast cancer cells that expressed csGRP78 and suppressed both primary tumor growth as well as lung and bone micrometastases, leading to prolonged disease-free survival [49]. Despite the promising antitumor effect of BMTP-78 in vitro and in preclinical cancer models, subsequent toxicology studies in nonhuman primates presented unexpected cardiac toxicity, leading to morbidity and mortality [50]. This cardiac toxicity reduced the optimism for BMTP78 to become an anticancer drug. Recently, BC71, a cyclic pentapeptide derivative of ISM1, was shown to bind specifically to GRP78 and trigger apoptosis in cultured endothelial cells [51]. BC71 has the unique ability to both bind to csGRP78 and trigger apoptosis by itself. In vivo, BC71 preferentially accumulated in the tumor and suppressed xenograft tumor growth in mice. Hence, BC71 can be useful as a prototype peptide to develop further modified peptides with higher GRP78-binding affinity and more potent proapoptotic activity for anticancer drug development.

6. Conclusions and Future Perspectives

Due to the preferential presence of csGRP78 on cancer cells, csGRP78 has emerged as an attractive target for anticancer drug development. Proapoptotic ligands of csGRP78, including natural proteins, Mabs, and synthetic peptides, have the potential to become effective anticancer drugs. Although no anticancer drugs targeting csGRP78 have reached the clinic as of now, the Mab PAT-SM6 has shown promising results in early-stage clinical trials [46,47]. We envisage that a csGRP78-targeted proapoptotic anticancer drug is likely to emerge in the coming years. Nevertheless, how csGRP78 initiates the intracellular death signaling pathway remains poorly understood, especially because it sits on cancer cells preferentially as an external peripheral protein [20]. One hypothesis is that csGRP78 forms complexes with other cell surface transmembrane proteins to transmit the death signal to the intracellular environment. Future research in this interesting area is highly warranted. A more in-depth understanding of how csGRP78 functions as a cell surface signal receptor will greatly facilitate targeted cancer drug development.

Author Contributions: R.G. conceptualized and supervised the writing of this perspective. Both R.G. and C.K. contributed to writing of this perspective.

References

1. Shiu, R.P.; Pouyssegur, J.; Pastan, I. Glucose depletion accounts for the induction of two transformation-sensitive membrane proteinsin rous sarcoma virus-transformed chick embryo fibroblasts. *Proc. Natl. Acad. Sci. USA* **1977**, *74*, 3840–3844. [CrossRef] [PubMed]
2. Zala, C.A.; Salas-Prato, M.; Yan, W.T.; Banjo, B.; Perdue, J.F. In cultured chick embryo fibroblasts the hexose transport components are not the 75 000 and 95 000 dalton polypeptides synthesized following glucose deprivation. *Can. J. Biochem.* **1980**, *58*, 1179–1188. [CrossRef] [PubMed]
3. Lee, A.S. The glucose-regulated proteins: Stress induction and clinical applications. *Trends Biochem. Sci.* **2001**, *26*, 504–510. [CrossRef]
4. Lee, A.S. Grp78 induction in cancer: Therapeutic and prognostic implications. *Cancer Res.* **2007**, *67*, 3496–3499. [CrossRef]
5. Ni, M.; Zhang, Y.; Lee, A.S. Beyond the endoplasmic reticulum: Atypical grp78 in cell viability, signalling and therapeutic targeting. *Biochem. J.* **2011**, *434*, 181–188. [CrossRef]
6. Vig, S.; Buitinga, M.; Rondas, D.; Crevecoeur, I.; van Zandvoort, M.; Waelkens, E.; Eizirik, D.L.; Gysemans, C.; Baatsen, P.; Mathieu, C.; et al. Cytokine-induced translocation of grp78 to the plasma membrane triggers a pro-apoptotic feedback loop in pancreatic beta cells. *Cell Death Dis.* **2019**, *10*, 309. [CrossRef]
7. Shani, G.; Fischer, W.H.; Justice, N.J.; Kelber, J.A.; Vale, W.; Gray, P.C. Grp78 and cripto form a complex at the cell surface and collaborate to inhibit transforming growth factor beta signaling and enhance cell growth. *Mol. Cell Biol.* **2008**, *28*, 666–677. [CrossRef]
8. Tsai, Y.L.; Ha, D.P.; Zhao, H.; Carlos, A.J.; Wei, S.; Pun, T.K.; Wu, K.; Zandi, E.; Kelly, K.; Lee, A.S. Endoplasmic reticulum stress activates src, relocating chaperones to the cell surface where grp78/cd109 blocks tgf-beta signaling. *Proc. Natl. Acad. Sci. USA* **2018**, *115*, E4245–E4254. [CrossRef]
9. Philippova, M.; Ivanov, D.; Joshi, M.B.; Kyriakakis, E.; Rupp, K.; Afonyushkin, T.; Bochkov, V.; Erne, P.; Resink, T.J. Identification of proteins associating with glycosylphosphatidylinositol- anchored t-cadherin on the surface of vascular endothelial cells: Role for grp78/bip in t-cadherin-dependent cell survival. *Mol. Cell Biol.* **2008**, *28*, 4004–4017. [CrossRef]
10. Quinones, Q.J.; de Ridder, G.G.; Pizzo, S.V. Grp78: A chaperone with diverse roles beyond the endoplasmic reticulum. *Histol. Histopathol.* **2008**, *23*, 1409–1416.
11. Gonzalez-Gronow, M.; Selim, M.A.; Papalas, J.; Pizzo, S.V. Grp78: A multifunctional receptor on the cell surface. *Antioxid. Redox Signal.* **2009**, *11*, 2299–2306. [CrossRef] [PubMed]
12. Sato, M.; Yao, V.J.; Arap, W.; Pasqualini, R. Grp78 signaling hub a receptor for targeted tumor therapy. *Adv. Genet.* **2010**, *69*, 97–114. [PubMed]
13. Pizzo, S.V. *Cell Surface Grp78, a New Paradigm in Signal Transduction Biology*, 1st ed.; Pizzo, S.V., Ed.; Academic Press: Cambridge, MS, USA, 2018; Chapters 1–3; pp. 12–41.
14. Ibrahim, I.M.; Abdelmalek, D.H.; Elfiky, A.A. Grp78: A cell's response to stress. *Life Sci.* **2019**, *226*, 156–163. [CrossRef] [PubMed]
15. Gifford, J.B.; Hill, R. Grp78 influences chemoresistance and prognosis in cancer. *Curr. Drug Targets* **2018**, *19*, 701–708. [CrossRef]
16. Casas, C. Grp78 at the centre of the stage in cancer and neuroprotection. *Front. Neurosci.* **2017**, *11*, 177. [CrossRef]
17. Cook, K.L.; Clarke, R. Role of grp78 in promoting therapeutic-resistant breast cancer. *Future Med. Chem.* **2015**, *7*, 1529–1534. [CrossRef]
18. Bailly, C.; Waring, M.J. Pharmacological effectors of grp78 chaperone in cancers. *Biochem. Pharmacol.* **2019**, *163*, 269–278. [CrossRef]
19. Guicciardi, M.E.; Gores, G.J. Life and death by death receptors. *FASEB J.* **2009**, *23*, 1625–1637. [CrossRef]
20. Tsai, Y.L.; Zhang, Y.; Tseng, C.C.; Stanciauskas, R.; Pinaud, F.; Lee, A.S. Characterization and mechanism of stress-induced translocation of 78-kilodalton glucose-regulated protein (grp78) to the cell surface. *J. Biol. Chem.* **2015**, *290*, 8049–8064. [CrossRef]
21. Burikhanov, R.; Zhao, Y.; Goswami, A.; Qiu, S.; Schwarze, S.R.; Rangnekar, V.M. The tumor suppressor par-4 activates an extrinsic pathway for apoptosis. *Cell* **2009**, *138*, 377–388. [CrossRef]
22. Irby, R.B.; Kline, C.L. Par-4 as a potential target for cancer therapy. *Expert Opin. Ther. Targets* **2013**, *17*, 77–87. [CrossRef] [PubMed]

23. Lee, A.S. The par-4-grp78 trail, more twists and turns. *Cancer Biol. Ther.* **2009**, *8*, 2103–2105. [CrossRef] [PubMed]
24. Zhao, Y.; Burikhanov, R.; Brandon, J.; Qiu, S.; Shelton, B.J.; Spear, B.; Bondada, S.; Bryson, S.; Rangnekar, V.M. Systemic par-4 inhibits non-autochthonous tumor growth. *Cancer Biol. Ther.* **2011**, *12*, 152–157. [CrossRef]
25. Xiang, W.; Ke, Z.; Zhang, Y.; Cheng, G.H.; Irwan, I.D.; Sulochana, K.N.; Potturi, P.; Wang, Z.; Yang, H.; Wang, J.; et al. Isthmin is a novel secreted angiogenesis inhibitor that inhibits tumour growth in mice. *J. Cell Mol. Med.* **2011**, *15*, 359–374. [CrossRef] [PubMed]
26. Zhang, Y.; Chen, M.; Venugopal, S.; Zhou, Y.; Xiang, W.; Li, Y.H.; Lin, Q.; Kini, R.M.; Chong, Y.S.; Ge, R. Isthmin exerts pro-survival and death-promoting effect on endothelial cells through alphavbeta5 integrin depending on its physical state. *Cell Death Dis.* **2011**, *2*. [CrossRef] [PubMed]
27. Chen, M.; Zhang, Y.; Yu, V.C.; Chong, Y.S.; Yoshioka, T.; Ge, R. Isthmin targets cell-surface grp78 and triggers apoptosis via induction of mitochondrial dysfunction. *Cell Death Differ.* **2014**, *21*, 797–810. [CrossRef] [PubMed]
28. Chen, M.; Qiu, T.; Wu, J.; Yang, Y.; Wright, G.D.; Wu, M.; Ge, R. Extracellular anti-angiogenic proteins augment an endosomal protein trafficking pathway to reach mitochondria and execute apoptosis in huvecs. *Cell Death Differ.* **2018**, *25*, 1905–1920. [CrossRef]
29. Cao, Y.; Chen, A.; An, S.S.; Ji, R.W.; Davidson, D.; Llinas, M. Kringle 5 of plasminogen is a novel inhibitor of endothelial cell growth. *J. Biol. Chem.* **1997**, *272*, 22924–22928. [CrossRef]
30. Davidson, D.J.; Haskell, C.; Majest, S.; Kherzai, A.; Egan, D.A.; Walter, K.A.; Schneider, A.; Gubbins, E.F.; Solomon, L.; Chen, Z.; et al. Kringle 5 of human plasminogen induces apoptosis of endothelial and tumor cells through surface-expressed glucose-regulated protein 78. *Cancer Res.* **2005**, *65*, 4663–4672. [CrossRef]
31. McFarland, B.C.; Stewart, J., Jr.; Hamza, A.; Nordal, R.; Davidson, D.J.; Henkin, J.; Gladson, C.L. Plasminogen kringle 5 induces apoptosis of brain microvessel endothelial cells: Sensitization by radiation and requirement for grp78 and lrp1. *Cancer Res.* **2009**, *69*, 5537–5545. [CrossRef]
32. Nakatsuka, A.; Wada, J.; Iseda, I.; Teshigawara, S.; Higashio, K.; Murakami, K.; Kanzaki, M.; Inoue, K.; Terami, T.; Katayama, A.; et al. Visceral adipose tissue-derived serine proteinase inhibitor inhibits apoptosis of endothelial cells as a ligand for the cell-surface grp78/voltage-dependent anion channel complex. *Circ. Res.* **2013**, *112*, 771–780. [CrossRef] [PubMed]
33. Fang, S.; Hong, H.; Li, L.; He, D.; Xu, Z.; Zuo, S.; Han, J.; Wu, Q.; Dai, Z.; Cai, W.; et al. Plasminogen kringle 5 suppresses gastric cancer via regulating hif-1alpha and grp78. *Cell Death Dis.* **2017**, *8*, e3144. [CrossRef] [PubMed]
34. Rondas, D.; Crevecoeur, I.; D'Hertog, W.; Ferreira, G.B.; Staes, A.; Garg, A.D.; Eizirik, D.L.; Agostinis, P.; Gevaert, K.; Overbergh, L.; et al. Citrullinated glucose-regulated protein 78 is an autoantigen in type 1 diabetes. *Diabetes* **2015**, *64*, 573–586. [CrossRef] [PubMed]
35. Misra, U.K.; Mowery, Y.; Kaczowka, S.; Pizzo, S.V. Ligation of cancer cell surface grp78 with antibodies directed against its cooh-terminal domain up-regulates p53 activity and promotes apoptosis. *Mol. Cancer Ther.* **2009**, *8*, 1350–1362. [CrossRef]
36. Misra, U.K.; Pizzo, S.V. Modulation of the unfolded protein response in prostate cancer cells by antibody-directed against the carboxyl-terminal domain of grp78. *Apoptosis* **2010**, *15*, 173–182. [CrossRef]
37. de Ridder, G.G.; Ray, R.; Pizzo, S.V. A murine monoclonal antibody directed against the carboxyl-terminal domain of grp78 suppresses melanoma growth in mice. *Melanoma Res.* **2012**, *22*, 225–235. [CrossRef]
38. Mo, L.; Bachelder, R.E.; Kennedy, M.; Chen, P.H.; Chi, J.T.; Berchuck, A.; Cianciolo, G.; Pizzo, S.V. Syngeneic murine ovarian cancer model reveals that ascites enriches for ovarian cancer stem-like cells expressing membrane grp78. *Mol. Cancer Ther.* **2015**, *14*, 747–756. [CrossRef]
39. Lee, A.S. The er chaperone and signaling regulator grp78/bip as a monitor of endoplasmic reticulum stress. *Methods* **2005**, *35*, 373–381. [CrossRef]
40. Jakobsen, C.G.; Rasmussen, N.; Laenkholm, A.V.; Ditzel, H.J. Phage display derived human monoclonal antibodies isolated by binding to the surface of live primary breast cancer cells recognize grp78. *Cancer Res.* **2007**, *67*, 9507–9517. [CrossRef]
41. Liu, R.; Li, X.; Gao, W.; Zhou, Y.; Wey, S.; Mitra, S.K.; Krasnoperov, V.; Dong, D.; Liu, S.; Li, D.; et al. Monoclonal antibody against cell surface grp78 as a novel agent in suppressing pi3k/akt signaling, tumor growth, and metastasis. *Clin. Cancer Res.* **2013**, *19*, 6802–6811. [CrossRef]

42. Lee, A.S. Glucose-regulated proteins in cancer: Molecular mechanisms and therapeutic potential. *Nat. Rev. Cancer* **2014**, *14*, 263–276. [CrossRef] [PubMed]
43. Hensel, F.; Eckstein, M.; Rosenwald, A.; Brandlein, S. Early development of pat-sm6 for the treatment of melanoma. *Melanoma Res.* **2013**, *23*, 264–275. [CrossRef] [PubMed]
44. Rasche, L.; Duell, J.; Morgner, C.; Chatterjee, M.; Hensel, F.; Rosenwald, A.; Einsele, H.; Topp, M.S.; Brandlein, S. The natural human igm antibody pat-sm6 induces apoptosis in primary human multiple myeloma cells by targeting heat shock protein grp78. *PLoS ONE* **2013**, *8*, e63414. [CrossRef] [PubMed]
45. Rauschert, N.; Brandlein, S.; Holzinger, E.; Hensel, F.; Muller-Hermelink, H.K.; Vollmers, H.P. A new tumor-specific variant of grp78 as target for antibody-based therapy. *Lab. Invest.* **2008**, *88*, 375–386. [CrossRef] [PubMed]
46. Rasche, L.; Duell, J.; Castro, I.C.; Dubljevic, V.; Chatterjee, M.; Knop, S.; Hensel, F.; Rosenwald, A.; Einsele, H.; Topp, M.S.; et al. Grp78-directed immunotherapy in relapsed or refractory multiple myeloma - results from a phase 1 trial with the monoclonal immunoglobulin m antibody pat-sm6. *Haematologica* **2015**, *100*, 377–384. [CrossRef] [PubMed]
47. Rasche, L.; Menoret, E.; Dubljevic, V.; Menu, E.; Vanderkerken, K.; Lapa, C.; Steinbrunn, T.; Chatterjee, M.; Knop, S.; Dull, J.; et al. A grp78-directed monoclonal antibody recaptures response in refractory multiple myeloma with extramedullary involvement. *Clin. Cancer Res.* **2016**, *22*, 4341–4349. [CrossRef]
48. Arap, M.A.; Lahdenranta, J.; Mintz, P.J.; Hajitou, A.; Sarkis, A.S.; Arap, W.; Pasqualini, R. Cell surface expression of the stress response chaperone grp78 enables tumor targeting by circulating ligands. *Cancer Cell* **2004**, *6*, 275–284. [CrossRef]
49. Miao, Y.R.; Eckhardt, B.L.; Cao, Y.; Pasqualini, R.; Argani, P.; Arap, W.; Ramsay, R.G.; Anderson, R.L. Inhibition of established micrometastases by targeted drug delivery via cell surface-associated grp78. *Clin. Cancer Res.* **2013**, *19*, 2107–2116. [CrossRef]
50. Staquicini, D.I.; D'Angelo, S.; Ferrara, F.; Karjalainen, K.; Sharma, G.; Smith, T.L.; Tarleton, C.A.; Jaalouk, D.E.; Kuniyasu, A.; Baze, W.B.; et al. Therapeutic targeting of membrane-associated grp78 in leukemia and lymphoma: Preclinical efficacy in vitro and formal toxicity study of bmtp-78 in rodents and primates. *Pharmacogenomics J.* **2018**, *18*, 436–443. [CrossRef]
51. Kao, C.; Chandna, R.; Ghode, A.; Dsouza, C.; Chen, M.; Larsson, A.; Lim, S.H.; Wang, M.; Cao, Z.; Zhu, Y.; et al. Proapoptotic cyclic peptide bc71 targets cell-surface grp78 and functions as an anticancer therapeutic in mice. *EBioMedicine* **2018**, *33*, 22–32. [CrossRef]

3

Effective Delivery of Anti-Cancer Drug Molecules with Shape Transforming Liquid Metal Particles

Dasom Kim, Jangsun Hwang, Yonghyun Choi, Yejin Kwon, Jaehee Jang, Semi Yoon and Jonghoon Choi *

School of Integrative Engineering, Chung-Ang University, Seoul 06974, Korea; stvg54@gmail.com (D.K.); isnickawesome@gmail.com (J.H.); dydgus5057@gmail.com (Y.C.); angang1027@gmail.com (Y.K.); jjaeh95@gmail.com (J.J.); semi103306@gmail.com (S.Y.)

* Correspondence: nanomed@cau.ac.kr

Abstract: Liquid metals are being studied intensively because of their potential as a drug delivery system. Eutectic gallium–indium (EGaIn) alloy liquid metals have a low melting point, low toxicity, and excellent tissue permeability. These properties may enable them to be vascular embolic agents that can be deformed by light or heat. In this study, we developed EGaIn particles that can deliver anticancer drugs to tumor cells in vitro and change their shapes in response to external stimuli. These particles were prepared by sonicating a solution containing EGaIn and amphiphilic lipids. The liquid metal (LM)/amphiphilic lipid (DSPC, 1,2-distearoyl-sn-glycero-3-phosphocholin) particles formed a vehicle for doxorubicin, an anticancer drug, which was released (up to 50%) when the shape of the particles was deformed by light or heat treatment. LM/DSPC particles are non-toxic and LM/DSPC/doxorubicin particles have anticancer effects (resulting in a cell viability of less than 50%). LM/DSPC/doxorubicin particles were also able to mimic blood vessel embolisms by modifying their shape using precisely controlled light and heat in engineered microchannels. The purpose of this study was to examine the potential of EGaIn materials to treat tumor tissues that cannot be removed by surgery.

Keywords: liquid metal; EGaIn; photothermal; drug delivery system; vascular embolism; doxorubicin

---

1. Introduction

The development of new and effective drug carriers to treat cancer is crucial and ongoing [1]. These carriers are usually comprised of biomaterials and are designed to transport small molecules, proteins, DNA, and RNA [2]. When designing drug carriers, aspects such as biocompatibility and biodegradation are carefully considered [3]. Also, they should have low cytotoxicity, and they should be readily absorbed by cells. Drug carriers using metal particles have been widely studied because they are stable, their surface is easy to modify, they are accessible to various drugs, and they are easy to image with MRI or X-ray scanning [4,5].

Metals that are liquid at room temperature are known for their fluidity and conductivity. Mercury, a well-known room temperature liquid metal, is difficult to use in bioresearch because of its toxicity [6]. Alloys such as liquid metals (LM), gallium, gallium–indium common alloys (EGaIn, 75% Ga, 25% In), and galinstan (a liquid metal alloy composed from a family of eutectic alloys mainly consisting of gallium, indium, and tin) are promising alternatives to mercury because of their relatively low toxicity [7,8]. Gallium-based liquid metals have gained the attention of researchers because they are easily formable, deformable, and stretchable. They are also chemically stable and do not react with water at room temperature [9–11]. In contrast to mercury, unique properties such as high surface tension, good mobility, high electrical conductivity, good biocompatibility, and low toxicity make LM an attractive material for biomedical applications, as well as microfluidic systems such as circuits, pumps, electrodes, and sensors [12–16]. In particular, colloids of liquid metals are applied to pumps, sensors, catalysts, and drug delivery systems [17]. LM particles are easily produced by sonication, and can also cause vascular embolisms [18]. They have excellent photochemical and photothermal conversion properties, which can be applied to photothermal conversion agents (PTA) and the photothermal therapy (PTT) of tumors [19–22]. LM particles, however, possess drawbacks that require further research to address. They may cause embolisms in normal tissues; therefore, they must be administered directly to the target vessel using a catheter or stent. Also, their size can be difficult to control after inducing them to change. Furthermore, because no in vivo experiments were performed in this study, a toxicity assessment could not be conducted, and the potential toxicity of the LM particles was not characterized.

Tumor cell proliferation and differentiation are caused by a variety of growth factors, as well as a rich supply of oxygen and nutrients from blood vessels [23]. As tumor growth depends on blood vessels, starving tumors with vascular target therapy is a promising area of study, and research on angiogenesis inhibitors is ongoing [24–26]. However, because tumors become resistant to inhibitors, a new focus of research is on vascular blockage [27]. Several agents that can block blood vessels, including small molecule materials, have been studied along with several physical embolic methods such as coils, balloons, and nanoparticle embolics [28,29].

In this study, engineered liquid metal particles caused in vitro cancer cell necrosis through vascular embolization and conventional drug delivery methods (Figure 1). Using simple sonication techniques, liquid metal particles carrying doxorubicin, an anticancer agent, were formed, and their efficacy was verified. Furthermore, the shape of the liquid metal particles was modified to mimic vascular embolism and verify their potential as a vascular embolizing agent.

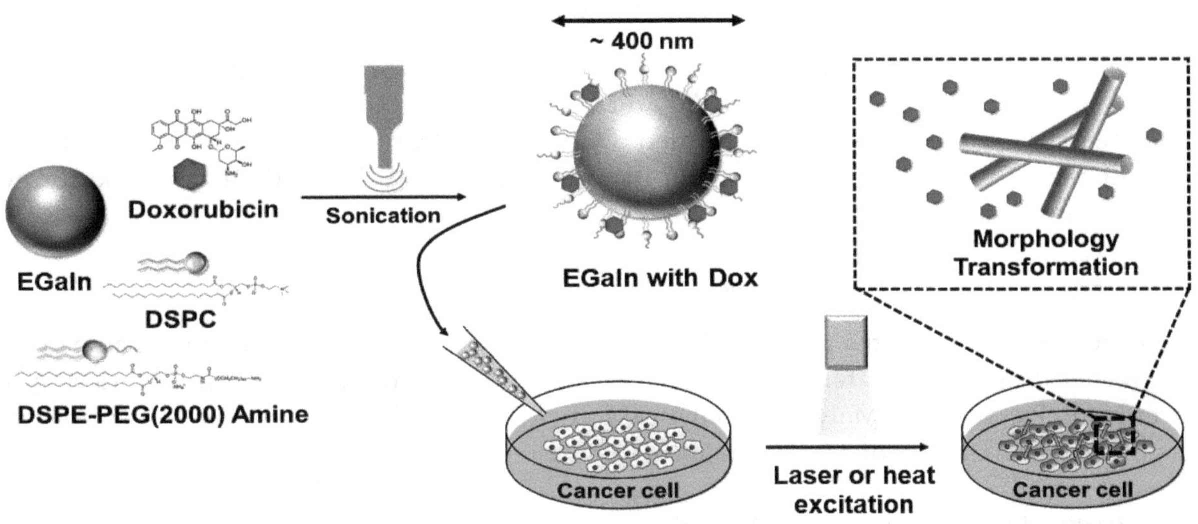

Figure 1. Schematic illustration showing the synthesis of doxorubicin-loaded core-shell liquid metal particles (liquid metal (LM)/1,2-distearoyl-sn-glycero-3-phosphocholin (DSPC)/doxorubicin (DOX)). DSPE-PEG-2000 Amine, 1,2-distearoyl-sn-glycero-3-phosphoethanolamine-N-[amino (polyethylene glycol)-2000]; EGaIn, eutectic gallium–indium.

2. Materials and Methods

2.1. Materials

All reagents, unless otherwise specified, were purchased from Sigma-Aldrich (St. Louis, MO, USA). 1,2-distearoyl-sn-glycero-3-phosphoethanolamine-N-[amino (polyethylene glycol)-2000] (DSPE-PEG-2000 Amine) and 1,2-distearoyl-sn-glycero-3-phosphocholin (DSPC), which were used to synthesize the particles, were purchased from Avanti Polar Lipids (Alabaster, AL, USA). MDA-MB-231 breast cancer cells, Hs578T breast cancer cells, and MIA-Paca-2 pancreatic cancer cells were purchased from ATCC (HTB-26, HTB-126, and CRL-1420) (Manassas, VA, USA). A LIVE/DEAD® Viability/Cytotoxicity Kit was used to analyze cell viability (Invitrogen, Carlsbad, CA, USA), and a Cell Counting Kit-8 (CCK-8) was obtained from Dojindo (Rockville, MD, USA). A dialysis bag (MW cut-off of 6–8 kDa) was purchased from Spectrumlabs (Piraeus, Greece) to investigate the drug release behavior of the metal particles.

2.2. Preparation of the LM/DSPC/Doxorubicin (DOX) Particles

As a general particle synthesis method, we added 10 mg of eutectic gallium–indium (EGaIn) into a 50 mL disposable sample vial and added 80 μL of DSPC (25 mg/mL in chloroform) and 400 μL of DSPE-PEG-2000 Amine (25 mg/mL in chloroform) [7,20,30]. We then placed the vial in a bath sonicator (2501E-DTH, BRANSON) and processed it for 10 min at 50 °C. Next, the chloroform was removed in a dry oven, leaving a powder behind. Then, 10 mL of deionized (DI) water was added to the powder, mixed, and dispersed using probe sonication (VCX750, SONICS) for one hour with an amplitude of 26% and a pulse of 5 s on/5 s pause. The samples were then centrifuged at 15,000× *g* for 10 min, washed twice with 10 mL of DI water, and left for one hour to remove large particles by gravity. To load the doxorubicin, 4 mg of doxorubicin was dissolved in 4 mL of DMSO, 2 μL of triethanolamine (TEA) was added, and the mixture was incubated at room temperature for 12 h. After the reaction, doxorubicin (1 mg/mL) was added to the sonicated sample particles so that the ratio of EGaIn and doxorubicin was 10:1 and rocked at 4 °C for 12 h. After rocking, the samples were centrifuged at 15,000× *g* for 10 min to remove free doxorubicin and rehydrated in 10 mL of DI water or 1× Dulbecco's phosphate buffered saline (DPBS, pH 7.5). The final product was stored at 4 °C.

2.3. Transmission Electron Microscopy (TEM) and Energy Dispersive X-ray Spectroscopy (EDS)

To analyze the shape of the synthesized LM/DSPC/DOX particles, the sample was placed on a copper grid and dried. Then, TEM (Talos L120C, FEI, FEI, Hillsboro, OR, USA) analysis was performed at 120 kV. Negative staining was not performed owing to the clear brightness difference of the metal particles. EDS imaging and mapping of gallium and indium (JEM-F2000, JEOL) were performed to analyze the composition of the particles.

2.4. Dynamic Light Scattering (DLS) Analysis

To determine the size of the particles that contained DSPC and DSPE-PEG-2000-Amine in EGaIn, samples were diluted with water at a ratio of 20:1 and analyzed by dynamic light scattering (DLS) (Zetasizer Nano Zs, Malvern, Malvern Panalytical Ltd., Malvern, UK). The samples were measured six times with a reflective index of 3.9 and an absorption intensity of 0.13.

2.5. Ultraviolet and Visible Spectroscopy Analysis

The absorption wavelength of the LM particles, particles synthesized with DSPC and DSPE-PEG-2000-Amine, and LM particles loaded with doxorubicin was measured with a UV/vis spectrophotometer (BIOMATE 3S, Thermo, Thermo, Waltham, MA, USA). The samples were measured in a 12.5 × 12.5 × 45 mm cuvette at 300 nm and 900 nm. DI water was used as the blank.

2.6. DOX-Loading Efficiency and In Vitro Release Test

To quantitatively analyze the doxorubicin, a standard curve was established using serial dilutions of a stock solution containing 50 μg/mL of doxorubicin in DI water. The fluorescence of each dilution was measured using an excitation wavelength of 480 nm and an emission wavelength of 560 nm.

The drug loading efficiency during the synthesis of the LM/DSPC/DOX particles was confirmed by centrifuging the samples for 10 min at 15,000× *g* and removing the remaining doxorubicin that was not loaded by taking out the supernatant. Using the doxorubicin standard curve as a reference, the fluorescence values of free doxorubicin were analyzed using a multi-plate reader (Synergy H1, BioTek, BioTek, Winooski, VT, USA) at λex 480 nm and λem 560 nm. The drug-loading efficiency was calculated by measuring the free DOX concentrations. In addition, to confirm the release behavior of the drug from the LM/DSPC/DOX particles, 1 mL of the sample was placed into a dialysis bag and stored in 5 mL of 1× DPBS. Then, 1 mL of the diffused drug was sampled at various time points during the incubation (e.g., 1 h, 2 h, 3 h, 6 h, 9 h, 12 h, 24 h, 48 h, and 72 h) at 37 °C to measure the fluorescence, and 1 mL of 1× DPBS was added back to perform an accumulative release.

2.7. *Confocal Laser Scanning Microscopy*

MDA-MB-231 breast cancer cells were used to confirm the behavior, intracellular penetration, and anticancer effects of the LM/DSPC/DOX particles. MDA-MB-231 cells (1.0×10^5 cells/well in an eight-well glass bottom chamber) were incubated in high glucose (Dulbecco's Modified Eagle Medium) DMEM containing 5% (Fetal Bovine Serum) FBS and 1% penicillin/streptomycin in a 37 °C incubator at 5% CO_2. After seeding the cells, they were incubated for one day. LM/DSPC/DOX particles were then added at a concentration of 3 μg/mL. The control group was treated with 3 μg/mL of doxorubicin. The samples were incubated for eight hours, washed with 1× DPBS, and fixed with 4% paraformaldehyde. The cells were stained with (4′,6-Diamidine-2′-phenylindole dihydrochloride) DAPI and analyzed using a confocal laser scanning microscope (LSM710, Carl Zeiss, Oberkochen, Germany) at a λ_{ex} of 405 nm (DAPI) and at a λ_{ex} of 488 nm (DOX).

2.8. *Live/Dead Assays*

MDA-MB-231 breast cancer cells were used to determine the cell delivery rate and cell death caused by the LM/DSPC/DOX particles. The cells were seeded at a concentration of 5.0×10^3 cells/well in a 96-well culture plate and incubated at 37 °C with 5% CO_2 for one day. Subsequently, the LM/DSPC/DOX particles were added to the cells at a low (1 μg/mL) and high (20 μg/mL) concentration and incubated for eight hours. After washing with 1× DPBS, 100 μL of each live/dead assay reagent was added, and the cells were incubated at room temperature for 30 min. After the reagent was removed, the cells were washed again with 1× DPBS and observed using a fluorescence microscope (OX.2053-PLPH, Euromex, Arnhem, The Netherlands).

2.9. *Cytotoxicity Assays*

MDA-MB-231 breast cancer cells, Hs578T breast cancer cells, and MIA-Paca pancreatic cancer cells were used to analyze the time- and concentration-specific cytotoxicity of the LM/DSPC particles. Each cell type was seeded at a concentration of 5×10^3 cells/well in a 96-well culture plate and incubated at 37 °C with 5% CO_2 for one day. In the hourly cytotoxicity test, MDA-MD-231 cells were treated with control and LM/DSPC/DOX particles using a doxorubicin concentration of 3 μg/mL. After washing with 1× DPBS, the cells were treated with 10% CCK-8 reagent and incubated at 37 °C for two hours. The absorbance was then measured at 450 nm using a multi plate reader.

2.10. *Light- and Heat-Driven Morphology Changes of LM/DSPC/DOX Particles*

The photothermal/thermal characteristics of the LM/DSPC/DOX particles were observed using laser irradiation or 70 °C heat treatment. Laser irradiation used a repetition rate of 100 kHz, pulse width of 200 ns, scan speed of 100 mm/s, loop of 10, and power of 2 W. To conduct the heat treatment, the particles were incubated in a dry oven for 30 min at 50, 60, or 70 °C. Morphological changes were analyzed using TEM according to the experimental conditions outlined above. DLS was used before and after the light/heat treatment to analyze particle sizes according to the particle shape change.

2.11. Membrane Blockage Caused by the Shape Transformation of LM/DSPC/DOX Particles

In order to evaluate the blood vessel embolization potential of LM particles, a membrane perfusion experiment using LM/DSPC particles before and after heat treatment was performed. The membrane was a 40 μm pore size nylon cell strainer and the volume of LM/DSPC particles used in this experiment was 1 mL. The absorbance of the particles was measured between 300 nm and 900 nm wavelengths before and after passing through the membrane. After the light and temperature treatment (70 °C, 30 min), the same measurement was performed. The area of the absorbance range was used to analyze the membrane passage rates altered by the shape variations of particles after the light and temperature treatment.

2.12. Microfluidic Chip Embolization

Embolization experiments were carried out using a microfluidic chip introduced to LM/DSPC/DOX particles. A (Polydimethylsiloxane) PDMS chip 20 mm in length, 10 μm in depth, and 10 μm in width was fabricated, treated with O_2 plasma (FEMTO SCIENCE, Gyeonggi-Do, Korea) at 80 W for three minutes, and attached to slide glass. Then, 10 μL of LM/DSPC/DOX particles at a concentration of 5 mg/mL were introduced to the microfluidic chip. They then blocked the channel in the chip after heating it to 70 °C for 30 min. The shape changes and channel blocking behavior of the LM/DSPC/DOX particles were observed using a phase contrast microscope.

3. Results and Discussion

3.1. The Physiological Properties of LM/DSPC/DOX Particles

The LM/DSPC/DOX particles formed a reddish-gray solution after sonication and were analyzed by TEM. They had a core-shell form of lipids with an EGaIn core (Figure 2a–c). Core-shell particles of various sizes were identified (Supplementary Figure S1). The particles consisted of 75% gallium, 20% indium, and 5% oxygen, which maintained their initial content (Figure 2d,e). The average diameter of the particles was 500 nm with a size distribution ranging from tens to hundreds of nanometers (Figure 2f and Supplementary Figure S1). Surface analysis using (Field Emission Scanning Electron Microsope) FE-SEM also showed spherical particles and various size distributions (Supplementary Figure S2). When the absorbance of the synthesized particles was measured, they had a very broad absorbance value in all wavelength ranges measured (from UV to near-infrared regions (NIR)) (Figure 2g). At a wavelength of 808 nm, the mass extinction coefficient of the particles was higher than that of gold nanorods, which are often used as photothermal conversion agents [31]. Therefore, an 808 nm laser was chosen to increase the local temperature and for its biocompatibility in the in vivo light processing experiments. Free doxorubicin not loaded onto the particles was removed to confirm a loading efficiency of approximately 30%. In a drug release test of LM/DSPC/DOX particles loaded with 10 μg/mL of DOX, the drug was released continuously at a rate of up to 60% discharge over 72 h (Figure 2h).

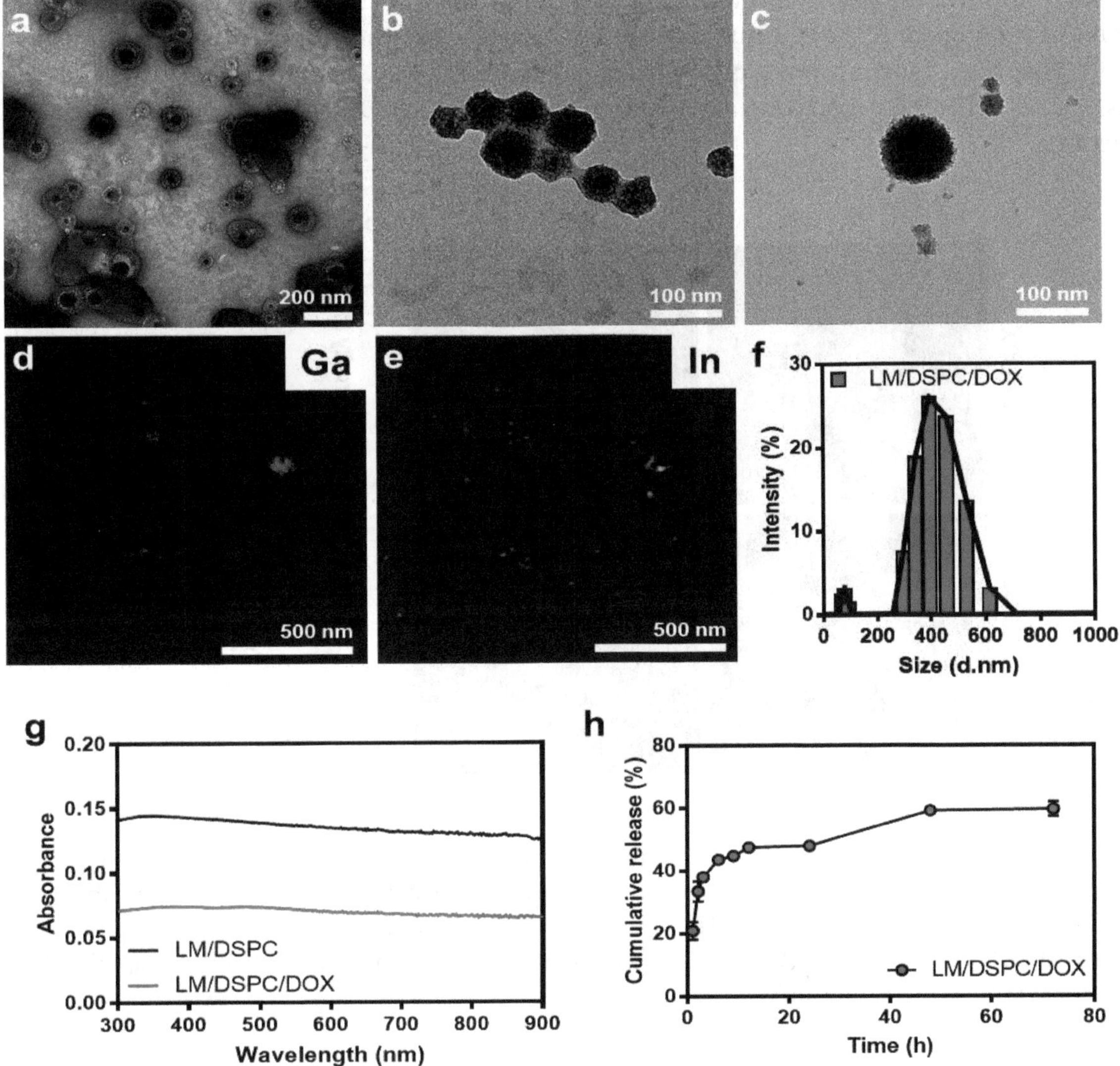

Figure 2. Characteristics of the LM/DSPC/DOX particles. (**a**–**c**) Morphology analysis of the LM/DSPC/DOX particles using transmission electron microscopy (TEM) and (**d**,**e**) energy dispersive X-ray spectroscopy (EDS) mapping. (**f**) Size distribution of the LM/DSPC/DOX particles. (**g**) UV spectroscopy of the LM/DSPC and LM/DSPC/DOX particles. (**h**) Cumulative doxorubicin release of the LM/DSPC/DOX particles.

3.2. Cellular Uptake of LM/DSPC/DOX

After LM/DSPC/DOX particles were introduced to MBA-MD-231 cells, it was confirmed that they were taken up by the cells, the drug molecules were released, and the drug was transported into the nucleus. As a result, the fluorescence intensity appeared higher in the experimental group treated with LM/DSPC/DOX particles when compared with the control group treated with the same concentration (3 μg/mL) of free doxorubicin. The drug penetration into the cells was significant (Figure 3a). Comparing the fluorescence intensity of the cells with image J showed that there was no statistically significant difference between the control group and the experimental group ($n = 10$, $p = 0.2748$, Figure 3b). However, the enlarged images in Figure 3a show that the drug was delivered to the nucleus of the cell in the experimental group. Larger aggregated particles remain around the cytoplasm of the cell (yellow arrow), suggesting that the smaller particulates effectively migrated into the cell. The particles can be observed around the cytoplasm of the cell even in cells treated with LM/DSPC particles (Supplementary Figure S3a,b). Furthermore, when LM/DSPC/DOX particles were analyzed using confocal microscopy, doxorubicin fluorescence was observed on the particles themselves or around the particles, indicating that the drug had, in fact, been loaded onto the particles (Supplementary Figure S3c,d). Thus, it was confirmed that the liquid metal nanoparticles were effectively absorbed by the cancer cells and that doxorubicin was effectively transported into the nucleus of cells within a given time. These data show that LM/DSPC/DOX particles can be used as drug carriers.

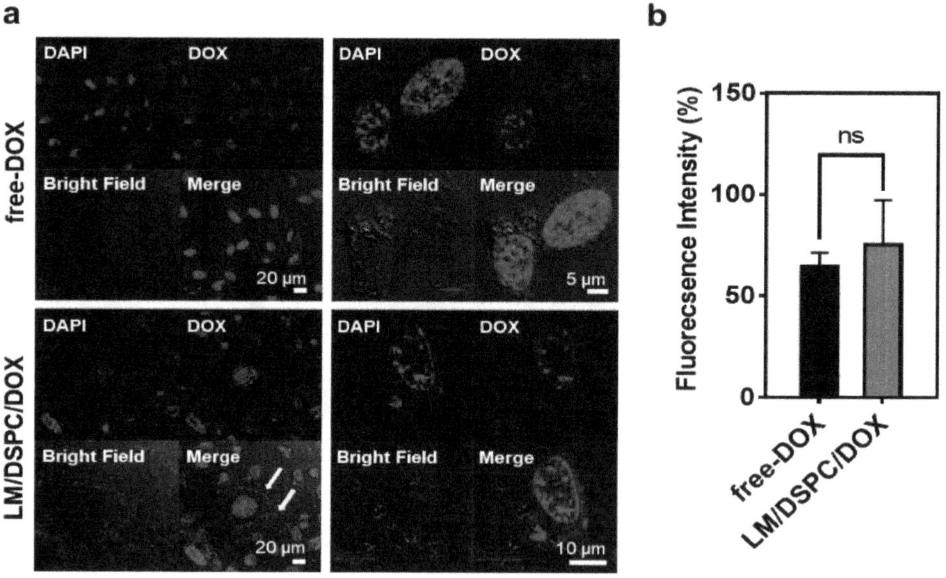

Figure 3. The cellular uptake of doxorubicin (3 μg/mL) and LM/DSPC/DOX particles. (**a**) Confocal microscopy of MDA-MB-231 breast cancer cells after an 8 h incubation with doxorubicin (red) and LM/DSPC/DOX particles (red). The nuclei were stained with (4′,6-Diamidine-2′-phenylindole dihydrochloride) DAPI (blue). (**b**) Fluorescence intensity comparison verifying cellular uptake efficacy ($p = 0.2748$). (ns = no significant).

3.3. The Effect of LM/DSPC/DOX Particle Drug Delivery on Cell Death

A live/dead assay was used on cancer cells to determine the drug delivery rate of the synthesized LM/DSPC/DOX particles and to determine any anti-cancer effects. MDA-MB-231 breast cancer cells were treated with nanoparticles containing the same concentration of doxorubicin as the control. After eight hours of incubation, the low (1 μg/mL) and high (20 μg/mL) concentrations of DOX-loaded experimental groups showed the same cancer cell killing capacity as the control group treated with free doxorubicin (Figure 4a, Supplementary Figure S4). This demonstrates that doxorubicin was effectively delivered to the cells by the LM/DSPC/DOX particles and that the LM/DSPC/DOX particles are more effective at causing cancer cell necrosis than free doxorubicin.

3.4. Cell Viability Test Using LM/DSPC and LM/DSPC/DOX Particles

As most metal particles are toxic, we performed cytotoxicity experiments in cells treated with LM/DSPC particles without DOX loading. LM/DSPC particles did not exhibit cytotoxicity in the three types of cancer cells evaluated (Figure 4b–e). Several types of cancer cells were treated with LM/DSPC/DOX particles using various concentrations of doxorubicin, and cell viability was analyzed. Particles added to Hs548T cancer cells showed statistically insignificant anti-cancer effects when compared with the cytotoxicity caused by free doxorubicin (Figure 4b). Treatment of MIA-Paca-2 cells and MDA-MB-231 cells showed similar results (Figure 4c,d).

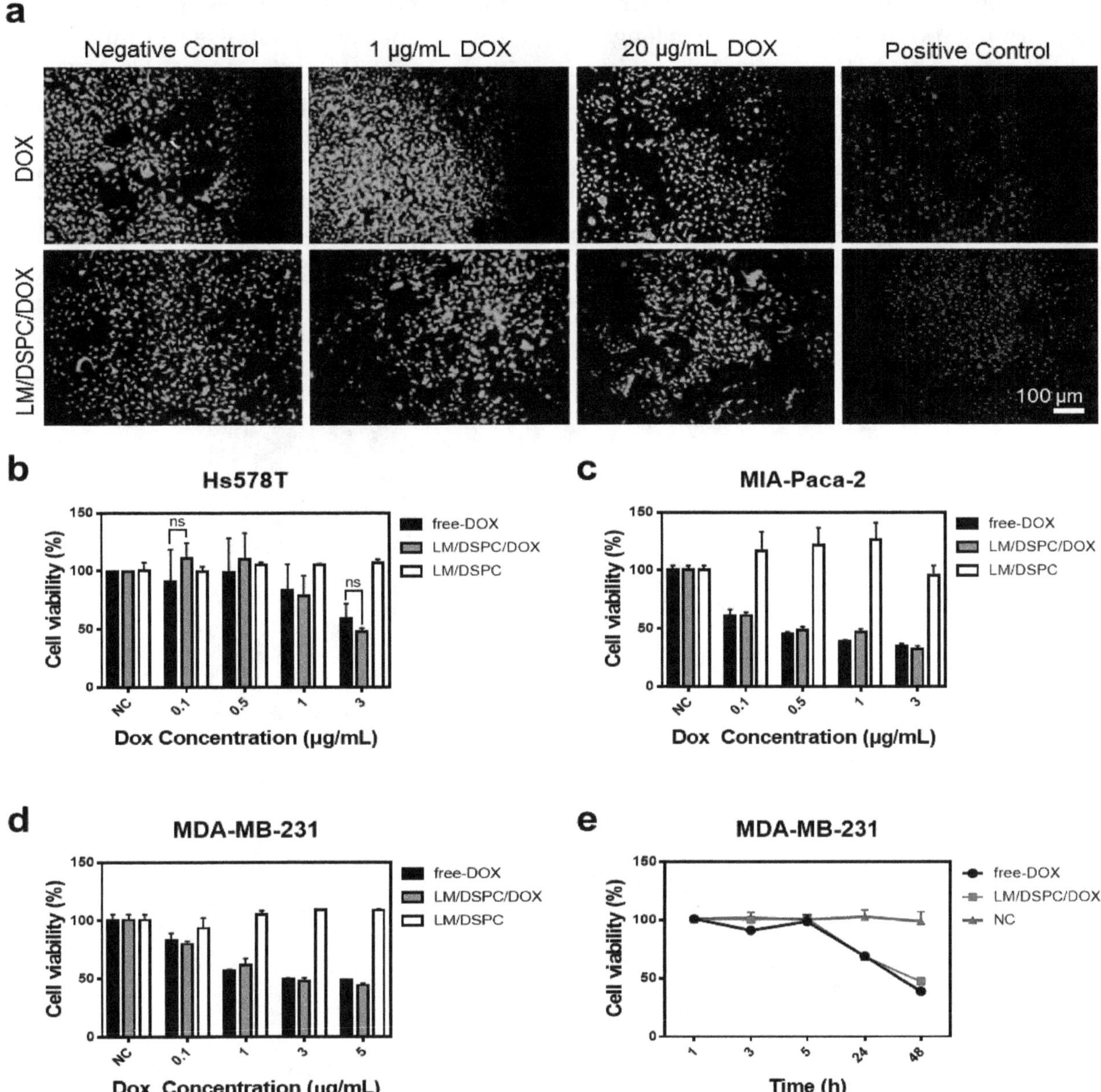

Figure 4. The effect of LM/DSPC/DOX particles on cell viability. (**a**) A live/dead cell viability assay showing live cells stained with calcein-AM (green) and dead cells stained with EthD-1 (red). (**b**) Viability of pancreatic cancer cells treated with LM/DSPC/DOX particles loaded with increasing concentrations of doxorubicin. (**c**,**d**) Viability of breast cancer cells treated with LM/DSPC/DOX particles loaded with increasing concentrations of doxorubicin. (**e**) The cytotoxicity of the nanoparticles on MDA-MB-231 cells depends on time (NC = negative control).

MDA-MB-231 cancer cells were used to investigate the hourly drug delivery of LM/DSPC/DOX particles. The cell survival rate was similar to that of the control group. After 24 h of particle and drug treatment, 40% of the cells died, and after 48 h, 60% of the cells died (Figure 4e). These results indicate that LM/DPSC/DOX particles, per se, are not cytotoxic, are efficiently absorbed into cells, and have the same anticancer effects as free DOX in several types of cancer cells.

3.5. Shape Transition of LM/DSPC Particles Caused by Light and Heat Treatment

The photothermal characteristics and temperature-dependent changes of the LM/DSPC and LM/DSPD/DOX particles were confirmed by TEM after laser irradiation and heat treatment (Figure 5,

Supplementary Figure S5). Upon laser treatment, the shape of the two particles changes in a similar fashion, forming rods of around 500 nm in length (Figure 5a,b). The particles showed a similar tendency upon heat treatment, indicating that their change in shape is due to temperature (Figure 5c,d). In Supplementary Figure S5g–i, the shape change at 50, 60, and 70 °C is shown. However, because it takes a long time to reach a temperature that can cause shape deformation, it will be necessary to design particles that can change their shape more rapidly. In addition, when the size of the particles before and after the heat treatment was measured by DLS and compared, the average diameter of the particles before the heat treatment was 400 nm, but the average particle size after the heat treatment increased to 600 nm. Also, the overall size distribution shifted toward larger diameters (Supplementary Figure S6). Owing to these changes in the shape of LM/DSPC particles, they are a potential vascular embolic material.

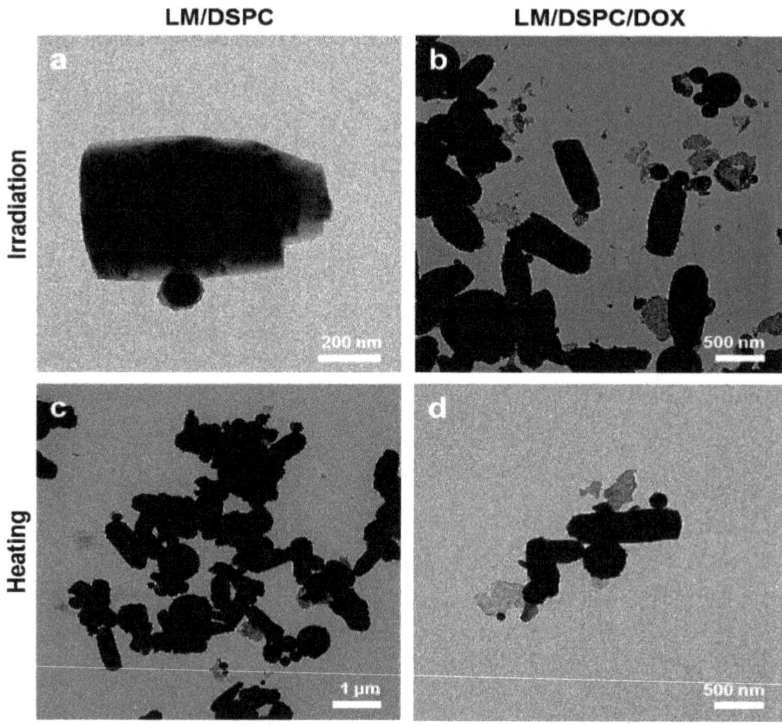

Figure 5. Morphological transformation of LM/DSPC and LM/DSPC/DOX particles. (**a**,**b**) TEM images of LM/DSPC and LM/DSPC/DOX particles after laser exposure. (**c**,**d**) TEM images of LM/DSPC and LM/DSPC/DOX particles after heating them to 70 °C.

3.6. *Transforming the Shape of LM/DSPC Particles Causes Membrane Occlusion*

To determine whether LM/DSPC particles can cause a vascular embolism, a membrane passage experiment quantified the perfusion of the particles before and after temperature treatment via absorbance with a spectrophotometer (Supplementary Figure S7). The absorbance decreased 49%, indicating that LM/DSPC particles could pass through the membrane. After applying heat, the LM/DSPC particles agglomerated and failed to cross the membrane because of changes in their size and shape. These data illustrate their potential for blood vessel embolization.

3.7. *Mimicking Vascular Embolization*

Experiments were performed to simulate vascular embolism by flowing LM/DSPC/DOX particles into a microfluidic chip (Figure 6). The particles were dispersed and flowed freely through the channel before heat treatment, but heat treatment caused the particles to change their shape, aggregate, and block the channel (Figure 6c,d). For a more detailed observation, the same experiment was conducted using 10 µL of LM/DSPC/DOX particles on a microfluidic chip with a depth of 50 µm and a width of 100 μm. At room temperature, the particles gathered via evaporation, but the particles did not block the channel. Upon heat treatment, however, the particles blocked the microchannel in the same way as the microfluidic chip with the smaller sized channels (Supplementary Figure S8). This verifies that LM/DSPC/DOX particles change their shape with heat and, consequentially, may be capable of inducing vascular embolism.

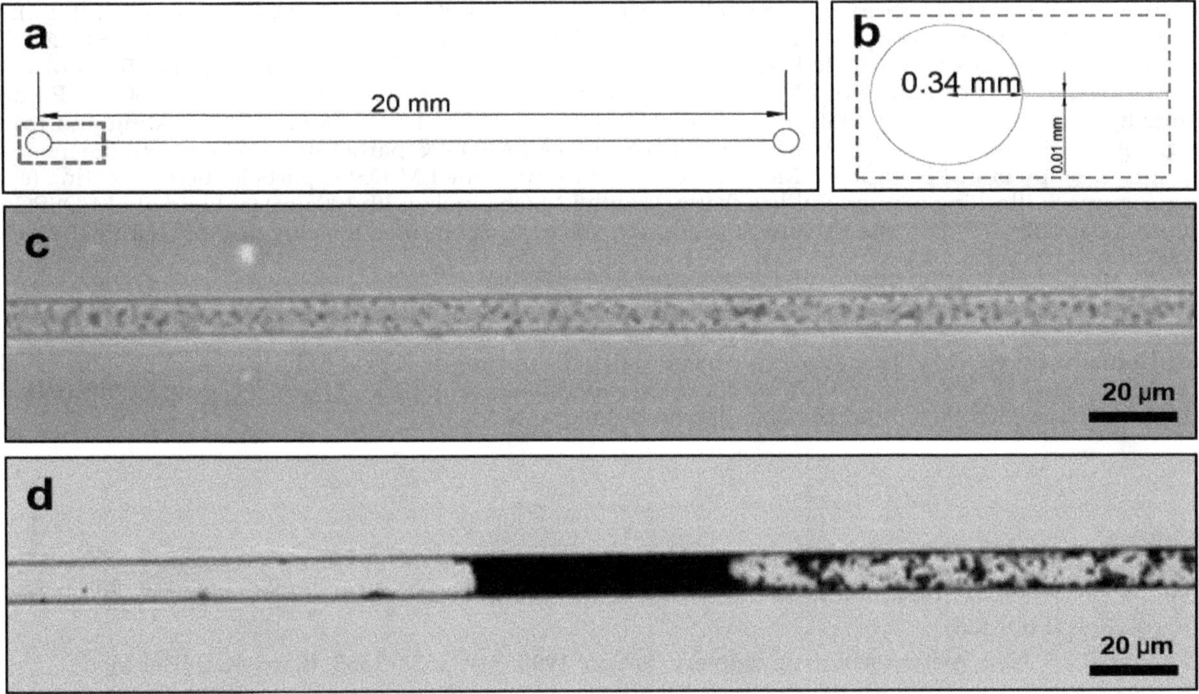

Figure 6. LM/DSPC/DOX particles tested on microfluidic chips as an embolism model. (**a**,**b**) The design of the PDMS microfluidic chip. (**c**) Fluid containing LM/DSPC/DOX particles in a micro channel. (**d**) Blocking the micro channel with heat induced transformation of LM/DSPC/DOX particles.

4. Conclusions

In this study, we developed a nanoparticle drug carrier and vascular embolic agent that can be applied to tumors that cannot be removed by surgery. The nanoparticles contained an EGaIn core and a lipid DSPC-containing surfactant (DSPE-PEG-2000) containing the anticancer drug doxorubicin. They absorb light at all wavelengths, similar to EGaIn, and have a diameter of approximately 500 nm. This allows them to be treated with infrared light, which is more suitable for in vivo applications. When cancer cells were treated with LM/DSPC/DOX particles, it was confirmed that the particles located to the cell periphery because of their lipid component, and the drug penetrated the cells and was transported to the nucleus. LM/DSPC/DOX particles showed similar anticancer effects to doxorubicin, alone, in several cancer cell types. In particular, the anti-cancer effects of free-dox and LM/DSPC/Dox were the same (approximately 50%) after 24 h of Dox (3 μg/mL) treatment. The potential of LM/DSPC/DOX particles as a vascular embolic agent was also demonstrated by their ability to block microfluidic channels after heat treatment. After 10 μL of particles (5 mg/mL) was injected and processed at 70 °C for 30 min, they successfully blocked the channel flow.

One major limitation of working with LM particles is that changing their shapes in a uniform fashion is difficult to achieve with a laser because it does not evenly transfer heat to the particles. In future experiments, it will be necessary to study methods that add polymers or nanoparticles to LM. Polymers and nanoparticles increase the efficiency of light/heat transfer, which causes LM particles to change their shape. In addition, the drug delivery properties of LM particles should be verified using 3D cell cultures to ensure the particles can efficiently change their shape at in vivo temperatures. LM particles should be tested in future animal experiments as a vascular embolizer for tumor tissues that cannot be treated surgically.

Supplementary Materials:

Figure S1: Transmission electron microscopy (TEM) images of LM/DSPC, Figure S2: Field Emission Scanning Electron Microscope (FE-SEM) images of (a–c) LM/DSPC and (d–f) LM/DSPC/DOX, Figure S3: (a,b) Confocal microscopy of MDA-MB-231 breast cancer cell after incubation for 8 h with LM/DSPC and nuclei (blue). (c,d) Confocal laser scanning microscopy (CLSM) images of LM/DSPC/DOX and doxorubicin (red), Figure S4: Live/Dead cell viability assay. Cells were treated with (a) doxorubicin and (b) LM/DSPC/DOX, Figure S5: TEM images of morphological transformation of LM/DSPC after heating at (a–g) 70 °C, (h) 60 °C and (i) 50 °C, Figure S6: Dynamic light scattering (DLS) analysis. Size distribution of (a) LM/DSPC/DOX before heating and (b) after heating, Figure S7: Changes in absorbance of LM/DSPC, when LM/DSPC particles passed through the membrane. (a) UV spectroscopy of LM/DSPCs. (b) Membrane passed through the LM/DSPC particles before heating (c) after heating, Figure S8: Blocking of microfluidics channels with LM (channel width 100 μm) (a) Fluid of LM/DSPC/DOX micro/nano particles. (b) Dry the solvent at room temperature. (c) Induce the clogging of channel by heating LM/DSPC/DOX particles.

Author Contributions: D.K., J.H. and J.C. conceptualized the project. D.K., J.H., Y.C., and J.C. designed the experiments. D.K., J.H., Y.K., J.J., and S.Y. executed the experiments. D.K., Y.K., J.J. and SY analyzed the data. D.K., J.H., Y.C. and J.C. wrote the manuscript. J.C. acquired the grants.

References

1. Allen, T.M.; Cullis, P.R.J.S. Drug delivery systems: Entering the mainstream. *Science* **2004**, *303*, 1818–1822. [CrossRef] [PubMed]
2. Langer, R.J.S. New methods of drug delivery. *Science* **1990**, *249*, 1527–1533. [CrossRef] [PubMed]
3. Nicolas, J.; Mura, S.; Brambilla, D.; Mackiewicz, N.; Couvreur, P.; Patrick, C. Design, functionalization strategies and biomedical applications of targeted biodegradable/biocompatible polymer-based nanocarriers for drug delivery. *Chem. Soc. Rev.* **2013**, *42*, 1147–1235. [CrossRef]
4. Rocca, J.D.; Liu, D.; Lin, W. Nanoscale Metal–Organic Frameworks for Biomedical Imaging and Drug Delivery. *Acc. Chem. Res.* **2011**, *44*, 957–968. [CrossRef] [PubMed]
5. Sun, C.-Y.; Qin, C.; Wang, X.-L.; Su, Z.-M. Metal-organic frameworks as potential drug delivery systems. *Expert Opin. Drug Deliv.* **2013**, *10*, 89–101. [CrossRef]
6. Clarkson, T.W.; Magos, L. The Toxicology of Mercury and Its Chemical Compounds. *Crit. Rev. Toxicol.* **2006**, *36*, 609–662. [CrossRef]
7. Lu, Y.; Hu, Q.; Lin, Y.; Pacardo, D.B.; Wang, C.; Sun, W.; Ligler, F.S.; Dickey, M.D.; Gu, Z. Transformable liquid-metal nanomedicine. *Nat. Commun.* **2015**, *6*, 10066. [CrossRef]
8. Dickey, M.D.; Chiechi, R.C.; Larsen, R.J.; Weiss, E.A.; Weitz, D.A.; Whitesides, G.M. Eutectic Gallium-Indium (EGaIn): A Liquid Metal Alloy for the Formation of Stable Structures in Microchannels at Room Temperature. *Adv. Funct. Mater.* **2008**, *18*, 1097–1104. [CrossRef]
9. Hohman, J.N.; Kim, M.; Wadsworth, G.A.; Bednar, H.R.; Jiang, J.; LeThai, M.A.; Weiss, P.S. Directing Substrate Morphology via Self-Assembly: Ligand-Mediated Scission of Gallium–Indium Microspheres to the Nanoscale. *Nano Lett.* **2011**, *11*, 5104–5110. [CrossRef]
10. Yamaguchi, A.; Mashima, Y.; Iyoda, T. Reversible Size Control of Liquid-Metal Nanoparticles under Ultrasonication. *Angew. Chem. Int. Ed.* **2015**, *54*, 12809–12813. [CrossRef]
11. Sheng, L.; Zhang, J.; Liu, J. Diverse Transformations of Liquid Metals Between Different Morphologies. *Adv. Mater.* **2014**, *26*, 6036–6042. [CrossRef] [PubMed]
12. Tang, S.Y.; Khoshmanesh, K.; Sivan, V.; Petersen, P.; O'Mullane, A.P.; Abbott, D.; Kalantar-zadeh, K. Liquid metal enabled pump. *Proc. Natl. Acad. Sci. USA* **2014**, *111*, 3304–3309. [CrossRef] [PubMed]
13. Zhang, J.; Yao, Y.; Sheng, L.; Liu, J. Self-Fueled Biomimetic Liquid Metal Mollusk. *Adv. Mater.* **2015**, *27*, 2648–2655. [CrossRef] [PubMed]

14. Boley, J.W.; White, E.L.; Chiu, G.T.-C.; Kramer, R.K. Direct Writing of Gallium-Indium Alloy for Stretchable Electronics. *Adv. Funct. Mater.* **2014**, *24*, 3501–3507. [CrossRef]
15. So, J.-H.; Dickey, M.D. Inherently aligned microfluidic electrodes composed of liquid metal. *Lab Chip* **2011**, *11*, 905–911. [CrossRef]
16. Liu, T.; Sen, P.; Kim, C.-J. Characterization of Nontoxic Liquid-Metal Alloy Galinstan for Applications in Microdevices. *J. Microelectromech. Syst.* **2011**, *21*, 443–450. [CrossRef]
17. Gao, M.; Gui, L. A handy liquid metal based electroosmotic flow pump. *Lab Chip* **2014**, *14*, 1866–1872. [CrossRef]
18. Wang, Q.; Yu, Y.; Liu, J. Delivery of Liquid Metal to the Target Vessels as Vascular Embolic Agent to Starve Diseased Tissues or Tumors to Death. 2014. Available online: https://arxiv.org/ftp/arxiv/papers/1408/1408.0989.pdf (accessed on 4 August 2014).
19. Yi, L.; Liu, J. Liquid metal biomaterials: A newly emerging area to tackle modern biomedical challenges. *Int. Mater. Rev.* **2017**, *62*, 415–440. [CrossRef]
20. Lu, Y.; Lin, Y.; Chen, Z.; Hu, Q.; Liu, Y.; Yu, S.; Gao, W.; Dickey, M.D.; Gu, Z. Enhanced Endosomal Escape by Light-Fueled Liquid-Metal Transformer. *Nano Lett.* **2017**, *17*, 2138–2145. [CrossRef]
21. Wang, X.; Yao, W.; Guo, R.; Yang, X.; Tang, J.; Zhang, J.; Gao, W.; Timchenko, V.; Liu, J. Soft and Moldable Mg-Doped Liquid Metal for Conformable Skin Tumor Photothermal Therapy. *Adv. Health Mater.* **2018**, *7*, 1800318. [CrossRef]
22. Sun, X.; Sun, M.; Liu, M.; Yuan, B.; Gao, W.; Rao, W.; Liu, J. Shape tunable gallium nanorods mediated tumor enhanced ablation through near-infrared photothermal therapy. *Nanoscale* **2019**, *11*, 2655–2667. [CrossRef] [PubMed]
23. Witsch, E.; Sela, M.; Yarden, Y. Roles for growth factors in cancer progression. *Physiology* **2010**, *25*, 85–101. [CrossRef]
24. Folkman, J. *Advances in Cancer Research*; Elsevier: Amsterdam, The Netherlands, 1974; Volume 19331–19358.
25. Jain, R.K. Vascular and interstitial barriers to delivery of therapeutic agents in tumors. *Cancer Metastasis Rev.* **1990**, *9*, 253–266. [CrossRef] [PubMed]
26. Thorpe, P.E. Vascular targeting agents as cancer therapeutics. *Clin. Cancer Res.* **2004**, *10*, 415–427. [CrossRef]
27. Thorpe, P.E.; Chaplin, D.J.; Blakey, D.C. The first international conference on vascular targeting: meeting overview. *Cancer Res.* **2003**, *63*, 1144–1147. [PubMed]
28. Denekamp, J. Commentary: The tumour microcirculation as a target in cancer therapy: A clearer perspective. *Eur. J. Clin. Investig.* **1999**, *29*, 733–736. [CrossRef]
29. Hori, K.; Saito, S.; Kubota, K. A novel combretastatin A-4 derivative, AC7700, strongly stanches tumour blood flow and inhibits growth of tumours developing in various tissues and organs. *Br. J. Cancer* **2002**, *86*, 1604–1614. [CrossRef]
30. Chechetka, S.A.; Yu, Y.; Zhen, X.; Pramanik, M.; Pu, K.; Miyako, E. Light-driven liquid metal nanotransformers for biomedical theranostics. *Nat. Commun.* **2017**, *8*, 15432. [CrossRef]
31. Hu, J.J.; Liu, M.D.; Chen, Y.; Gao, F.; Peng, S.Y.; Xie, B.R.; Zhang, X.Z. Immobilized liquid metal nanoparticles with improved stability and photothermal performance for combinational therapy of tumor. *Biomaterials* **2019**, *207*, 76–88. [CrossRef]

4

The Oncogene AF1Q is Associated with WNT and STAT Signaling and Offers a Novel Independent Prognostic Marker in Patients with Resectable Esophageal Cancer

Elisabeth S. Gruber [1], Georg Oberhuber [2,3], Peter Birner [2], Michaela Schlederer [2], Michael Kenn [4], Wolfgang Schreiner [4], Gerd Jomrich [1], Sebastian F. Schoppmann [1], Michael Gnant [1], William Tse [5,6,*] and Lukas Kenner [2,7,8,9,*]

1 Division of General Surgery, Department of Surgery, Comprehensive Cancer Center, Medical University of Vienna, 1090 Vienna, Austria; elisabeth.s.gruber@meduniwien.ac.at (E.S.G.); gerd.jomrich@meduniwien.ac.at (G.J.); sebastian.schoppmann@meduniwien.ac.at (S.F.S.); michael.gnant@meduniwien.ac.at (M.G.)

2 Institute of Pathology, Department of Experimental and Translational Pathology, Medical University of Vienna, 1090 Vienna, Austria; georg.oberhuber@patho.at (G.O.); peter.birner@meduniwien.ac.at (P.B.); michaela.schlederer@meduniwien.ac.at (M.S.)

3 PIZ—Patho im Zentrum GmbH, 3100 St. Poelten, Lower Austria, Austria

4 Section of Biosimulation and Bioinformatics, Center for Medical Statistics, Informatics and Intelligent Systems (CeMSIIS), Medical University of Vienna, 1090 Vienna, Austria; michael.kenn@meduniwien.ac.at (M.K.); wolfgang.schreiner@meduniwien.ac.at (W.S.)

5 James Graham Brown Cancer Center, University of Louisville School of Medicine, Louisville, KY 40202, USA

6 Division of Blood and Bone Marrow Transplantation, Department of Medicine, University of Louisville School of Medicine, Louisville, KY 40202, USA

7 Christian Doppler Laboratory for Applied Metabolomics (CDL-AM), Medical University of Vienna, 1090 Vienna, Austria

8 Institute of Laboratory Animal Pathology, University of Veterinary Medicine Vienna, 1210 Vienna, Austria

9 CBmed Core Lab 2, Medical University of Vienna, 1090 Vienna, Austria

* Correspondence: william.tse@louisville.edu (W.T.); lukas.kenner@meduniwien.ac.at (L.K.);

Abstract: AF1q impairs survival in hematologic and solid malignancies. AF1q expression is associated with tumor progression, migration and chemoresistance and acts as a transcriptional co-activator in WNT and STAT signaling. This study evaluates the role of AF1q in patients with resectable esophageal cancer (EC). A total of 278 patients operated on for EC were retrospectively included and the expression of AF1q, CD44 and pYSTAT3 was analyzed following immunostaining. Quantified data were processed to correlational and survival analysis. In EC tissue samples, an elevated expression of AF1q was associated with the expression of CD44 ($p = 0.004$) and pYSTAT3 ($p = 0.0002$). High AF1q expression in primary tumors showed high AF1q expression in the corresponding lymph nodes ($p = 0.016$). AF1q expression was higher after neoadjuvant therapy ($p = 0.0002$). Patients with AF1q-positive EC relapsed and died earlier compared to patients with AF1q-negative EC (disease-free survival (DFS), $p = 0.0005$; disease-specific survival (DSS), $p = 0.003$); in the multivariable Cox regression model, AF1q proved to be an independent prognostic marker (DFS, $p = 0.01$; DSS, $p = 0.03$). AF1q is associated with WNT and STAT signaling; it impairs and independently predicts DFS and DSS in patients with resectable EC. Testing AF1q could facilitate prognosis estimation and provide a possibility of identifying the patients responsive to the therapeutic blockade of its oncogenic downstream targets.

Keywords: AF1Q; MLLT11; WNT; STAT; esophageal cancer; prognosis

1. Introduction

AF1Q was originally identified as an *MLL* fusion partner in acute myeloid leukemia patients with a t(1; 11)(q21; q23) translocation (*MLLT11*); here, multiple chromosomal translocations of the AF1q locus have been described [1]. Enhanced AF1q expression is associated with poor clinical outcome in hematologic and several solid malignancies, such as breast, thyroid as well as testicular cancer and neuroblastoma [2–9]. Further on, AF1q plays a role in cell differentiation and maintenance during neuronal development [10], and is involved in stem cell differentiation. Here, it promotes T cell development, and at the same time impairs B cell differentiation; in addition, CD34-enriched stem cells show high AF1q levels, which are diminished during cell differentiation [11]. We delineated the precise oncogenic function of AF1q in breast cancer models, where AF1q functions as transcriptional co-factor and interacts with the T-cell factor/lymphoid enhancer factor (TCF/LEF) transcriptional complex in the wingless-type MMTV integration site family (WNT) [3] and signal transducer and activator of transcription 3 (STAT3) [12] signaling pathway. These two core cancer pathways play a pivotal role in tumors of the gastrointestinal tract and are involved in tumor initiation, progression, metastases, and chemoresistance [13,14]. In colorectal cancer, WNT signaling is a major driver of oncogenicity, and AF1q has been reported to drive proliferation, migration, and invasion in vitro and in vivo [5,15]. Recently, the suppression of breast cancer dissemination has been subscribed to GATA3-driven miR29b induction, which reportedly inhibits AF1q [16]. Controversly, some studies reported γ-irradiation or doxorubicin-induced pro-apoptotic effects through Blc-2-antagonist of cell death (BAD) in liver and ovarian cancer cells that were mediated by AF1q [7,8]. However, the exact mechanisms that AF1q involves to promote cancer are largely unidentified.

Esophageal cancer (EC) is one of the 10 most common types of cancer and is responsible for more than half a million deaths worldwide [17]. Surgery is the treatment of choice in locally limited resectable disease, and surgical techniques have been extended recently to meet the resection challenges. For locally advanced stage cancers, preoperative treatment is recommended [18]. At the time of diagnosis, half of the patients are metastasized and might benefit from targeted therapies; still, randomized data in EC are scarce [18]. Since EC's genetic landscape is very distinct and driver mutations differ largely among subgroups, the definition of therapeutic targets on the basis of a genetic analysis is challenging. However, several targets for blocking the proposed AF1q downstream pathways WNT and STAT have demonstrated satisfying tumor response in cancer patients [12,13,19–22].

The aim of this study was to elucidate the role of AF1q in resectable EC, which to date remains unclear. By correlating tumoral AF1q expression with the expression of downstream targets CD44 and STAT3 as well as clinciopathological parameters, we wanted to evaluate the oncogenic potential of AF1q and its prognostic value for postoperative survival. Our data provide evidence that AF1q is associated with both WNT and STAT signaling and serves as a prognostic factor in EC patients.

2. Materials and Methods

2.1. Study Population

Patients diagnosed with cancer of the esophagus and the esophagogastric junction who had undergone surgery between 1992 and 2002 at the Division of General Surgery, Medical University of Vienna were included into the study under ethical approval from the local review board ('Ethikkommission') of the Medical University of Vienna, #1197/2019). In case of locally advanced stage cancer, patients received neoadjuvant treatment according to the latest clinical practice guidelines at the time of diagnosis followed by surgery. Histopathological staging was conducted according to the AJCC/UICC staging system [23]. Surgical specimens were processed to tissue microarrays (TMAs), in which each tumor was represented by triplicate core biopsies. The location of the tumors was assessed according to the rules published in the fourth edition of the World Health Organization (WHO) classification of gastrointestinal tumors [24]. In brief, all squamous carcinomas from the tubular esophagus and from the area of the esophagogastric junction were considered to be carcinomas of the esophagus. The proximal extent of the gastric folds was used as the landmark for the esophagogastric junction. Due to similar initiating factors and prognosis of adenocarcinomas of the distal esophagus and adenocarcinomas of the esophagogastric junction (AEG) as well as challenges in clear clinical and histopathological distinction, these two groups were merged before analysis [18]. Histological response to neoadjuvant chemotherapy was graded according to Mandard [25].

2.2. *Immunohistochemistry*

The expression of AF1q as well as CD44 (as bona fide WNT target gene) as a possible AF1q downstream target was evaluated in resected human EC specimens; pySTAT3 expression was available from previous studies [26]. Immunostainings were performed using a standard protocol. Paraffin sections were de-waxed, and for the antigen retrieval, a citrate buffer pH 6 (CD44) or a Tris/Ethylenediaminetetraacetic acid (EDTA) buffer pH 9 (AF1q) was used. After endogenous peroxidase blocking, avidin and biotin blocking steps were performed. The antibodies were incubated overnight at 4 °C in PBS+1% bovine serum albumin (BSA). The following antibodies were used: CD44 (Santa Cruz, sc-9960) in a 1:200 dilution and AF1q (Abcam, ab109016) in a 1:200 dilution. Slides were washed with phosphate buffered saline (PBS) the following day and incubated with polyvalent-secondary antibody (IDetect Super Stain System HRP, ID laboratories) and horseradish peroxidase (HRP; IDetect Super Stain System HRP, ID laboratories). Signals were visualized with 3-amino-9-ethylcarbazole (ID laboratories). After counterstaining with hemalaun, the slides were mounted. The specimen were analyzed by a board-certified pathologist. A specimen was considered as positive when at least 50% of tumor cells showed moderate or strong cytoplasmic marker expression. Antibody specificity has been confirmed in previous studies [3,12,26–29].

2.3. *Statistical Analysis*

In terms of experimental characteristics, data were described by mean (± standard deviation). Statistical differences were analyzed by a Student's t-test. A two-sided *p*-value less than 0.05 was considered statistically significant.

In terms of patient and tumor characteristics, numerical data were described by median (range) and categorical variables were described by frequencies. In order to compare AF1q expression with patient and tumor characteristics, the chi-square test was applied as appropriate. In order to describe the correlation between AF1q and ordinal or continuous variables, the Spearman rank correlation coefficient (r_s) was calculated. The inverse Kaplan–Meier method was used to estimate the median follow-up time [30]. Survival estimates were calculated by the Kaplan–Meier method with the log-rank test for group comparisons. DSS was defined as time from esophageal surgery until death from EC. DFS was defined as time from esophageal surgery until EC recurrence. In order to identify independent predictive factors for survival, established prognostic factors such as neoadjuvant therapy and histological tumor subtype, as well as TNM staging, tumor grading, and resection margin [18,31], were entered into a multivariable Cox regression model in addition to AF1q. MATLAB Version 9.6/R2019a (MathWorks) was used for all statistical calculations. For all analyses, a two-sided *p*-value less than 0.05 was considered statistically significant.

3. Results

3.1. AF1q Expression Analysis in Human Esophageal Cancer Samples

In total, 278 patients with cancer of the esophagus and the esophagogastric junction as well as corresponding fully annotated tumor samples were retrospectively defined for analysis. The cohort consisted of 118 patients with esophageal squamous cell carcinoma (ESCC, 42.2%), 67 patients with esophageal adenocarcinoma (EAC, 24.1%) and 93 patients with adenocarcinoma of the esophagogastric junction (AEG, 33.5%); out of those, 138 tumor samples (49.6%) showed significant AF1q expression (ESCC, n = 54, 45.8%; EAC, n = 42, 62.7%; AEG, n = 42, 45.2%). An example of positive tumoral AF1q expression in EC is shown in Figure 1. Patient and tumor characteristics compared between AF1q-positive and AF1q-negative tumors are compiled in Table 1. In short, patients who received neoadjuvant therapy showed higher tumoral AF1q expression compared to patients who were resected upfront (p = 0.0002); histological response to neoadjuvant therapy did not correlate with AF1q expression (r_s = 0.22, p = 0.09). Patients with AF1q-positive tumors suffered from a higher rate of positive resection margins (R1) compared to patients with AF1q-negative tumors (p = 0.004).

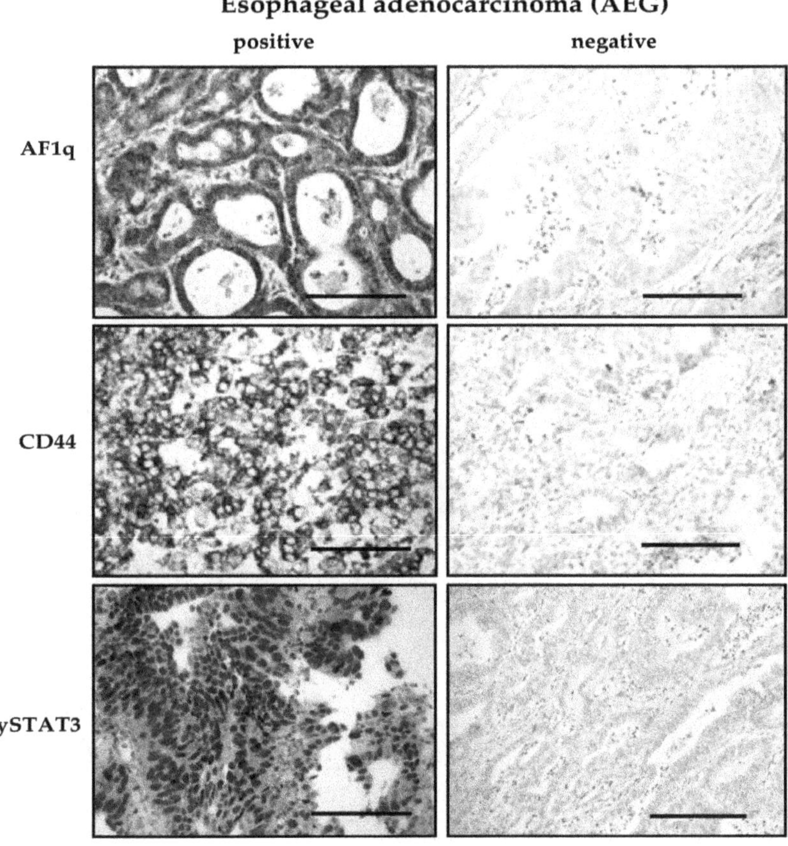

Figure 1. Examples of immunohistochemical (IHC) stained esophageal adenocarcinoma. Examples of AF1q expression in high-risk esophageal adenocarcinoma: Right example showing enhanced AF1q expression in high-risk adenocarcinoma vs. left example showing no AF1q expression in low-risk esophageal adenocarcinoma, size bar 100 µm.

Table 1. Patient and tumor characteristics compared between patients with AF1q-positive and AF1q-negative EC.

Factor	Patients with EC, n = 278 (100.0)	Patients with AF1q-positive EC, n = 138 (49.6)	Patients with AF1q-negative EC, n = 140 (50.4)	*p*-value
Female sex	65 (23.4)	28 (43.1)	37 (56.9)	0.23 *
Male sex	213 (76.6)	110 (51.6)	103 (48.4)	
Age	63.3 (34–90)	63.8 (38–90)	63.9 (34–90)	rs = 0.03 ** (0.65)
Adiposity	16 (5.8)	10 (62.5)	6 (37.5)	0.11 *
Reflux	5 (1.8)	2 (40.0)	3 (60)	0.22 *
Neoadjuvant therapy	68 (24.5)	47 (69.1)	21 (30.9)	0.0002 *
Factor	**Patients with EC, n = 278 (100.0)**	**Patients with AF1q-positive EC, n = 138 (49.6)**	**Patients with AF1q-negative EC, n = 140 (50.4)**	***p*-value**
		Histological tumor subtype		
ESCC	118 (42.4)	54 (45.8)	64 (54.2)	rs = 0.02 ** (0.88)
AC	160 (57.6)	84 (52.5)	76 (47.5)	
EAC	67 (24.1)	42 (62.7)	25 (37.3)	n.a.
AEG	93 (33.5)	42 (45.2)	51 (54.8)	
		AJCC/UICC tumor staging ESCC n = 118 (42.4)		
IB	3 (2.5)	0 (0.0)	3 (100.0)	rs = 0.06 ** (0.55)
IIA	32 (27.1)	15 (46.9)	17 (53.1)	
IIIA	13 (11.0)	6 (46.2)	7 (53.8)	
IIIB	45 (38.1)	20 (44.4)	25 (55.6)	
IVA	19 (15.3)	10 (55.6)	8 (44.4)	
IVB	7 (5.9)	3 (42.9)	4 (57.1)	
		AJCC/UICC tumor staging EAC n = 67 (24.1)/AEG n = 93 (33.5)		
IC	8 (5.0)	4 (50.0)	4 (50.0)	rs = 0.12 ** (0.14)
IIA	3 (1.9)	0 (0.0)	3 (100.0)	
IIB	21 (13.1.)	10 (47.6)	11 (32.4)	
IIIA	8 (5.0)	2 (25.0)	6 (75.0)	
IIIB	59 (36.9)	33 (55.9)	26 (44.1)	
IVA	61 (38.1)	35 (57.4)	26 (42.6)	
		Regional lymph nodes pN		
N1	119 (44.1)	65 (54.6)	54 (45.4)	0.18 *
		Tumor grading G		
G1	11 (4.0)	4 (36.4)	7 (63.6)	rs = 0.02 ** (0.69)
G2	132 (47.5)	66 (50.0)	66 (50.0)	
G3	135 (48.6)	68 (50.4)	67 (49.6)	
		Resection margin R		
R0	228 (82.0)	104 (45.6)	124 (54.5)	0.004 *
R1	50 (18.0)	34 (68.0)	16 (32.0)	

Table 1. *Cont.*

Factor	Patients with EC, n = 278 (100.0)	Patients with AF1q-positive EC, n = 138 (49.6)	Patients with AF1q-negative EC, n = 140 (50.4)	*p*-value
		Histological response to neoadjuvant therapy		
none	7 (10.3)	7 (10.3)	0 (0.0)	rs = 0.22 ** (0.09)
poor	30 (44.1)	21 (70.0)	9 (30.0)	
moderate	17 (25.0)	11 (64.7)	6 (35.3)	
good	4 (5.9)	2 (50.0)	2 (50.0)	

Note. Continuous variables are shown as median and range, categorical variables are expressed as absolute and relative numbers, n (%); adiposity is defined as BMI >30 kg/m2; EC—esophageal cancer; ESCC—esophageal squamous cell carcinoma; AC—adenocarcinomas; EAC—esophageal adenocarcinoma; AEG—adenocarcinomas of the esophagogastric junction; AJCC/UICC—American Joint Committee on Cancer/Union for International Cancer Control (https://cancerstaging.org/Pages/default.aspx; https://www.uicc.org); n.a.—not applicable; * chi-square test, ** Spearman correlation coefficient.

In order to evaluate an association of AF1q with WNT and STAT signaling, we correlated immunohistochemical (IHC) expression levels of CD44 (as bona fide WNT target gene) and tyrosine phosphorylated STAT3 (pYSTAT3) as possible AF1q downstream targets; we found a strong association of AF1q expression with both CD44 (n = 268, $p = 0.004$) as well as pYSTAT3 (n = 227, $p = 0.0002$) levels in EC (Table 2). Examples of positive tumoral CD44 as well as pYSTAT3 expression in EC are shown in Figure 1.

Table 2. Correlation of AF1q expression with proposed downstream target expression (CD44, pYSTAT3) in tumors of EC patients.

Factor	Patients with AF1q-positive EC, n = 133 (49.6)	Patients with AF1q-negative EC, n = 135 (50.4)	*p*-value
	CD44, n = 268 (100)		
positive, n = 94 (35.1)	58 (21.6)	36 (13.5)	0.004
negative, n = 174 (74.9)	75 (28.0)	99 (36.9)	
Factor	**Patients with AF1q-positive EC, n = 117 (51.5)**	**Patients with AF1q-negative EC, n = 110 (48.5)**	***p*-value**
	pYSTAT3, n = 227 (100)		
positive, n = 101 (44.5)	66 (29.1)	35 (15.4)	0.0002
negative, n = 126 (55.5)	51 (22.4)	75 (33.1)	

Note. EC—esophageal cancer; variables are expressed as absolute and relative numbers, n (%).

In order to explore AF1q-mediated dissemination features, we compared AF1q expression in lymph node metastases (n = 32) to AF1q expression in corresponding primary tumors and found a significant correlation ($p = 0.016$; Table 3).

Table 3. Correlation of enhanced AF1q expression in primary tumors and lymph node metastases of EC patients.

Factor	AF1q-positive local EC, n = 18 (56.3)	AF1q-negative local EC, n = 14 (43.7)	*p*-value
	Lymph node metastases, n = 32 (100)		
AF1q positive, n = 19 (59.4)	14 (43.8)	5 (15.6)	0.016
AF1q negative, n = 13 (40.6)	4 (12.5)	9 (28.1)	

Note. EC—esophageal cancer; variables are expressed as absolute and relative numbers, n (%).

3.2. *Survival Analysis*

During a median postoperative follow-up period of 71 months (range 52–90 months), 156 out of 278 (56.1%) patients relapsed, and 185 out of 278 (66.5%) patients had died of EC. The median DFS time was 17 months (range 13–20 months), and the median DSS time was 21 months (range 15–25 months). In patients with a high tumoral AF1q expression, the median DFS was 13 months (range 10–16 months) and the median DSS was 22 months (range 18–27 months) compared to 23 months (range 16–31 months) median DFS and 26 months (range 18–24 months) median DSS in patients with a low tumoral AF1q expression. Enhanced AF1q expression in the tumor proper resulted in significantly decreased DFS (Kaplan Meier/log rank; $p = 0.0005$; Figure 2) and DSS (Kaplan Meier/log rank, $p = 0.003$; Figure 3).

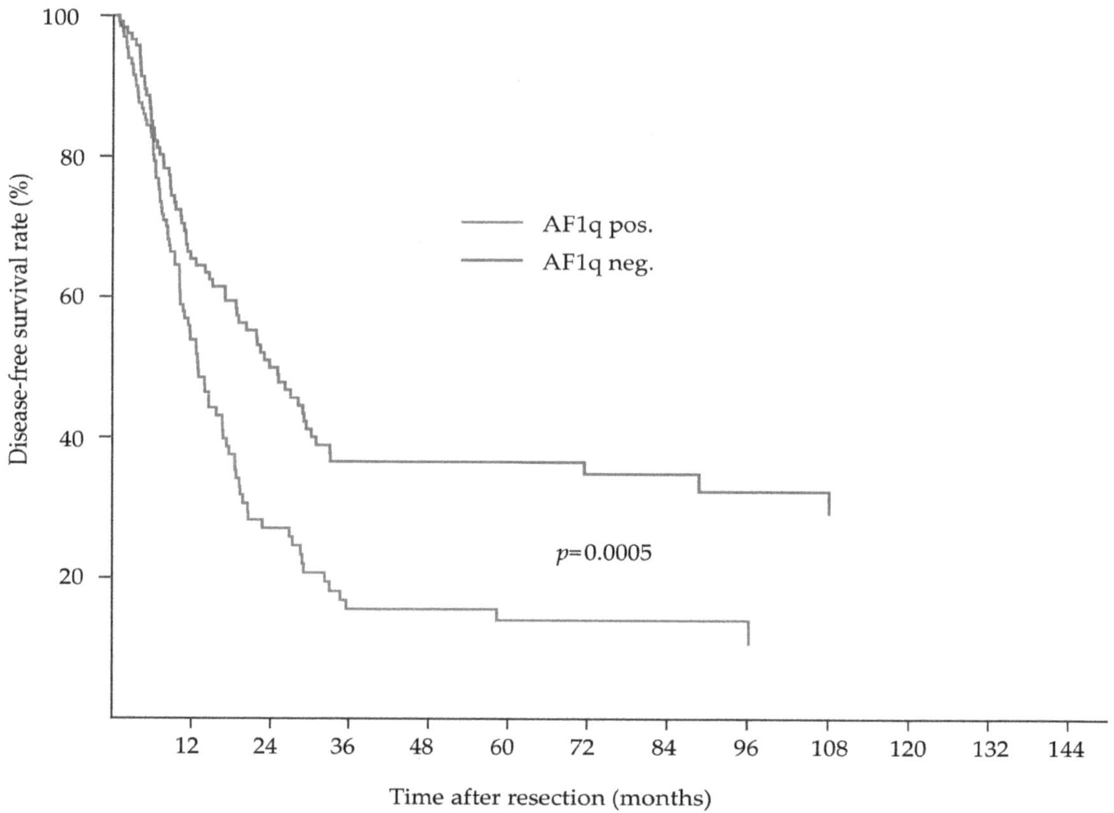

Figure 2. Kaplan–Meier analysis for disease-free survival in esophageal cancer (EC) patients. EC patients with high tumoral AF1q levels relapse earlier compared to patients with low or no tumoral AF1q expression (disease-free survival (DFS), log rank: $p = 0.0005$).

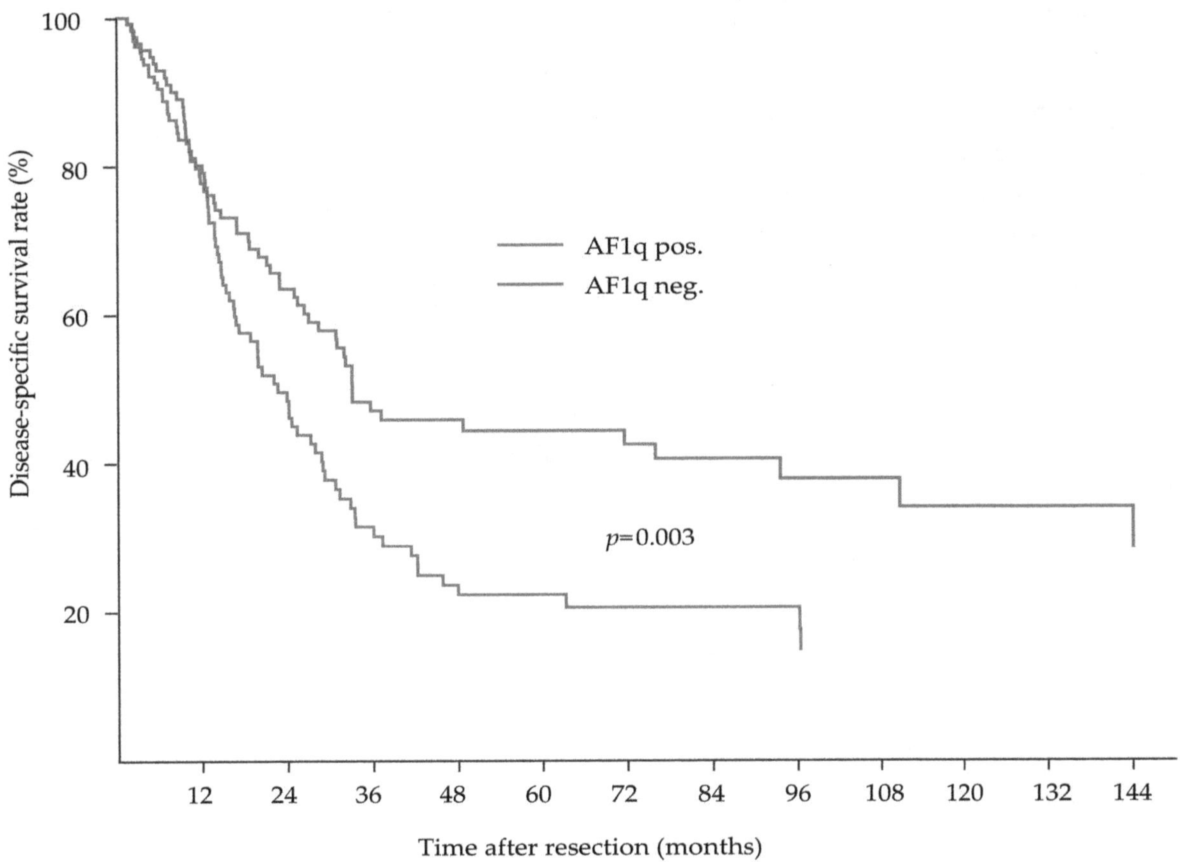

Figure 3. Kaplan–Meier analysis for disease-specific survival in esophageal cancer (EC) patients. EC patients with high tumoral AF1q die earlier compared to patients with low or no tumoral AF1q expression (disease-specific survival (DSS), log rank; $p = 0.003$).

Cox regression analysis showed a 1.5 times higher risk for both disease recurrence and disease-specific death in patients with a high tumoral AF1q expression. Further prognostic factors were neoadjuvant therapy in regard to DFS ($p = 0.0002$), local tumor stage (DFS, $p = 0.001$ and DSS, $p = 0.0004$, respectively), regional lymph node metastases (DFS, $p < 0.0001$ and DSS, $p < 0.0001$, respectively), and resection margin (DFS, $p = 0.02$ and DSS, $p = 0.01$, respectively). In a multivariable Cox regression model, AF1q proved to be an independent factor for survival (DFS $p = 0.01$; DSS $p = 0.03$) next to the local tumor stage in regard to DSS ($p = 0.007$, respectively), regional lymph node metastases (DFS, $p < 0.0001$ and DSS, $p < 0.0001$, respectively), and histological tumor subtype (DFS $p = 0.0004$ and DSS, $p = 0.003$) as well as neoadjuvant therapy in regard to DFS ($p = 0.005$). The data of univariate and multivariable Cox regression analysis are compiled in Table 4.

Table 4. Univariable and multivariable Cox regression analysis in EC patients.

Factor	Univariate *p*-Value	Multivariable *p*-Value	HR	95% CI Low	95% CI High
		Disease-free survival			
AF1q	0.0005	0.01	1.5	1.1	2.2
Neoadjuvant therapy	0.0002	0.005	1.7	1.2	2.6
Histological tumor subtype *	0.16	0.0004	1.9	1.3	2.7
Local tumor stage pT	0.001	0.07		n.a.	
Regional lymph nodes pN	<0.0001	<0.0001	2.3	1.6	3.2
Tumor grading G	0.13	0.30		n.a.	
Resection margin R	0.02	0.50		n.a.	
		Disease-specific survival			
AF1q	0.003	0.03	1.5	1.0	2.1
Neoadjuvant therapy	0.10	0.83		n.a.	
Histological tumor subtype *	0.30	0.003	1.8	1.2	2.7
Local tumor stage pT	0.0004	0.007	1.9	1.2	3.0
Regional lymph nodes pN	<0.0001	<0.0001	2.2	1.5	3.2
Tumor grading G	0.22	0.48		n.a.	
Resection margin R	0.01	0.31		n.a.	

Note. EC—esophageal cancer; HR—hazard ratio; CI—confidence interval; HR and CR refer to multivariable model; * adenocarcinoma and squamous cell carcinoma.

4. Discussion

We show here for the first time the oncogenic potential as well as the utility of AF1q as a prognostic marker in esophageal cancer (EC). We demonstrate a significant association of AF1q expression with WNT as well as STAT3 signaling pathways, and show that tumoral AF1q expression impairs survival and serves as an independent prognostic factor in patients with resectable EC.

Well known for exerting multiple oncogenic functions, WNT and STAT3 have been shown to be of prognostic value in EC [13,14,26,32]. Both signaling pathways promote intestinal tumor growth and regeneration; interestingly, this can be reversed through gp130-JAK-STAT3 blockade [33]. These data imply that there might be a link between these two core cancer pathways. In fact, what WNT and STAT3 seem to share is AF1q as an activator of their target gene transcription. We previously reported that AF1q physically binds TCF/LEF and STAT3 and boosts their target gene transcription [3,12]. In breast cancer patients, the cooperation of AF1q with TCF7 led to the transcription of CD44 [3], which is a WNT target gene that is essentially involved in tumor progression and epithelial-to-mesenchymal transition [34,35]. In invasive breast cancer cells, AF1q further induced pYSTAT3 levels through the Src kinase-driven PDGFB/PDGFRB cascade [12]. Similarily to the findings in breast cancer, we here demonstrate an association of AF1q with both WNT and STAT signaling in the sense that the patients with AF1q-positive EC show enhanced tumoral levels of both proposed downstream targets CD44 and pYSTAT3.

AF1q expression is reportedly associated with metastatic spread in colorectal, lung, and breast cancer [5,12,36,37]. Since HER-2 is commonly expressed in EC, lung, and breast cancer [38–41], HER-2 might be another signaling pathway AF1q interacts with. However, further studies are needed to prove this concept.

We here demonstrate a correlation of AF1q expression in the local tumor with AF1q expression in the lymph node metastases of EC patients. In addition, AF1q-positive ECs show higher rates of positive resection margins compared to AF1q-negative ECs. We believe that the AF1q-induced co-activation of

WNT and STAT signaling plays a key role in EC initiation, proliferation, and dissemination. Recently, Src kinase and JAK phosphorylation have been shown to facilitate STAT3 signaling [42], which further results in excessive proliferation and the malignant transformation of intestinal epithelial cells [43]. In invasive breast cancer cells, enhanced AF1q expression induced pYSTAT3 levels through the Src kinase-driven platelet-derived growth factor beta (PDGFB)/platelet-derived growth factor receptor beta (PDGFRB) cascade, which was reversible upon Src kinase blockade with protein phosphate 1 (PP1) or PDGFRB blockade using imatinib [12]. Consequently, patients with AF1q-positive EC are at exceptional risk to develop rapid disease progression that might respond to CD44 and STAT3 inhibition [13,19–22].

Conversely, AF1q has been reported to mediate the pro-apoptotic effects of cytotoxic agents such as doxorubicin, retinoic acid, or γ-irradiation through activation of the Blc-2-antagonist of cell death (BAD) [7–9]. In advanced stage EC, neoadjuvant (radio-)chemotherapy is applied to facilitate tumor shrinkage and consecutive R0 resection rates, and prevent recurrence [18,44]. Consistent with other findings, we showed an increased AF1q expression in patients treated with neoadjuvant therapy compared to treatment-naïve patients [7,8,12]. These findings support the fact that AF1q induction can be at least partly triggered by external factors such as cytotoxic agents and/or γ-irradiation [18]. Paradoxically, these data also indiciate that patients with AF1q-positive EC might suffer a disadvantage from currently applied oncologic treatment protocols due to fact that an enhanced induction of AF1q expression not only promotes EC dissemination, but might rather enforce EC's metastic potential.

For a prognosis estimation of esophageal cancer, all staging efforts are recommended to be based on neoadjuvant therapy, histological tumor subtype, and TNM staging, as well as tumor grading and resection margin as important prognostic factors [18,31]. In this cohort of patients, AF1q proved to have a highly significant prognostic impact on both DFS and DSS in the univariate analysis. In fact, neoadjuvant therapy, histological tumor subtype, and regional lymph node status remained as independent prognostic factors for DFS and histological tumor subtype, local tumor stage, as well as regional lymph node status remained as independent prognostic factors for DSS in the model next to AF1q, respectively. Although none of these established prognostic factors correlated with tumoral AF1q expression, they demonstrate predominant importance for survival estimation in this selected cohort of patients with resectable esophageal cancer.

5. Conclusions

Our data underline the potency of AF1q to enforce and link the two major oncogenic pathways WNT and STAT3 involved in tumor initiation, progression, and dissemination. We demonstrate here for the first time a positive correlation between the expression of AF1q and the WNT and the STAT3 target genes CD44 and pYSTAT3 in EC, suggesting that AF1q may act as a cofactor for boosting the transcription of CD44 and pYSTAT3 in EC. Consequently, we demonstrate that patients with AF1q-positive EC relapse and die earlier. The association of AF1q with WNT and STAT3 signaling implicates various (combinatorial) targeting options such as CD44 and STAT3, JAK, and Src, as well as tyrosine kinases. Particularly, blockade of the AF1q/TCF7/CD44 regulatory axis as well as PDGF-B might hold therapeutic promise for patients with EC. Importantly, AF1q serves as an independent prognostic marker, and might add value to the estimation of resectability and disease progression. This study should prompt future clinical studies to validate these findings.

Author Contributions: Conception and design: E.S.G., G.O., M.S., P.B., L.K.; development of methodology: E.S.G., P.B., M.K., W.S.; acquisition of data: P.B., S.F.S., G.J.; analysis and interpretation of data: E.S.G., G.O., M.S., P.B., L.K.; Writing, review and/or revision of the manuscript: E.S.G., G.O., S.F.S., M.G., W.T., L.K.; administrative, technical or material support: none; study supervision: W.T., L.K.

Acknowledgments: We thank Gertrude Krainz for her support in spelling and phraseology.

References

1. Tse, W.; Zhu, W.; Chen, H.S.; Cohen, A. A novel gene, AF1q, fused to MLL in t(1;11) (q21;q23), is specifically expressed in leukemic and immature hematopoietic cells. *Blood* **1995**, *85*, 650–656. [CrossRef] [PubMed]
2. Strunk, C.J.; Platzbecker, U.; Thiede, C.; Schaich, M.; Illmer, T.; Kang, Z.; Leahy, P.; Li, C.; Xie, X.; Laughlin, M.J.; et al. Elevated AF1q expression is a poor prognostic marker for adult acute myeloid leukemia patients with normal cytogenetics. *Am. J. Hematol.* **2009**, *84*, 308–309. [CrossRef] [PubMed]
3. Park, J.; Schlederer, M.; Schreiber, M.; Ice, R.; Merkel, O.; Bilban, M.; Hofbauer, S.; Kim, S.; Addison, J.; Zou, J.; et al. AF1q is a novel TCF7 co-factor which activates CD44 and promotes breast cancer metastasis. *Oncotarget* **2015**, *6*, 20697–20710. [CrossRef] [PubMed]
4. Tse, W.; Meshinchi, S.; Alonzo, T.A.; Stirewalt, D.L.; Gerbing, R.B.; Woods, W.G.; Appelbaum, F.R.; Radich, J.P. Elevated expression of the AF1q gene, an MLL fusion partner, is an independent adverse prognostic factor in pediatric acute myeloid leukemia. *Blood* **2004**, *104*, 3058–3063. [CrossRef] [PubMed]
5. Hu, J.; Li, G.; Liu, L.; Wang, Y.; Li, X.; Gong, J. AF1q Mediates Tumor Progression in Colorectal Cancer by Regulating AKT Signaling. *Int. J. Mol. Sci.* **2017**, *18*, 987. [CrossRef]
6. Liu, T.; Bohlken, A.; Kuljaca, S.; Lee, M.; Nguyen, T.; Smith, S.; Cheung, B.; Norris, M.D.; Haber, M.; Holloway, A.J.; et al. The retinoid anticancer signal: Mechanisms of target gene regulation. *Br. J. Cancer* **2005**, *93*, 310–318. [CrossRef]
7. Co, N.; Tsang, W.; Wong, T.; Cheung, H.; Tsang, T.; Kong, S.; Kwok, T. Oncogene AF1q enhances doxorubicin-induced apoptosis through BAD-mediated mitochondrial apoptotic pathway. *Mol. Cancer Ther.* **2008**, *7*, 3160–3168. [CrossRef]
8. Co, N.; Tsang, W.; Tsang, T.; Yeung, H.; Yau, P.; Kong, S.K.; Kwok, T.T. AF1q enhancement of γ irradiation-induced apoptosis by up-regulation of BAD expression via NF-κB in human squamous carcinoma A431 cells. *Oncol. Rep.* **2010**, *24*, 547–554. [CrossRef]
9. Tiberio, P.; Cavadini, E.; Callari, M.; Daidone, M.G.; Appierto, V. AF1q: A novel mediator of basal and 4-HPR-induced apoptosis in ovarian cancer cells. *PLoS ONE* **2012**, *7*, e39968. [CrossRef]
10. Lin, H.; Shaffer, K.; Sun, Z.; Jay, G.; He, W.; Ma, W. AF1q, a differentially expressed gene during neuronal differentiation, transforms HEK cells into neuron-like cells. *Mol. Brain Res.* **2004**, *131*, 126–130. [CrossRef]
11. Tse, W.; Deeg, H.; Stirewalt, D.; Appelbaum, F.; Radich, J.; Gooley, T. Increased AF1q gene expression in high-risk myelodysplastic syndrome. *Br. J. Haematol.* **2005**, *128*, 218–220. [CrossRef] [PubMed]
12. Park, J.; Kim, S.; Joh, J.; Remick, S.C.; Miller, D.M.; Yan, J.; Kanaan, Z.; Chao, J.-H.; Krem, M.M.; Basu, S.K.; et al. MLLT11/AF1q boosts oncogenic STAT3 activity through Src-PDGFR tyrosine kinase signaling. *Oncotarget* **2016**, *7*, 43960–43973. [CrossRef] [PubMed]
13. Anastas, J.N.; Moon, R.T. WNT signalling pathways as therapeutic targets in cancer. *Nat. Rev. Cancer* **2013**, *13*, 11–26. [CrossRef] [PubMed]
14. Yu, H.; Lee, H.; Herrmann, A.; Buettner, R.; Jove, R. Revisiting STAT3 signalling in cancer: New and unexpected biological functions. *Nat. Rev. Cancer* **2014**, *14*, 736–746. [CrossRef] [PubMed]
15. Vacante, M.; Borzì, A.M.; Basile, F.; Biondi, A. Biomarkers in colorectal cancer: Current clinical utility and future perspectives. *World J. Clin. Cases* **2018**, *6*, 869–881. [CrossRef] [PubMed]
16. Xiong, Y.; Li, Z.; Ji, M.; Tan, A.; Bemis, J.; Tse, J.; Huang, G.; Park, J.; Ji, C.; Chen, J.; et al. MIR29B regulates expression of MLLT11 (AF1Q), an MLL fusion partner, and low MIR29B expression associates with adverse cytogenetics and poor overall survival in AML. *Br. J. Haematol.* **2011**, *153*, 753–757. [CrossRef]
17. Bray, F.; Ferlay, J.; Soerjomataram, I.; Siegel, R.L.; Torre, L.A.; Jemal, A. Global cancer statistics 2018: GLOBOCAN estimates of incidence and mortality worldwide for 36 cancers in 185 countries. *CA Cancer J. Clin.* **2018**, *68*, 394–424. [CrossRef]
18. Lordick, F.; Mariette, C.; Haustermans, K.; Obermannova, R.; Arnold, D.; Committee, E.G. Oesophageal cancer: ESMO Clinical Practice Guidelines for diagnosis, treatment and follow-up. *Ann. Oncol.* **2016**, *27*, v50–v57. [CrossRef]
19. Buchert, M.; Burns, C.J.; Ernst, M. Targeting JAK kinase in solid tumors: Emerging opportunities and challenges. *Oncogene* **2016**, *35*, 939–951. [CrossRef]
20. Hubbard, J.M.; Grothey, A. Napabucasin: An Update on the First-in-Class Cancer Stemness Inhibitor. *Drugs* **2017**, *77*, 1091–1103. [CrossRef]

21. Dembowsky, K. A Safety and Pharmacokinetic Phase I/Ib Study of AMC303 in Patients With Solid Tumours. 2016. Available online: https://clinicaltrials.gov/ct2/show/NCT03009214 (accessed on 1 August 2016).
22. Menke-van der Houven, C.W.; van Oordt, C.G.R.; van Herpen, C.; Coveler, A.L.; Mahalingam, D.; Verheul, H.M.; van der Graaf, W.T.; Christen, R.; Rüttinger, D.; Weigand, S.; et al. First-in-human phase I clinical trial of RG7356, an anti-CD44 humanized antibody, in patients with advanced, CD44-expressing solid tumors. *Oncotarget* **2016**, *7*, 80046–80058.
23. Rice, T.W.; Patil, D.T.; Blackstone, E.H. 8th edition AJCC/UICC staging of cancers of the esophagus and esophagogastric junction: Application to clinical practice. *Ann. Cardiothorac. Surg.* **2017**, *6*, 119–130. [CrossRef] [PubMed]
24. Odze, R.; Flejou, J.; Boffetta, P.; Hofler, H.; Montgomery, E.; Spechler, S. Adenocarcinoma of the oesophgogastric junction. In *WHO Classification of Tumours of the Digestive System, World Health Organization Classification of Tumours*; Bosman, F., Carneiro, F., Hruban, R., Theise, N., Eds.; IARC Press: Lyon, Paris, 2010; pp. 39–44.
25. Mandard, A.M.; Dalibard, F.; Mandard, J.C.; Marnay, J.; Henry-Amar, M.; Petiot, J.F.; Roussel, A.; Jacob, J.H.; Segol, P.; Samama, G.; et al. Pathologic assessment of tumor regression after preoperative chemoradiotherapy of esophageal carcinoma. Clinicopathologic correlations. *Cancer* **1994**, *73*, 2680–2686. [CrossRef]
26. Schoppmann, S.F.; Jesch, B.; Friedrich, J.; Jomrich, G.; Maroske, F.; Birner, P. Phosphorylation of signal transducer and activator of transcription 3 (STAT3) correlates with Her-2 status, carbonic anhydrase 9 expression and prognosis in esophageal cancer. *Clin. Exp. Metastasis* **2012**, *29*, 615–624. [CrossRef] [PubMed]
27. Addison, J.B.; Koontz, C.; Fugett, J.H.; Creighton, C.J.; Chen, D.; Farrugia, M.K.; Padon, R.R.; Voronkova, M.A.; McLaughlin, S.L.; Livengood, R.H.; et al. KAP1 Promotes Proliferation and Metastatic Progression of Breast Cancer Cells. *Cancer Res.* **2015**, *75*, 344–355. [CrossRef] [PubMed]
28. Chu, T.-H.; Chan, H.-H.; Hu, T.-H.; Wang, E.M.; Ma, Y.-L.; Huang, S.-C.; Wu, J.-C.; Chang, Y.-C.; Weng, W.-T.; Wen, Z.-H.; et al. Celecoxib enhances the therapeutic efficacy of epirubicin for Novikoff hepatoma in rats. *Cancer Med.* **2018**, *7*, 2567–2580. [CrossRef]
29. Jin, H.; Sun, W.; Zhang, Y.; Yan, H.; Liufu, H.; Wang, S.; Chen, C.; Gu, J.; Hua, X.; Zhou, L.; et al. MicroRNA-411 Downregulation Enhances Tumor Growth by Upregulating MLLT11 Expression in Human Bladder Cancer. *Mol. Ther. Nucleic Acids* **2018**, *11*, 312–322. [CrossRef]
30. Schemper, M.; Smith, T.L. A Note on Quantifying Follow-up in Studies of Failure Time. *Control. Clin. Trials* **1996**, *17*, 343–346. [CrossRef]
31. Rice, T.; Kelsen, D.; Blackstone, E.; Ishwaran, H.; Patil, D.; Bass, A.; Erasmus, J.; Gerdes, H.; Hofstetter, W. Esophagus and Esophagogastric Junction. In *AJCC Cancer Staging Manual*, 8th ed.; Springer International Publishing: New York, NY, USA, 2017. [CrossRef]
32. Yu, H.; Kortylewski, M.; Pardoll, D. Crosstalk between cancer and immune cells: Role of STAT3 in the tumour microenvironment. *Nat. Rev. Immunol.* **2007**, *7*, 41–51. [CrossRef]
33. Phesse, T.J.; Buchert, M.; Stuart, E.; Flanagan, D.J.; Faux, M.; Afshar-Sterle, S.; Walker, F.; Zhang, H.H.; Nowell, C.J.; Jorissen, R. Partial inhibition of gp130-Jak-Stat3 signaling prevents Wnt–b-catenin–mediated intestinal tumor growth and regeneration. *Cancer Biol.* **2014**, *7*, 1–11. [CrossRef]
34. Naor, D.; Wallach-Dayan, S.B.; Zahalka, M.A.; Sionov, R.V. Involvement of CD44, a molecule with a thousand faces, in cancer dissemination. *Semin. Cancer Biol.* **2008**, *18*, 260–267. [CrossRef] [PubMed]
35. Zoller, M. CD44: Can a cancer-initiating cell profit from an abundantly expressed molecule? *Nat. Rev. Cancer* **2011**, *11*, 254–267. [CrossRef] [PubMed]
36. Chang, X.Z.; Li, D.Q.; Hou, Y.F.; Wu, J.; Lu, J.S.; Di, G.H.; Jin, W.; Ou, Z.L.; Shen, Z.Z.; Shao, Z.M. Identification of the functional role of AF1Q in the progression of breast cancer. *Breast Cancer Res. Treat.* **2008**, *111*, 65–78. [CrossRef] [PubMed]
37. Yang, S.; Dong, Q.; Yao, M.; Shi, M.; Ye, J.; Zhao, L.; Su, J.; Gu, W.; Xie, W.; Wang, K.; et al. Establishment of an experimental human lung adenocarcinoma cell line SPC-A-1BM with high bone metastases potency by (99m)Tc-MDP bone scintigraphy. *Nucl. Med. Biol.* **2009**, *36*, 313–321. [CrossRef] [PubMed]
38. Bartley, A.N.; Washington, M.K.; Ventura, C.B.; Ismaila, N.; Colasacco, C.; Benson, A.B., III; Carrato, A.; Gulley, M.L.; Jain, D.; Kakar, S.; et al. HER2 Testing and Clinical Decision Making in Gastroesophageal Adenocarcinoma: Guideline From the College of American Pathologists, American Society for Clinical Pathology, and American Society of Clinical Oncology. *Am. J. Clin. Pathol.* **2016**, *146*, 647–669. [CrossRef]

39. Schoppmann, S.F.; Jesch, B.; Friedrich, J.; Wrba, F.; Schultheis, A.; Pluschnig, U.; Maresch, J.; Zacherl, J.; Hejna, M.; Birner, P. Expression of Her-2 in carcinomas of the esophagus. *Am. J. Surg. Pathol.* **2010**, *34*, 1868–1873. [CrossRef]
40. Cardoso, F.; Kyriakides, S.; Ohno, S.; Penault-Llorca, F.; Poortmans, P.; Rubio, I.T.; Zackrisson, S.; Senkus, E. Early Breast Cancer: ESMO Clinical Practice Guidelines. *Ann. Oncol.* **2019**, *30*, 1194–1220. [CrossRef]
41. Kerr, K.; Bubendorf, L.; Edelman, M.; Marchetti, A.; Mok, T.; Novello, S.; O'Byrne, K.; Stahel, R.; Peters, S.; Felip, E. ESMO Consensus Guidelines: Pathology and molecular biomarkers for non-small-cell lung cancer. *Ann. Oncol.* **2014**, *25*, 1681–1690. [CrossRef]
42. Qing, Y.; Stark, G.R. Alternative activation of STAT1 and STAT3 in response to interferon-gamma. *J. Biol. Chem.* **2004**, *279*, 41679–41685. [CrossRef]
43. Peterson, L.W.; Artis, D. Intestinal epithelial cells: Regulators of barrier function and immune homeostasis. *Nat. Rev. Immunol.* **2014**, *14*, 141–153. [CrossRef]
44. Smyth, E.C.; Verheij, M.; Allum, W.; Cunningham, D.; Cervantes, A.; Arnold, D.; Committee, E.G. Gastric cancer: ESMO Clinical Practice Guidelines for diagnosis, treatment and follow-up. *Ann. Oncol.* **2016**, *27*, v38–v49. [CrossRef] [PubMed]

5

Zinc Finger Transcription Factor MZF1—A Specific Regulator of Cancer Invasion

Ditte Marie Brix [1,2], Knut Kristoffer Bundgaard Clemmensen [1] and Tuula Kallunki [1,3,*]

[1] Cell Death and Metabolism, Center for Autophagy, Recycling and Disease, Danish Cancer Society Research Center, 2100 Copenhagen, Denmark; dittemariebrix@gmail.com (D.M.B.); knucle@cancer.dk (K.K.B.C.)
[2] Danish Medicines Council, Dampfærgevej 27-29, 2100 Copenhagen, Denmark
[3] Department of Drug Design and Pharmacology, Faculty of Health Sciences, University of Copenhagen, 2200 Copenhagen, Denmark
* Correspondence: tk@cancer.dk

Abstract: Over 90% of cancer deaths are due to cancer cells metastasizing into other organs. Invasion is a prerequisite for metastasis formation. Thus, inhibition of invasion can be an efficient way to prevent disease progression in these patients. This could be achieved by targeting the molecules regulating invasion. One of these is an oncogenic transcription factor, Myeloid Zinc Finger 1 (MZF1). Dysregulated transcription factors represent a unique, increasing group of drug targets that are responsible for aberrant gene expression in cancer and are important nodes driving cancer malignancy. Recent studies report of a central involvement of MZF1 in the invasion and metastasis of various solid cancers. In this review, we summarize the research on MZF1 in cancer including its function and role in lysosome-mediated invasion and in the expression of genes involved in epithelial to mesenchymal transition. We also discuss possible means to target it on the basis of the current knowledge of its function in cancer.

Keywords: cancer therapy; EMT; lysosome; lysosome-mediated invasion; MZF1; phosphorylation; PAK4; SUMOylation; transcription factor; zinc finger

---

1. Transcription Factors as Drug Targets in Cancer

For a long time, steroid receptors, which are also known as ligand-activated transcription factors, have been the main group of transcription factors targeted in anti-cancer treatments. During recent years, other sequence-specific transcription factors have emerged as promising anti-cancer drug targets and consequently, transcription factors have lost their status of being "undruggable". This is especially the case for zinc finger transcription factors, which is a large group of proteins with their own specific DNA binding sequences. A good example of a cancer drug that targets a transcription factor is thalidomide, an antiemetic drug from the 1950s that has been repurposed as a novel treatment against hematological malignancies and which functions by inactivating zinc finger transcription factors Ikarios (IKZF1) and Aiolos (IKZF3) through their destabilization [1,2]. Here we will summarize the recent literature on the role and function of another cancer-relevant zinc finger transcription factor, Myeloid Zinc Finger 1 (MZF1), and present reasoning for its potential targeting in cancer and discuss the possibilities of how to target it.

2. What Is MZF1?

2.1. MZF1 Is a Sequence-Specific, Oncogenic Transcription Factor Involved in Myeloid Differentiation

MZF1 is a member of the SCAN domain-containing zinc finger transcription factor (SCAN-ZFP) family, a subfamily of zinc finger proteins (ZFPs)[3]. SCAN-ZFPs represent a class of DNA-binding proteins, many of which are known to regulate transcription during different developmental processes. MZF1 was first isolated from the peripheral blood from a patient with chronic myeloid leukemia and was described as a novel zinc finger protein involved in transcriptional regulation of hematopoietic development [4]. A few years later it was shown to regulate the expression of hematopoiesis-specific genes influencing differentiation, proliferation and programmed cell death and its aberrant expression was found to result in the development of hematopoietic cancers [5,6]. During the last decade, MZF1 was shown to be implicated in the development of various types of solid cancers by enhancing cancer cell growth, migration and invasion [7–15]. Knowledge on the detailed mechanisms by which MZF1 activity is regulated and the central target genes it activates has steadily increased and is still emerging due to active research on the topic.

2.2. MZF1 Transcript Variants and Functional Domains

MZF1 is encoded by a single-copy gene located at chromosome 19q13.4, which is the sub-telomeric region of the chromosome 19q, containing a large number zinc finger genes [4]. Full-length MZF1 protein is estimated to be about 82 kD without post translational modifications. *MZF1* gene supposedly encodes three transcript variants, which are predicted to result from alternative use of two transcription initiation sites and from alternative splicing [16,17]. MZF1 gene is composed of six exons [16,17]. Early work on *MZF1* transcripts lead to the identification of two human MZF1 isoforms: one full-length 734 amino acid isoform containing a SCAN domain in the N-terminus; 13 zinc finger DNA-binding domains in the C-terminus; and one N-terminally truncated, 485 amino acid isoform containing the 13 zinc finger DNA-binding domains and a short N-terminal fragment [16,17] (Figure 1).

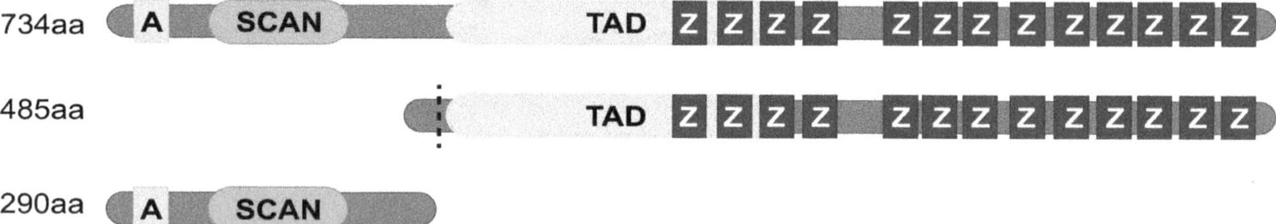

Figure 1. MZF1 protein isoforms. Top: Domain structure of the full-length (734 amino acid) MZF1 isoform containing five distinct domains: acidic domain (A), SCAN domain (SCAN), transactivation domain (TAD), and 13 highly conserved Krüppel-like zinc finger motifs (Z) arranged in two domains. Middle: Domain structure of the putative (485 amino acid) "zinc finger only"-form of MZF1, that in addition to 13 zinc fingers also has the TAD domain. The amino terminus of the new, recently identified 450 kD zinc finger only isoform is marked with a dashed black line. Bottom: Domain structure of the 290 amino acids "SCAN domain only" form of MZF1 that in addition to the SCAN domain also has the acidic domain (A).

Because the smaller 485 amino acid MZF1 isoform (the so-called zinc finger only isoform) was isolated and characterized first, it was for some years believed to be the full-length MZF1. Only when a novel mouse isoform of MZF1, then denoted as Mzf-2, was identified [16,18], was it discovered that also human MZF1 exists in a larger form, containing several additional structural and functional domains [17]. Soon after, these full-length MZF1 isoforms, Mzf-2a (mouse) and MZF1B/C (human), were collectively denoted as MZF1. A third MZF1 isoform of 290 amino acids containing only the SCAN domain in the N-terminus was later identified by the National Institutes of Health Mammalian Gene Collection Program (http://genecollections.nci.nih.gov/MGC/) (Figure 1). This so-called "SCAN domain only" isoform belongs to a group of proteins known as SCAND proteins. SCAND proteins are expected to function as regulators of other SCAN domain-containing proteins [19,20]. The tissue-specific expression and function of this isoform has not been elucidated. It also needs to be noted that the 485 amino acid "zinc finger only" isoform of MZF1 has been recently deleted from the human NBCI sequences and replaced with the predicted sequence of 450 amino acids "zinc finger only" form, where the N-terminus is slightly shorter than in the 485 amino acids form (Figure 1).

Full-length MZF1 consists of five distinctive domains (Figure 1). The domain furthest towards the N-terminus is called an acidic domain (A), which is rich in glutamic and aspartic acid [16,21]. This domain is involved in transcriptional activation and contains regulatory SUMO and phospho-sites [22]. It can also mediate interactions between MZF1 and other transcription factors [22–24]. Downstream of the acidic domain is the SCAN domain of 84 amino acids, a leucine-rich region known to mediate protein–protein interactions [16,17,25,26]. The SCAN domain is found in the SCAN-ZFP family of zinc finger proteins and it mediates homo- and heterodimer formation between SCAN domain containing zinc finger proteins [25–28]. Following the highly conserved SCAN domain there is a so-called transcriptional activation domain (TAD). It is a serine and threonine rich region that is involved in the transcriptional activation of MZF1 [18,21]. This MZF1 domain was identified as a TAD by a classical study by Ogawa and co-workers [21]. In the study, they showed that in murine MZF1 this domain is phosphorylated by mitogen-activated protein kinase ERK and p38 in three of its serines, serine 257, 275 and 295, leading to transcriptional inactivation of Mzf-2a. Consequently, substitution of all of these serines with alanines resulted in strong enhancement of its transcriptional activity in murine myeloid cell line LGM-1[21]. The corresponding sites are conserved in human MZF1, where they are represented as serine 256, 274 and 294. Later on, post-translational modifications in both the acidic domain and the SCAN domain were found to contribute to the transcriptional activity of human MZF1 [22]. In the C-terminal region of MZF1 are the 13 highly conserved Krüppel-like zinc finger motifs arranged in two domains. The first four zinc-finger motifs form one zinc-finger domain and the last nine motifs form another zinc-finger domain, separated from the first one by a glycine-proline-rich region of 24 amino acid residues [4] (Figure 1). The two zinc-finger domains of MZF1 bind to two distinct, yet similar DNA consensus sequences with a common core sequence of four or five guanines, which allows MZF1 to bind more than one DNA sequence at the same time [29], or to bind stronger in genomic sites containing binding sites for both motifs.

3. MZF1 and Cancer

3.1. *MZF1 and Hematological Malignancies*

MZF1 was originally isolated from chronic myeloid leukemia and was shown to be involved in hematopoietic differentiation due to its ability to control the expression of genes involved in hematopoiesis such as *CD34* and *MYB* [4–6]. Due to these reasons, most of the earliest studies on the function of MZF1 were done in hematopoietic cells. Some of the results concerning the actual role and function of MZF1 in hematopoietic malignancies are contradictory. This is because during the earliest studies of MZF1, the knowledge of MZF1 isoforms was not complete. Thus, many studies were done using overexpression of the so-called zinc-finger-only isoform of MZF1, that was the 485 amino acid isoform (Figure 1), which is practically missing most of the N-terminal regulatory domains. As mentioned, this zinc-finger-only isoform was later deleted from the human NBCI sequences, suggesting that it may be a cloning artifact. It has, however, been replaced with a slightly shorter, 450 amino acid isoform, which is a predicted alternative MZF1 transcript that can theoretically exist. In brief, early experiments involving overexpression of the 485 amino acid zinc-finger-only isoform in myeloid cells showed that it inhibits hematopoietic differentiation of mouse embryonic stem cells and delays retinoic acid-induced granulocytic differentiation and apoptosis by inducing proliferation in human promyeloblasts [6,30]. Contrary to what would be expected from these overexpression studies, silencing of MZF1 with antisense oligodeoxynucleotides (AOS) significantly inhibited granulocyte development in vitro from granulocyte colony-stimulating factor-induced cells originating from normal bone marrow, which was evident from granulocyte colony formation assays [31]. This result coincides with the results obtained from Mzf1 knockout mice, which accumulate highly proliferating myeloid cells in their bone marrow and liver, disturbing the tissue architecture, indicating that Mzf1 may function as a tumor suppressor in the hematopoietic compartment [32]. Since AOS and knockout studies target the full-length MZF1, it is understandable that the results obtained when downregulating or inhibiting MZF1 expression would not necessarily be the opposite of the results obtained when overexpressing the MZF1 zinc-finger-only isoform. The zinc-finger-only-isoform, by lacking the N-terminus that contains most of the regulatory domains of MZF1, would have impaired regulation of its activity and would be unable to dimerize with SCAN domain-containing proteins. However, it could mimic MZF1 in a potential state where it is void of its upstream regulation. This could be achieved for example via cancer-induced aberrant expression of MZF1. Thus, it can be concluded that aberrant expression and regulation of MZF1 can make it oncogenic, which is also supported by the fact that mouse embryonic fibroblasts that overexpress the zinc-finger-only MZF1 isoform form aggressive tumors in athymic mice and lose their contact inhibition and upregulate their growth ex vivo [33].

3.2. *MZF1 Acts as an Oncogene in Solid Cancers*

Several studies demonstrate that MZF1 can promote tumorigenesis of various solid cancers. These include breast, cervical, colorectal, liver, lung, and prostate cancer [7–9,11–15,34]. Many MZF1 target genes have a central role in cancer, and increased expression and/or activation of MZF1 induces cell growth, migration and invasion [7–15]. Below we will summarize most of the results obtained on MZF1 in some common solid cancers.

3.2.1. MZF1 in Breast Cancer

MZF1 is needed for the invasion of ErbB2-expressing breast cancer cells [7]. In a study by Rafn and co-workers, ErbB2 activation was shown to induce the invasion of breast cancer cell spheroids via activation of a signaling network that involves TGFβ receptor 1 and 2 (*TGFBR1* and 2), ERK2 (*MAPK1*), PAK4, PAK5 and PAK6 (*PAK4, PAK5* and *PAK6*), cdc42 binding protein kinase beta (*CDC42BPB*), and protein kinase Cα (PKCα; *PRKCA*). Activation of this signaling network leads to activation of MZF1 and MZF1-mediated induction of expression of lysosomal cysteine cathepsins B and L (*CTSB* and *CTSL1*). This work implied for the first-time involvement of lysosomes in the invasion of ErbB2-expressing cancer cells. It showed that MZF1, upon activation by ErbB2 signaling, can induce the pericellular accumulation of lysosomes at the invadosome-like cellular protrusions in invasive ErbB2 expressing breast cancer cells, thereby initiating and promoting their invasion [7]. Once lysosomes have travelled to the cell periphery, their hydrolytic content can be secreted into the extracellular space (lysosomal exocytosis). This can initiate and induce invasion mainly via cathepsin B, which cleaves and thereby activates matrix metalloproteases (MMP) 2 and 3 and the urokinase plasminogen activator [35–37]. Consistently, ErbB2-positive primary breast tumors exhibit increased mRNA and protein expression of cathepsins B and L. Supporting the in vivo connection of ErbB2 activation and cathepsins B and L, the positive correlation between ErbB2 and cathepsin B and L expression in invasive breast cancer was found to be significant [7].

Interestingly, MZF1 regulates the expression of TGFβ1 gene (*TGFB1*) in response to osteopontin-induced integrin signaling in human mesenchymal stem cells, where increased TGFβ signaling induces them to differentiate and adapt a cancer-associated fibroblast phenotype, a process that leads to increased tumor growth and metastasis [14]. TGFβ1 is considered as one of the main regulators of epithelial mesenchymal transition (EMT) [38] and ErbB2 overexpression is connected to TGFβ overexpression, secretion and activation of TGFβ signaling [39]. TGFβ signaling amplifies oncogenic ErbB2 signaling and promotes invasion and metastasis of ErbB2 positive cancer cells [40–42]. Since ErbB2-induced activation of MZF1 is enhanced by TGFβ receptor signaling and *TGFB1* is a MZF1 target gene, increased TGFβ signaling can further induce ErbB2 signaling via a feedback loop involving MZF1 activation. This may additionally lead to enhanced activation of other MZF1 target genes that are important for amplification of breast cancer signaling networks and promoting breast cancer cell migration and invasion, such as *PRKCA* [11]. Interestingly, a complex formation between Elk-1 and MZF1 has been shown to enhance *PRKCA* expression in a synergistic manner and its expression correlates positively with the expression of Elk1 and MZF1 in various breast cancer cell lines [11]. Moreover, a high level of MZF1 in triple-negative breast cancer cell lines Hs578T and MDA-MB-231 is associated with a mesenchymal phenotype with increased cell migration and invasion, which is mediated via insulin-like growth factor receptor (IGF1) [24]. Consequently, destabilization of MZF1 by the IGF1R-driven p38MAPK-Erα-SLUG-E-cadherin pathway leads to conversion of the invasion-promoting mesenchymal phenotype to the less invasive epithelial phenotype. In osteoblasts, which are involved in osteolytic breast cancer metastasis, MZF1 has been shown to upregulate the expression of another EMT regulator, N-cadherin (*CDH2*) [43]. Moreover, a MZF1 target gene *AXL*, which can be activated upon lapatinib resistance in ErbB2 positive breast cancer cells [44], has been shown to induce EMT in breast cancer cells [45]. This all suggests that MZF1 has a role in the development of aggressive breast cancer.

3.2.2. MZF1 in Cervical and Colorectal Cancers

MZF1 activation has been implicated in the progression of cervical and colorectal cancer, where it increases invasion and metastasis, at least partially, via increased expression and activity of receptor tyrosine kinase AXL [8]. Increased expression of *AXL* has been connected to invasion and metastasis of many types of cancers [45–47]. Supportively, both MZF1 and AXL protein levels are considerably higher in colorectal tumors than in corresponding normal tissue [8]. MZF1 binds directly to the *AXL* promoter, leading to increased *AXL* mRNA and protein expression [8]. However, depletion of *AXL* by RNA interference only partially inhibits MZF1-induced migration and invasion of colorectal cancer cells, suggesting that additional MZF1-regulated genes are involved in this process. MZF1 is also central for the activation of the expression of Phosphoinositide -3-Kinase Regulatory Subunit 3 Gamma (*PIK3R3*), which is a regulatory subunit of PI3 kinase (PI3K) needed for PI3K signaling and is important for cancer cell proliferation [15]. In human papillomavirus infected cervical cancer, MZF1 induces the expression of another transcription factor, *NKX2-1*, which in turn upregulates a cancer stem cell regulator *FOXM1*, resulting in increased tumor growth and invasion [48]. In another study with SiHa human cervical cancer cells, MZF1 was shown to bind the matrix metalloprotease 2 (MMP2) promoter, and a bit surprisingly to suppress its expression, and thus was reported to function as a tumor suppressor in these cells [49].

3.2.3. MZF1 in Liver and Lung Cancer

MZF1 regulates the expression of the PKCα gene, *PRKCA*, in human hepatocellular carcinoma cells, where it binds directly to the MZF1 binding site in the *PRKCA* promoter region [9,12]. Depletion of MZF1 with specific antisense oligonucleotides reduces proliferation, migration and invasion of hepatocellular carcinoma cells [9,12] and suppresses the growth of the corresponding xenografts [10,12]. In lung cancer, MZF1 activates the expression of the c-Myc gene (*MYC*) upon loss of the liver kinase B1 (*LKB1*) [13]. This results in enhanced migration and invasion of lung cancer cells and facilitates their growth in soft agar [13]. In tumors from lung adenocarcinoma patients there is a positive correlation between high MYC and MZF1 and low LKB1 expression. Importantly, lung adenocarcinoma patients with low *LKB1* expression have a shorter overall survival than patients with high *LKB1* expression [13]. In lung cancer, MZF1 can upregulate the expression of *NKX2-1*, which in turn increases the expression of *FOXM1* resulting in facilitated tumor growth and invasion [48]. On the other hand, in lung adenocarcinomas, the loss of *LKB1* is associated with *NKX2-1* expression [50].

3.2.4. MZF1 in Prostate Cancer

The role of MZF1 in prostate cancer is somewhat more complicated. The expression of the cell division control 37 (*CDC37*) gene is increased in prostate cancer cells. Here, MZF1 was shown to bind to the promoter of *CDC37* and upregulate its expression [51]. As expected, depletion of MZF1 in prostate cancer cells decreases *CDC37* expression and reduces their tumorigenesis. Interestingly, SCAND1, a SCAN domain protein that can inhibit MZF1 by dimerizing with it, can upon overexpression accumulate at the MZF1 binding sites at the *CDC37* promoter and downregulate its expression-inhibiting tumorigenesis [51]. On the contrary, MZF1 was shown to have the opposite effect in PC3 and DU145 prostate cancer cells, where expression of MZF1 upregulated ferroportin (*FPN*), the only known mammalian iron exporter [52]. Depletion of MZF1 was found to decrease the expression of *FPN*, as expected, but in turn this was shown to result in enhanced cancer cell growth in addition to increased cytoplasmic iron retention [52]. Consequently, increase in the expression of MZF1 inhibited tumor growth, suggesting that in respect to *FPN* regulation in these prostate cancer cells, MZF1 can exhibit a tumor suppressor type of function.

3.2.5. MZF1 in Other Type of Cancers

In glioma cell lines, MZF1 binds directly to the LIM-only protein 3 (*LMO3*) promoter and induces the expression of *LMO3* [53], which is a transcriptional co-activator that can act as an oncogene in glioma, one of the most aggressive and most common tumors of the central nervous system. *LMO3* is often overexpressed in gliomas and its expression correlates positively with poor prognosis [53]. The 19q chromosomal deletions together with the deletion of 1p are used to define the oligodendroglioma, which is a specific type of glioma with favorable prognosis and good response to chemotherapy [54]. Interestingly, the 19q chromosomal deletions in oligodendroglioma include the MZF1 locus as well as the locus of genes coding for many other zinc-finger proteins. In esophageal squamous cell carcinoma samples of 13 patients, MZF1 was found to be co-activated with three other transcription factors, SPIB, MAFG and NFE2L1 when compared to their paired non-cancerous tissues using microarray analysis, where the expression of 17 other transcription factors was suppressed [55]. In gastric cancer cells, MZF1 upregulates *MMP14* expression by directly binding to its promoter [56]. In the same study it was shown that in the clinical samples, *MZF1* expression correlated positively with *MMP14* expression in gastric cancer. On the contrary to this, another study where human gastric cancer samples were analyzed indicated that MZF1 expression was decreased during gastric cancer progression, which correlated with increased invasiveness of gastric cancer [57].

3.2.6. Many MZF1 Target Genes Have a Role in Cancer

MZF1 exerts its activity via modulating the expression of its target genes. Aberrant MZF1 expression and activation results in transcriptional changes that increase cell growth, migration and invasion (see above and reviewed by Eguchi and co-workers [58]). In summary, MZF1 may promote invasion and migration partially by controlling the expression of kinases that are controlling these processes such as *AXL* and *PRKCA*. It can also increase expression of lysosomal, invasion-inducing and promoting hydrolases *CTSB* and *CTSL1*, which facilitate intra- and extracellular degradation of extracellular matrix components by their direct cleavage or by indirectly cleaving and activating matrix metalloproteases MMP2 and MMP3 and urokinase plasminogen activator, which in turn degrade the extracellular matrix [35,36]. MZF1 is also expected to have a role in EMT by controlling the expression of *TGFB1*, *CDH2* and *FOXM1*, and several other EMT-related genes. In Table 1, we have listed the known MZF1 target genes. However, it needs to be noticed that only the ones that are verified by chromatin immunoprecipitation can be considered definite direct targets of MZF1.

Table 1. MZF1 target genes; their method of identification (ChIP: chromatin immunoprecipitation; EMSA: electrophoretic mobility shift assay), reference, function (the role of MZF1) and their involvement generally in EMT (yes, if involvement has been reported).

Gene	Method	Reference	Function	EMT
AXL	ChIP, Luciferase	[8]	Activator	yes
CD14	EMSA,luciferase	[59]	Activator	yes
CD34	EMSA, Acetyltransferase activity	[6]	Activator	
CDC37	ChIP, Luciferase	[51]	Activator	

Table 1. *Cont.*

Gene	Method	Reference	Function	EMT
CDH2 (N-Cadherin)	EMSA	[43]	Activator	yes
CDH2 (N-Cadherin)	ChIP, Luciferase	[60]	Activator	
CK17	Luciferase, qPCR	[61]	Activator	
CTGF	ChIP	[62]	Activator	yes
CTSB	ChIP, Luciferase	[7]	Activator	
GAPDH	ChIP	[63]	Activator	yes
HK2	ChIP	[64]	Suppressor	
IGFIR	ChIP, Luciferase	[65]	Suppressor	yes
ITGAM (CD11b)	EMSA, luciferase	[59]	Activator	
LMO3	ChIP	[53]	Activator	
MMP2	ChIP, Luciferase	[49]	Suppressor	yes
Mtor	ChIP, EMSA, Luciferase	[66]	Suppressor	yes
MYB (c-myb)	EMSA, Acetyltransferase activity	[6]	Activator	
MYC	ChIP, Luciferase	[13]	Activator	
NFKB1A	ChIP	[67]	Activator	yes
NKX2-1	ChIP, Luciferase	[48]	Activator	yes
NKX2-5	ChIP, Luciferase	[68]	Activator	yes
NOV	ChIP	[61]	Activator	
OOCT4	Luciferase	[69]	Activator	yes
PAX2	Luciferase	[70]	Suppressor	yes
PIK3R3 (p55PIK)	ChIP, Luciferase	[15]	Activator	yes
PRAME	ChIP	[71]	Activator	yes
PRKCA (PKC alpha)	ChIP, Luciferase	[12]	Activator	
SLC40A1 (FPN)	ChIP, Luciferase	[52]	Activator	
SMAD4	ChIP, EMSA, Luciferase	[72]	Activator	
TGFB1	ChIP, Luciferase	[73]	Activator	yes
TNFRSF10B (DR5)	Luciferase	[74]	Activator	
YAP1	ChIP, EMSA, Luciferase	[75]	Activator	yes

4. How Does MZF1 Function?

In order to target the oncogenic functions of MZF1, we need to understand how MZF1 is regulated. The key to MZF1 function in cancer lies in its domain structure and in its post-translational modifications (Figure 2) that are regulating its association with other factors, its activation status and its availability.

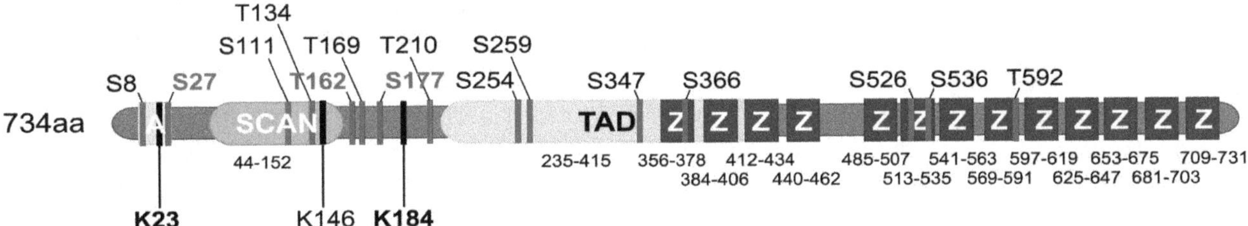

Figure 2. Schematic representation of the protein structure of full-length human MZF1 with reported SUMO-sites (K) and serine (S) and threonine (T) phosphorylation sites. The domain structure of MZF1 is presented as in Figure 1. The location of each indicated SUMO- and phospho-site is shown. The verified SUMO-sites are marked with bold font and the predicted SUMO-site (K146) is marked with regular font. The phospho-sites that are highlighted with red have been identified as ErbB2-responsive sites. Note that the serines 256, 274 and 294 corresponding to the ERK phosphorylation sites in the TAD of murine MZF1 have not yet been reported as phospho-sites in humans.

4.1. Regulation of MZF1 Expression

Relatively little is known about the transcriptional regulation of *MZF1*. Originally, MZF1 was identified as an important transcriptional regulator of myeloid differentiation, and its expression was believed to be myeloid-specific [76]. Later on, it was identified as an oncogenic transcription factor responsible for migratory and invasive phenotypes of various cancer cell lines. Analysis of TCGA website data indicates that there is a significant amplification of the *MZF1* gene in various solid cancers [58]. These include breast, bladder, lung, and uterine cancers. Indeed, increased expression of MZF1 protein levels has been detected in the study of 321 tissue microarray samples containing primary breast cancer and normal breast samples [77]. In these samples, MZF1 levels were shown to significantly increase from normal breast tissue to grade 1–2 tumors, which define invasive ductal carcinoma.

Non-coding RNAs have arisen as important regulators of gene expression. Several microRNAs (miRNAs) can regulate *MZF1* expression. Let-7 miRNAs belong to the group of miRNAs whose aberrant expression is most frequently associated with cancer [78]. Let-7 is upregulated during differentiation, and its expression is systematically downregulated in malignant cancers including breast cancer [79]. Let-7 binds to the 3′-untranslated region of *MZF1*, and ectopic expression of let-7 microRNAs let-7d and let-7e can efficiently downregulate *MZF1* and invasion of constitutively active ErbB2-expressing breast cancer cells [77]. MiR-492 is another microRNA that can bind to the 3′-untranslated region of *MZF1* [52]. MiR-492 regulates *MZF1* expression in prostate cancer cells, and in prostate tumors, miR-492 levels correlate reversibly with the levels of MZF1. Another study with glioma cell lines indicates that overexpression of miR-101 leads to a decrease in *MZF1* expression, without going further into detail in regard to its potential binding sites in *MZF1* [53]. MiRNA-337-3p inhibits gastric cancer progression by downregulating MZF1 activity via a specific mechanism, where miRNA-337-3p binds to the promoter region of *MMP14* adjacent to its MZF1 binding site and represses the MZF1-induced expression of *MMP14* [56]. Consequently, in the same study, miRNA-337-3p was shown to inhibit growth, invasion, metastasis, and angiogenesis of gastric cancer cells in vitro and in vivo via repression of MZF1 activity. Furthermore, miRNA-337-3p expression was found to be an independent prognostic factor for a favorable outcome in gastric cancer.

Interestingly, according to UCSC genome browser (https://genome.ucsc.edu), a validated long non-coding RNA exists that contains the whole MZF1 coding sequence resulting in 15,573 base pair antisense RNA (LOC100131691). Thus far, no studies exist of its actual regulation, expression or function, although it is tempting to speculate that it can have a regulatory role in the expression of MZF1.

4.2. Regulation of the Transcriptional Activity of MZF1

4.2.1. Interaction with Other Transcription Factors

MZF1 has to dimerize to function as a transcription factor. MZF1 utilizes its SCAN domain to form homo- and heterodimers with other SCAN-domain transcription factors [25–28]. The possibility of heterodimerization via the SCAN domain exposes MZF1 to an additional level of regulation, since depending on its dimerization partner, MZF1 may function as a transcriptional activator or repressor. Known SCAN domain-containing MZF1 dimerization partners include SCAN-ZFP family members RAZ1, ZNF24, ZNF174, and ZNF202 [3,26,80], which are all heterodimerizing with MZF1 via a SCAN–SCAN interaction. A recent computational study has tried to shed new light on MZF1 SCAN domain interactions by identification and analysis of cancer-specific mutations in the MZF1 SCAN domain [81]. In this study, 23 cancer-specific mutations were identified in the MZF1 SCAN domain, which could affect MZF1 function by changing its dimerization capacity directly or indirectly via gain or loss of possible post-translational modifications (Nygaard et al., 2016). This work identified cysteine 69 as a potential regulator of MZF1 SCAN–SCAN interactions. Moreover, simultaneous expression and appearance of other SCAN and SCAND domain-containing proteins and possible cancer-inducing mutations in them could also affect MZF1 function for example by directly or indirectly replacing the binding partners of MZF1. However, this type of exiting regulation scheme is still mostly theoretical, especially in the case of MZF1 heterodimers, since detailed biological information on the specific regulation of the transcriptional activity of MZF1 via heterodimeric SCAN–SCAN interactions is still missing.

In addition to SCAN-domain proteins, MZF1 can interact with proteins without the classical SCAN domain, which complicates the scenario of its regulation by binding partners. Moreover, MZF1 interaction with other proteins can even occur via other domains than the SCAN domain. Recent work has indicated that the acidic domain of MZF1 is an additional protein–protein interaction domain. The acidic domain of MZF1 is involved in its association with Elk1 in triple negative breast cancer [12,23,24]. Association of MZF1 and Elk1 via the acidic domain of MZF1 and the heparin-binding domain of Elk1 increases invasion, migration and mesenchymal phenotype of breast cancer cells. This occurs via increasing the expression of *PRKCA* and *IGF1R* by direct binding of MZF1 to their promoter regions. In non-invasive MCF7 breast cancer cells, MZF1 interacts with the CCCTC-binding factor (CTCF) via its acidic domain, which results in downregulation of the transcriptional activity of MZF1 [22]. Activation of ectopic ErbB2 signaling results in SUMO-directed (SUMOylation of lysine 23) phosphorylation of MZF1 serine 27 at its acidic domain, which dissociates MZF1 from its transcriptional repressor CTCF, allowing transcriptional activation of MZF1 [22].

4.2.2. SUMOylation of MZF1

The activity of transcription factors can be modulated by covalent attachment of small ubiquitin-related modifier (SUMO) proteins: SUMO1, SUMO2, SUMO3, and SUMO4 in their SUMO acceptor sites [82]. According to current knowledge of consensus SUMOylation sites, MZF1 has three predicted SUMOylation sites: lysine 23, 184 and 146 (Figure 2) [22,58]. An earlier study that was the first to report MZF1 SUMOylation, suggested that a SUMOylation site would reside in the amino terminus of MZF1 between amino acids 15–27 [80], which is a conserved sequence found in a subset of SCAN-ZFPs [19,80]. This site was identified by showing that overexpressed full-length MZF1 has the ability to accumulate into promyelocytic leukemia nuclear bodies (PML-NBs), a function which requires SUMOylation, and which could be abolished when this area was deleted from MZF1 [80].

SUMOylation of transcription factors and their cofactors may lead to transcriptional activation or inactivation [82,83]. Several studies suggest an important role of PML-NBs in transcriptional regulation [84,85]. Especially, PML-NBs has been presented as a site where SUMO-conjugation occurs and where SUMOylated nuclear proteins reside and accumulate [86]. PML-NBs usually associate to the areas of genomic regions with high transcriptional activity, and many transcription factors can be transiently recruited to PML-NBs. Since SUMOylation usually occurs in the nucleus [83], introduction of mutations in the nuclear SUMO-modified proteins that interfere with their SUMOylation can promote their translocation into the cytoplasm. Thus, MZF1 SUMOylation may be involved in its nuclear retention and its ability to function as a transcription factor.

MZF1 lysine 23 has been identified as a SUMOylation site that directly regulates the transcriptional activity of MZF1 [22]. Its occupation by SUMO groups exposes a nearby serine 27 for phosphorylation by PAK4 in response to ErbB2 activation, which in turn results in increased transcriptional activity of MZF1, indicating its importance for the transcriptional activation of MZF1 as well as defining a new mechanistic type of post-translational regulation, "SUMO-directed phosphorylation". In the same study, lysine 184 was mapped as an additional functional SUMO acceptor site. However, no biological function has yet been identified for it. It is tempting to speculate that MZF1 SUMOylation may be regulating its stability. However, in our studies of MZF1 post-translational modification and their effect on protein stability, we found that in ErbB2-expressing breast cancer cells, MZF1 is a very stable protein and its stability was not affected by mutating its SUMO sites (Brix and Kallunki, unpublished observations). Moreover, in the ErbB2-expressing breast cancer cells, no evidence of SUMOylation of lysine 146 was found [22]. It is possible that lysine 146 is not a functional SUMO acceptor site in MZF1. Supporting this, its probability as a SUMO acceptor site is much lower than that of lysine 23 and 184 [22,58].

4.2.3. Phosphorylation of MZF1

MZF1 is a phosphoprotein that contains several potential as well as functional phosphorylation sites. Even though its massive phosphorylation has been known for some time, thanks to the large amount of phosphorylation analysis done by Mass Spectrometry that has been deposited on the web (http://www.phosphosite.org), thus far no biological function has been shown for the majority of these sites. In a study conducted in MCF7 breast cancer cells with inducible expression of constitutively active ErbB2, ErbB2 activation was shown to increase the transcriptional activity of MZF1 via a signaling network that involves TGFβ receptors 1 and 2 (TGFBR1 and 2), ERK2, PAK4 (PAK5 and PAK6), cdc42 binding protein beta kinase (CDC42BPB), and PKCα (PRKCA) [7]. In a recent study that utilized ErbB2 positive breast cancer cells for phosphorylation analysis by Mass Spectrometry, 13 MZF1 phosphorylation sites were identified [22]. Only three of these were phosphorylated in response to ErbB2 activation. These were serine 27, serine 162 and threonine 177, other sites being constitutively phosphorylated. Of these three sites, only phosphorylation of serine 27 was shown to increase the transcriptional activity of MZF1, the two others having no significant effect on it [22]. Supporting the importance of this phospho-site in vivo, serine 27 phosphorylation was found in an ErbB2-positive breast tumor sample in a proteomics study covering 105 breast tumors that were characterized for TCGA [87]. Furthermore, MZF1 serine 27 phosphorylation was found to correlate positively and significantly with ErbB2 status in a breast tumor tissue microarray containing 225 tissue cores embedded as duplicates and enriched with primary invasive breast cancer samples [22]. The phosphorylation of serine 27 is tightly connected to the SUMOylation of lysine 23 through a mechanism where SUMOylation of lysine 23 is needed as a prerequisite for the phosphorylation of serine 27 by PAK4. In silico modelling of this activation mechanism suggests that SUMOylation of lysine 23 opens up and exposes the serine 27, which otherwise is masked and not approachable for PAK4 to dock to it and phosphorylate it (Figure 3). Phosphorylation of serine 27 will then dissociate MZF1 from the transcriptional repressor CTCF, allowing MZF1 to activate transcription of *CTSB* needed for the invasion of ErbB2-expressing cells. Interestingly, a recent study in human esophageal cancer cell lines demonstrated that phosphorylation of MZF1 serine 27 by constitutively active casein kinase 2 (CK2), which is often upregulated in cancers, mediates their epithelial to mesenchymal transition by inducing the expression of N-cadherin [60].

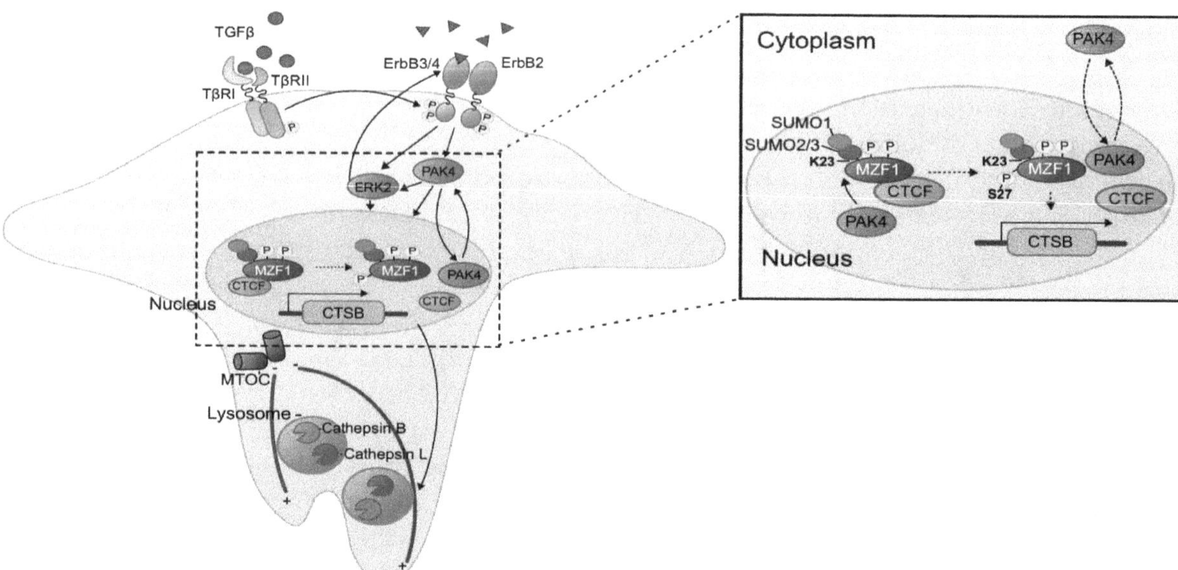

Figure 3. Graphical presentation of MZF1 activation and induction of *CTSB* expression in lysosome-mediated invasion as a response to ErbB2 signaling. ErbB2 activation, further supported by activation of TGFβ signaling, activates ERK2 and PAK4. Active PAK4 will phosphorylate MZF1 serine 27, if its adjacent lysine 23 is SUMOylated, which exposes MZF1 serine 27 to PAK4 phosphorylation. As a response to phosphorylation of serine 27, MZF1 association of its transcriptional repressors, e.g., CTCF, is prevented and MZF1 can now activate *CTSB* expression and lysosome redistribution, which leads to lysosome-mediated invasion.

4.2.4. Mutations Creating New MZF1 Binding Sites in the Genome

Cancer-induced somatic mutations can create new transcription factor binding sites at the regulatory regions of cancer genes [88]. Mutations at the promoter regions of genes that are important for cancer progression can create new transcription factor binding sites that can contribute to the overexpression of that particular gene. Tian and co-workers have identified a mechanism by which MZF1 can affect gene expression via cancer-induced allelic mutations that result in a novel transcription factor co-operation at the promoter of the hepatocyte growth factor gene *HGF* [89]. They have identified single-nucleotide polyformism (SNP) and single nucleotide variants (SNV) in multiple myeloma at the promoter region of *HGF* that result in its increased expression. These mutations resemble the wild-type sequences of the binding motifs of MZF1, nuclear factor kappa-B (NFκB) and nuclear factor erythroid 2-related factor 2 (NFR-2), which together can contribute to increased expression of *HGF*. Whether this is a single type of cancer and a gene where new MZF1 binding sites are gained through a cancer-induced mutation or if multiple cancers and promoters are involved, is not yet known.

5. How Does MZF1 Promote Cancer Invasion and Metastasis?

The mechanistical explanations of how MZF1 promotes cancer progression must rely on the activation of its specific target genes in cancer. Currently known MZF1 target genes have been mapped in individual functional studies, however, no genome-wide studies on MZF1 transcriptional targets have been reported. The majority of the known MZF1 target genes are known cancer genes, whose activation is expected to promote cancer progression (Table 1). Two of the invasive processes activated by MZF1 have been described in more detail. We will briefly present these below.

5.1. Lysosomes, MZF1 and Invasion

Lysosomes have a central role in the induction of invasion by ErbB2 in breast cancer cells [90]. Invasion of the MCF7 breast cancer spheroids expressing the trastuzumab-resistant p95 form of ErbB2 depends on the activation of a signaling network that culminates in the activation of MZF1 [7]. Here MZF1 regulates the function and activity of lysosomes by mediating ErbB2-induced, increased expression of lysosomal cysteine cathepsins B and L (*CTSB* and *CTSL1*), which is necessary for the invasion of these cells. Increased expression of *CTSB* and *CTSL1* leads to increased activity of cathepsins B and L, whose expression correlates positively ($p < 0.0001$) with high ErbB2 status in primary invasive breast cancer [7]. This is connected to the redistribution of lysosomes from a perinuclear to a peripheral position in invadosome-like cellular protrusions adjacent to the cell membrane, which is induced by phosphorylation of MZF1 serine 27 [22]. The appearance of the peripheral population of lysosomes correlates positively with the invasiveness of ErbB2 positive ovarian and breast cancer cells [7,91] and can contribute to extracellular matrix (ECM) degradation both internally and externally [34,36,37]. Peripheral lysosomes degrade the ECM components that have been internalized by the cell. Moreover, they can secrete their hydrolytic content, including cathepsin B, into the extracellular space to initiate and promote invasion. Secreted cathepsin B degrades the ECM components type IV collagen, laminin, and fibronectin and initiates the activation of the extracellular degradome by cleaving the pro-forms of urokinase plasminogen activator and MMP2 and MMP3 [92], which are activators of MMP9 and MMP13 (Figure 4). MZF1 seems to be a central regulator of invasion-associated pericellular lysosome distribution and lysosome-mediated invasion of ErbB2 expressing highly invasive cancer cells [7,22,90] (Figure 3).

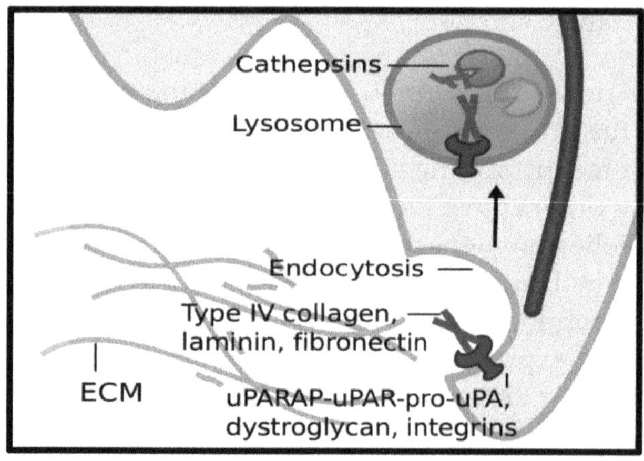

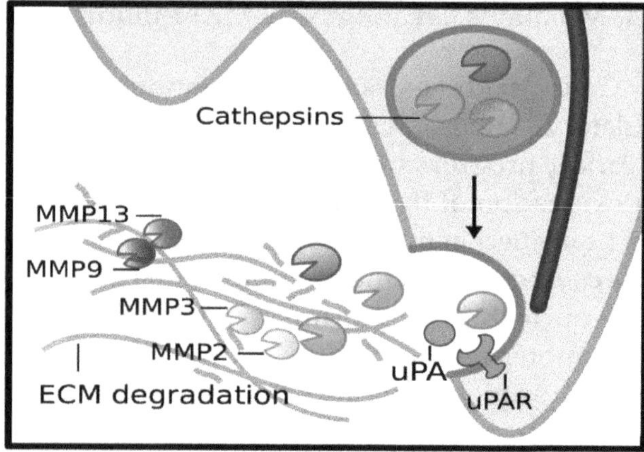

Figure 4. Graphical presentation of cellular mechanisms activated in lysosome-mediated invasion. Peripheral lysosomes contribute to extracellular matrix (ECM) degradation both internally (**left**) and externally (**right**). Peripheral lysosomes degrade the ECM components that have been internalized by the cell e.g., via endocytosis. Peripheral lysosomes can secrete their contents, including cathepsin B, into the extracellular space via lysosomal exocytosis, a process where the lysosome membrane fuses with the plasma membrane, which allows the secretion of the lysosomal contents to the extracellular space. Secreted cathepsin B degrades the ECM components: type IV collagen, laminin and fibronectin and initiates the activation of the extracellular degradome by cleaving the pro-forms of urokinase plasminogen activator and MMP2 and MMP3, which are activators of MMP9 and MMP13.

5.2. MZF1 and EMT

Recently, MZF1 has been connected to EMT, a biological process where epithelial cells lose their polarity and cell–cell adhesion capability and gain invasive and migratory properties by adapting a mesenchymal phenotype. In human esophageal cancer cell lines, phosphorylation of MZF1 serine 27 by CK2 initiates EMT by inducing the transcription of N-cadherin during the EMT-inducing switch from E-cadherin to N-cadherin [60]. Knockdown of MZF1 by specific shRNA reverses the mesenchymal phenotype of these cells into epithelial and downregulates the expression of N-cadherin. In triple-negative breast cancer cells, MZF1 activation can maintain the mesenchymal phenotype by interacting with Elk1 at the promoter region of *IGF1R* [24]. Even though evidence of the connection between MZF1 and EMT is increasing, it is still not clear if the role of MZF1 in EMT is cancer type-specific, or if MZF1 can have a more general role in the initiation and/or maintenance of EMT. Intriguingly, 17 of the 31 (55%) reported MZF1 target genes (Table 1) are somehow involved in EMT in other cancer studies.

6. Conclusions and Future Directions

The majority of studies on MZF1 in cancer report that MZF1 functions as an oncogene in various solid cancers by regulating the expression of genes involved in cancer progression, EMT, extracellular matrix degradation, invasion, and angiogenesis. Inhibition of MZF1 function could be a way to inhibit these processes. Different efficient approaches to inhibit transcription factor activity in cancer exist, including transcription factor destabilization by affecting the post-translational modifications that regulate stability or activity. Regarding MZF1, probably one of the most successful scenarios could be to inhibit its association with its specific co-transcription factors such as Elk1, which is needed for MZF1-induced activation of the expression of *PRKCA* and *IGF1R*, and which contributes to the stability of MZF1 in triple-negative breast cancer [24].

Specific post-translational modifications of MZF1 are induced in invasive cancer, as is the case for breast cancer harboring ErbB2 activation, and these are necessary for the invasive signaling mediated via MZF1 in response to ErbB2 activation in breast cancer cells [22]. Thus, another valid possibility would be to target the enzymes responsible for these post-translational modifications, namely SUMOylation of lysine 23 and/or phosphorylation of serine 27. It is not known what regulates the SUMOylation of lysine 23, which is a prerequisite of the phosphorylation of serine 27 by PAK4 [22]. However, a theory exists according to which the generally high phosphorylation status of MZF1, and especially the phosphorylation of serine 8 can bend the MZF1 molecule to a position where lysine 23 is exposed to SUMOylation [22,81]. Interestingly, increased SUMOylation is generally connected to cancer progression, and in breast cancer it is associated with poor prognosis [93,94]. The expression of SUMOylation-associated enzymes is often increased in cancer, and thus, numerous SUMO-pathway-targeting inhibitors have been developed, many of which can be considered as promising anti-cancer agents [95]. These could also target SUMOylation of MZF1 lysine 23 and thus prevent the activation of MZF1 by hindering the phosphorylation of serine 27.

PAK4, a kinase that can phosphorylate MZF1 serine 27 in response to ErbB2 activation, is considered as a good target for the treatment of a variety of solid cancers including breast cancer, and its inhibition for this purpose has been patented by Hoffman-La Roche and Genentech [96]. Although the resulting PAK4 inhibitor PF-3758309 failed in phase I clinical trials [97], a new PAK4 inhibitor, KPT-9274, has been developed (Karyopharm Therapeutics, USA), which is currently in phase I clinical trials [98]. Identification of MZF1 as an oncogenic target of PAK4, whose activity is important for invasiveness of ErbB2 positive breast cancer cells, suggests that PAK4 inhibitors might be useful for the treatment of cancers whose aggressiveness depends on MZF1.

Another possible way to target MZF1 could be by preventing its binding to the regulatory regions of its cancerous target genes. For this, more understanding of its DNA-binding specificity would be needed. For example, since it has two distinct zinc finger domains with divergent binding sequences, it would be useful to find out if either of them is a preferred binding domain for its target genes that are important in cancer. Interestingly, by using CRISPR-Cas9 gene editing technology, we have experienced that ErbB2-expressing breast cancer cell lines have developed dependency on *MZF1*, so that these cancer cells harboring full knockout of *MZF1* are not viable [22], suggesting that they could have developed oncogene addiction towards MZF1. If this is the case, efficient inhibition of MZF1 could result not only in inhibition of invasion but could also be lethal for them.

An increasing number of studies point to a central role for enhanced MZF1 expression and activation in the invasiveness of different solid cancers, making it an attractive therapeutic target. Several probabilities already exist for how its activity could be controlled, and at the same, interesting possibilities still remain to be studied. One potentially useful future approach would be to carry out an in silico screen to identify compounds that interfere with MZF1 DNA binding, dimerization with specific partners or with post-translational modifications that are important for its activation. Especially, its DNA binding domain as well as SUMOylation of lysine 23 and phosphorylation of serine 27 are well characterized. These modification sites are located in domains for which crystal structures are available and would thus already be suitable for such an approach. To use this approach to identify molecules that can prevent MZF1 heterodimerization, more research would be needed to understand which associations are beneficial for cancer. In general, more research is still needed to increase the understanding of the detailed function of MZF1 in cancer, of the cellular cancer-promoting programs it regulates, the cancers where its inhibition would be most beneficial, and how it should be achieved.

References

1. Gandhi, A.K.; Kang, J.; Havens, C.G.; Conklin, T.; Ning, Y.; Wu, L.; Ito, T.; Ando, H.; Waldman, M.F.; Thakurta, A.; et al. Immunomodulatory agents lenalidomide and pomalidomide co-stimulate T cells by inducing degradation of T cell repressors Ikaros and Aiolos via modulation of the E3 ubiquitin ligase complex CRL4(CRBN.). *Br. J. Haematol.* **2014**, *164*, 811–821. [CrossRef]
2. Licht, J.D.; Shortt, J.; Johnstone, R. From anecdote to targeted therapy: The curious case of thalidomide in multiple myeloma. *Cancer Cell* **2014**, *25*, 9–11. [CrossRef]
3. Peterson, F.C.; Hayes, P.L.; Waltner, J.K.; Heisner, A.K.; Jensen, D.R.; Sander, T.L.; Volkman, B.F. Structure of the SCAN domain from the tumor suppressor protein MZF1. *J. Mol. Biol.* **2006**, *363*, 137–147. [CrossRef]
4. Hromas, R.; Collins, S.J.; Hickstein, D.; Raskind, W.; Deaven, L.L.; O'Hara, P.; Hagen, F.S.; Kaushansky, K. A retinoic acid-responsive human zinc finger gene, MZF-1, preferentially expressed in myeloid cells. *J. Biol. Chem.* **1991**, *266*, 14183–14187.
5. Morris, J.F.; Rauscher, F.J., 3rd; Davis, B.; Klemsz, M.; Xu, D.; Tenen, D.; Hromas, R. The myeloid zinc finger gene, MZF-1, regulates the CD34 promoter in vitro. *Blood* **1995**, *86*, 3640–3647.
6. Perrotti, D.; Melotti, P.; Skorski, T.; Casella, I.; Peschle, C.; Calabretta, B. Overexpression of the zinc finger protein MZF1 inhibits hematopoietic development from embryonic stem cells: Correlation with negative regulation of CD34 and c-myb promoter activity. *Mol. Cell Biol.* **1995**, *15*, 6075–6087. [CrossRef]
7. Rafn, B.; Nielsen, C.F.; Andersen, S.H.; Szyniarowski, P.; Corcelle-Termeau, E.; Valo, E.; Fehrenbacher, N.; Olsen, C.J.; Daugaard, M.; Egebjerg, C.; et al. ErbB2-driven breast cancer cell invasion depends on a complex signaling network activating myeloid zinc finger-1-dependent cathepsin B expression. *Mol. Cell* **2012**, *45*, 764–776. [CrossRef] [PubMed]
8. Mudduluru, G.; Vajkoczy, P.; Allgayer, H. Myeloid zinc finger 1 induces migration, invasion, and in vivo metastasis through Axl gene expression in solid cancer. *Mol. Cancer Res.* **2010**, *8*, 159–169. [CrossRef] [PubMed]
9. Hsieh, Y.H.; Wu, T.T.; Tsai, J.H.; Huang, C.Y.; Hsieh, Y.S.; Liu, J.Y. PKCalpha expression regulated by Elk-1 and MZF-1 in human HCC cells. *Biochem. Biophys. Res. Commun.* **2006**, *339*, 217–225. [CrossRef] [PubMed]
10. Hsieh, Y.H.; Wu, T.T.; Huang, C.Y.; Hsieh, Y.S.; Liu, J.Y. Suppression of tumorigenicity of human hepatocellular carcinoma cells by antisense oligonucleotide MZF-1. *Chin. J. Physiol.* **2007**, *50*, 9–15. [PubMed]
11. Yue, C.H.; Chiu, Y.W.; Tung, J.N.; Tzang, B.S.; Shiu, J.J.; Huang, W.H.; Liu, J.Y.; Hwang, J.M. Expression of protein kinase C alpha and the MZF-1 and Elk-1 transcription factors in human breast cancer cells. *Chin. J. Physiol.* **2012**, *55*, 31–36. [CrossRef]
12. Yue, C.H.; Huang, C.Y.; Tsai, J.H.; Hsu, C.W.; Hsieh, Y.H.; Lin, H.; Liu, J.Y. MZF-1/Elk-1 Complex Binds to Protein Kinase Calpha Promoter and Is Involved in Hepatocellular Carcinoma. *PLoS ONE* **2015**, *10*, e0127420. [CrossRef]
13. Tsai, L.H.; Wu, J.Y.; Cheng, Y.W.; Chen, C.Y.; Sheu, G.T.; Wu, T.C.; Lee, H. The MZF1/c-MYC axis mediates lung adenocarcinoma progression caused by wild-type lkb1 loss. *Oncogene* **2015**, *34*, 1641–1649. [CrossRef] [PubMed]
14. Weber, C.E.; Kothari, A.N.; Wai, P.Y.; Li, N.Y.; Driver, J.; Zapf, M.A.; Franzen, C.A.; Gupta, G.N.; Osipo, C.; Zlobin, A.; et al. Osteopontin mediates an MZF1-TGF-beta1-dependent transformation of mesenchymal stem cells into cancer-associated fibroblasts in breast cancer. *Oncogene* **2015**, *34*, 4821–4833. [CrossRef] [PubMed]
15. Deng, Y.; Wang, J.; Wang, G.; Jin, Y.; Luo, X.; Xia, X.; Gong, J.; Hu, J. p55PIK transcriptionally activated by MZF1 promotes colorectal cancer cell proliferation. *Biomed. Res. Int.* **2013**, *2013*, 868131. [CrossRef] [PubMed]
16. Murai, K.; Murakami, H.; Nagata, S. A novel form of the myeloid-specific zinc finger protein (MZF-2). *Genes Cells* **1997**, *2*, 581–591. [CrossRef] [PubMed]
17. Peterson, M.J.; Morris, J.F. Human myeloid zinc finger gene MZF produces multiple transcripts and encodes a SCAN box protein. *Gene* **2000**, *254*, 105–118. [CrossRef]
18. Murai, K.; Murakami, H.; Nagata, S. Myeloid-specific transcriptional activation by murine myeloid zinc-finger protein 2. *Proc. Natl. Acad. Sci. USA* **1998**, *95*, 3461–3466. [CrossRef]
19. Sander, T.L.; Stringer, K.F.; Maki, J.L.; Szauter, P.; Stone, J.R.; Collins, T. The SCAN domain defines a large family of zinc finger transcription factors. *Gene* **2003**, *310*, 29–38. [CrossRef]

20. Edelstein, L.C.; Collins, T. The SCAN domain family of zinc finger transcription factors. *Gene* **2005**, *359*, 1–17. [CrossRef]
21. Ogawa, H.; Murayama, A.; Nagata, S.; Fukunaga, R. Regulation of myeloid zinc finger protein 2A transactivation activity through phosphorylation by mitogen-activated protein kinases. *J. Biol. Chem.* **2003**, *278*, 2921–2927. [CrossRef] [PubMed]
22. Brix, D.M.; Tvingsholm, S.A.; Hansen, M.B.; Clemmensen, K.B.; Ohman, T.; Siino, V.; Lambrughi, M.; Hansen, K.; Puustinen, P.; Gromova, I.; et al. Release of transcriptional repression via ErbB2-induced, SUMO-directed phosphorylation of myeloid zinc finger-1 serine 27 activates lysosome redistribution and invasion. *Oncogene* **2019**, *38*, 3170–3184. [CrossRef] [PubMed]
23. Lee, C.J.; Hsu, L.S.; Yue, C.H.; Lin, H.; Chiu, Y.W.; Lin, Y.Y.; Huang, C.Y.; Hung, M.C.; Liu, J.Y. MZF-1/Elk-1 interaction domain as therapeutic target for protein kinase Calpha-based triple-negative breast cancer cells. *Oncotarget* **2016**, *7*, 59845–59859. [CrossRef] [PubMed]
24. Yue, C.H.; Liu, J.Y.; Chi, C.S.; Hu, C.W.; Tan, K.T.; Huang, F.M.; Pan, Y.R.; Lin, K.I.; Lee, C.J. Myeloid Zinc Finger 1 (MZF1) Maintains the Mesenchymal Phenotype by Down-regulating IGF1R/p38 MAPK/ERalpha Signaling Pathway in High-level MZF1-expressing TNBC cells. *Anticancer Res.* **2019**, *39*, 4149–4164. [CrossRef]
25. Pengue, G.; Calabro, V.; Bartoli, P.C.; Pagliuca, A.; Lania, L. Repression of transcriptional activity at a distance by the evolutionarily conserved KRAB domain present in a subfamily of zinc finger proteins. *Nucleic Acids Res.* **1994**, *22*, 2908–2914. [CrossRef]
26. Sander, T.L.; Haas, A.L.; Peterson, M.J.; Morris, J.F. Identification of a novel SCAN box-related protein that interacts with MZF1B. The leucine-rich SCAN box mediates hetero- and homoprotein associations. *J. Biol. Chem.* **2000**, *275*, 12857–12867. [CrossRef]
27. Williams, A.J.; Khachigian, L.M.; Shows, T.; Collins, T. Isolation and characterization of a novel zinc-finger protein with transcription repressor activity. *J. Biol. Chem.* **1995**, *270*, 22143–22152. [CrossRef]
28. Williams, A.J.; Blacklow, S.C.; Collins, T. The zinc finger-associated SCAN box is a conserved oligomerization domain. *Mol. Cell Biol.* **1999**, *19*, 8526–8535. [CrossRef]
29. Morris, J.F.; Hromas, R.; Rauscher, F.J., 3rd. Characterization of the DNA-binding properties of the myeloid zinc finger protein MZF1: Two independent DNA-binding domains recognize two DNA consensus sequences with a common G-rich core. *Mol. Cell Biol.* **1994**, *14*, 1786–1795. [CrossRef]
30. Robertson, K.A.; Hill, D.P.; Kelley, M.R.; Tritt, R.; Crum, B.; Van Epps, S.; Srour, E.; Rice, S.; Hromas, R. The myeloid zinc finger gene (MZF-1) delays retinoic acid-induced apoptosis and differentiation in myeloid leukemia cells. *Leukemia* **1998**, *12*, 690–698. [CrossRef]
31. Bavisotto, L.; Kaushansky, K.; Lin, N.; Hromas, R. Antisense oligonucleotides from the stage-specific myeloid zinc finger gene MZF-1 inhibit granulopoiesis in vitro. *J. Exp. Med.* **1991**, *174*, 1097–1101. [CrossRef] [PubMed]
32. Gaboli, M.; Kotsi, P.A.; Gurrieri, C.; Cattoretti, G.; Ronchetti, S.; Cordon-Cardo, C.; Broxmeyer, H.E.; Hromas, R.; Pandolfi, P.P. Mzf1 controls cell proliferation and tumorigenesis. *Genes Dev.* **2001**, *15*, 1625–1630. [CrossRef] [PubMed]
33. Hromas, R.; Morris, J.; Cornetta, K.; Berebitsky, D.; Davidson, A.; Sha, M.; Sledge, G.; Rauscher, F., 3rd. Aberrant expression of the myeloid zinc finger gene, MZF-1, is oncogenic. *Cancer Res.* **1995**, *55*, 3610–3614.
34. Brix, D.M.; Clemmensen, K.K.; Kallunki, T. When Good Turns Bad: Regulation of Invasion and Metastasis by ErbB2 Receptor Tyrosine Kinase. *Cells* **2014**, *3*, 53–78. [CrossRef]
35. Mason, S.D.; Joyce, J.A. Proteolytic networks in cancer. *Trends Cell Biol.* **2011**, *21*, 228–237. [CrossRef]
36. Kallunki, T.; Olsen, O.D.; Jaattela, M. Cancer-associated lysosomal changes: Friends or foes? *Oncogene* **2013**, *32*, 1995–2004. [CrossRef]
37. Hamalisto, S.; Jaattela, M. Lysosomes in cancer-living on the edge (of the cell). *Curr. Opin. Cell Biol.* **2016**, *39*, 69–76. [CrossRef]
38. Imamura, T.; Hikita, A.; Inoue, Y. The roles of TGF-beta signaling in carcinogenesis and breast cancer metastasis. *Breast Cancer* **2012**, *19*, 118–124. [CrossRef]
39. Gupta, P.; Srivastava, S.K. HER2 mediated de novo production of TGFbeta leads to SNAIL driven epithelial-to-mesenchymal transition and metastasis of breast cancer. *Mol. Oncol.* **2014**, *8*, 1532–1547. [CrossRef]

40. Pradeep, C.R.; Zeisel, A.; Kostler, W.J.; Lauriola, M.; Jacob-Hirsch, J.; Haibe-Kains, B.; Amariglio, N.; Ben-Chetrit, N.; Emde, A.; Solomonov, I.; et al. Modeling invasive breast cancer: Growth factors propel progression of HER2-positive premalignant lesions. *Oncogene* **2012**, *31*, 3569–3583. [CrossRef]
41. Seton-Rogers, S.E.; Lu, Y.; Hines, L.M.; Koundinya, M.; LaBaer, J.; Muthuswamy, S.K.; Brugge, J.S. Cooperation of the ErbB2 receptor and transforming growth factor beta in induction of migration and invasion in mammary epithelial cells. *Proc. Natl. Acad. Sci. USA* **2004**, *101*, 1257–1262. [CrossRef] [PubMed]
42. Ueda, Y.; Wang, S.; Dumont, N.; Yi, J.Y.; Koh, Y.; Arteaga, C.L. Overexpression of HER2 (erbB2) in human breast epithelial cells unmasks transforming growth factor beta-induced cell motility. *J. Biol. Chem.* **2004**, *279*, 24505–24513. [CrossRef] [PubMed]
43. Le Mee, S.; Fromigue, O.; Marie, P.J. Sp1/Sp3 and the myeloid zinc finger gene MZF1 regulate the human N-cadherin promoter in osteoblasts. *Exp. Cell Res.* **2005**, *302*, 129–142. [CrossRef] [PubMed]
44. Liu, L.; Greger, J.; Shi, H.; Liu, Y.; Greshock, J.; Annan, R.; Halsey, W.; Sathe, G.M.; Martin, A.M.; Gilmer, T.M. Novel mechanism of lapatinib resistance in HER2-positive breast tumor cells: Activation of AXL. *Cancer Res.* **2009**, *69*, 6871–6878. [CrossRef]
45. Asiedu, M.K.; Beauchamp-Perez, F.D.; Ingle, J.N.; Behrens, M.D.; Radisky, D.C.; Knutson, K.L. AXL induces epithelial-to-mesenchymal transition and regulates the function of breast cancer stem cells. *Oncogene* **2014**, *33*, 1316–1324. [CrossRef]
46. Paccez, J.D.; Vogelsang, M.; Parker, M.I.; Zerbini, L.F. The receptor tyrosine kinase Axl in cancer: Biological functions and therapeutic implications. *Int. J. Cancer* **2014**, *134*, 1024–1033. [CrossRef]
47. Arteaga, C.L.; Engelman, J.A. ERBB receptors: From oncogene discovery to basic science to mechanism-based cancer therapeutics. *Cancer Cell* **2014**, *25*, 282–303. [CrossRef]
48. Chen, P.M.; Cheng, Y.W.; Wang, Y.C.; Wu, T.C.; Chen, C.Y.; Lee, H. Up-regulation of FOXM1 by E6 oncoprotein through the MZF1/NKX2-1 axis is required for human papillomavirus-associated tumorigenesis. *Neoplasia* **2014**, *16*, 961–971. [CrossRef]
49. Tsai, S.J.; Hwang, J.M.; Hsieh, S.C.; Ying, T.H.; Hsieh, Y.H. Overexpression of myeloid zinc finger 1 suppresses matrix metalloproteinase-2 expression and reduces invasiveness of SiHa human cervical cancer cells. *Biochem. Biophys. Res. Commun.* **2012**, *425*, 462–467. [CrossRef]
50. Tsai, L.H.; Chen, P.M.; Cheng, Y.W.; Chen, C.Y.; Sheu, G.T.; Wu, T.C.; Lee, H. LKB1 loss by alteration of the NKX2-1/p53 pathway promotes tumor malignancy and predicts poor survival and relapse in lung adenocarcinomas. *Oncogene* **2014**, *33*, 3851–3860. [CrossRef]
51. Eguchi, T.; Prince, T.L.; Tran, M.T.; Sogawa, C.; Lang, B.J.; Calderwood, S.K. MZF1 and SCAND1 Reciprocally Regulate CDC37 Gene Expression in Prostate Cancer. *Cancers* **2019**, *11*, 792. [CrossRef] [PubMed]
52. Chen, Y.; Zhang, Z.; Yang, K.; Du, J.; Xu, Y.; Liu, S. Myeloid zinc-finger 1 (MZF-1) suppresses prostate tumor growth through enforcing ferroportin-conducted iron egress. *Oncogene* **2015**, *34*, 3839–3847. [CrossRef] [PubMed]
53. Liu, X.; Lei, Q.; Yu, Z.; Xu, G.; Tang, H.; Wang, W.; Wang, Z.; Li, G.; Wu, M. MiR-101 reverses the hypomethylation of the LMO3 promoter in glioma cells. *Oncotarget* **2015**, *6*, 7930–7943. [CrossRef]
54. Sonabend, A.M.; Lesniak, M.S. Oligodendrogliomas: Clinical significance of 1p and 19q chromosomal deletions. *Expert. Rev. Neurother.* **2005**, *5*, 25–32. [CrossRef] [PubMed]
55. Zhao, Y.; Min, L.; Xu, C.; Shao, L.; Guo, S.; Cheng, R.; Xing, J.; Zhu, S.; Zhang, S. Construction of disease-specific transcriptional regulatory networks identifies co-activation of four gene in esophageal squamous cell carcinoma. *Oncol. Rep.* **2017**, *38*, 411–417. [CrossRef] [PubMed]
56. Zheng, L.; Jiao, W.; Mei, H.; Song, H.; Li, D.; Xiang, X.; Chen, Y.; Yang, F.; Li, H.; Huang, K.; et al. miRNA-337-3p inhibits gastric cancer progression through repressing myeloid zinc finger 1-facilitated expression of matrix metalloproteinase 14. *Oncotarget* **2016**, *7*, 40314–40328. [CrossRef] [PubMed]
57. Li, G.Q.; He, Q.; Yang, L.; Wang, S.B.; Yu, D.D.; He, Y.Q.; Hu, J.; Pan, Y.M.; Wu, Y. Clinical Significance of Myeloid Zinc Finger 1 Expression in the Progression of Gastric Tumourigenesis. *Cell Physiol. Biochem.* **2017**, *44*, 1242–1250. [CrossRef]
58. Eguchi, T.; Prince, T.; Wegiel, B.; Calderwood, S.K. Role and Regulation of Myeloid Zinc Finger Protein 1 in Cancer. *J. Cell Biochem.* **2015**, *116*, 2146–2154. [CrossRef]
59. Moeenrezakhanlou, A.; Shephard, L.; Lam, L.; Reiner, N.E. Myeloid cell differentiation in response to calcitriol for expression CD11b and CD14 is regulated by myeloid zinc finger-1 protein downstream of phosphatidylinositol 3-kinase. *J. Leukoc. Biol.* **2008**, *84*, 519–528. [CrossRef] [PubMed]

60. Ko, H.; Kim, S.; Yang, K.; Kim, K. Phosphorylation-dependent stabilization of MZF1 upregulates N-cadherin expression during protein kinase CK2-mediated epithelial-mesenchymal transition. *Oncogenesis* **2018**, *7*, 27. [CrossRef] [PubMed]
61. Wu, L.; Han, L.; Zhou, C.; Wei, W.; Chen, X.; Yi, H.; Wu, X.; Bai, X.; Guo, S.; Yu, Y.; et al. TGF-beta1-induced CK17 enhances cancer stem cell-like properties rather than EMT in promoting cervical cancer metastasis via the ERK1/2-MZF1 signaling pathway. *FEBS J.* **2017**, *284*, 3000–3017. [CrossRef] [PubMed]
62. Piszczatowski, R.T.; Rafferty, B.J.; Rozado, A.; Parziale, J.V.; Lents, N.H. Myeloid Zinc Finger 1 (MZF-1) Regulates Expression of the CCN2/CTGF and CCN3/NOV Genes in the Hematopoietic Compartment. *J. Cell Physiol.* **2015**, *230*, 2634–2639. [CrossRef] [PubMed]
63. Piszczatowski, R.T.; Rafferty, B.J.; Rozado, A.; Tobak, S.; Lents, N.H. The glyceraldehyde 3-phosphate dehydrogenase gene (GAPDH) is regulated by myeloid zinc finger 1 (MZF-1) and is induced by calcitriol. *Biochem. Biophys. Res. Commun.* **2014**, *451*, 137–141. [CrossRef] [PubMed]
64. Gupta, P.; Sheikh, T.; Sen, E. SIRT6 regulated nucleosomal occupancy affects Hexokinase 2 expression. *Exp. Cell Res.* **2017**, *357*, 98–106. [CrossRef]
65. Vishwamitra, D.; Curry, C.V.; Alkan, S.; Song, Y.H.; Gallick, G.E.; Kaseb, A.O.; Shi, P.; Amin, H.M. The transcription factors Ik-1 and MZF1 downregulate IGF-IR expression in NPM-ALK(+) T-cell lymphoma. *Mol. Cancer* **2015**, *14*, 53. [CrossRef]
66. Zhang, S.; Shi, W.; Ramsay, E.S.; Bliskovsky, V.; Eiden, A.M.; Connors, D.; Steinsaltz, M.; DuBois, W.; Mock, B.A. The transcription factor MZF1 differentially regulates murine Mtor promoter variants linked to tumor susceptibility. *J. Biol. Chem.* **2019**, *294*, 16756–16764. [CrossRef]
67. Lin, S.; Wang, X.; Pan, Y.; Tian, R.; Lin, B.; Jiang, G.; Chen, K.; He, Y.; Zhang, L.; Zhai, W.; et al. Transcription Factor Myeloid Zinc-Finger 1 Suppresses Human Gastric Carcinogenesis by Interacting with Metallothionein 2A. *Clin. Cancer Res.* **2019**, *25*, 1050–1062. [CrossRef]
68. Doppler, S.A.; Werner, A.; Barz, M.; Lahm, H.; Deutsch, M.A.; Dressen, M.; Schiemann, M.; Voss, B.; Gregoire, S.; Kuppusamy, R.; et al. Myeloid zinc finger 1 (Mzf1) differentially modulates murine cardiogenesis by interacting with an Nkx2.5 cardiac enhancer. *PLoS ONE* **2014**, *9*, e113775. [CrossRef]
69. Chen, H.; Zuo, Q.; Wang, Y.; Song, J.; Yang, H.; Zhang, Y.; Li, B. Inducing goat pluripotent stem cells with four transcription factor mRNAs that activate endogenous promoters. *BMC Biotechnol.* **2017**, *17*, 11. [CrossRef]
70. Jia, N.; Wang, J.; Li, Q.; Tao, X.; Chang, K.; Hua, K.; Yu, Y.; Wong, K.K.; Feng, W. DNA methylation promotes paired box 2 expression via myeloid zinc finger 1 in endometrial cancer. *Oncotarget* **2016**, *7*, 84785–84797. [CrossRef]
71. Lee, Y.K.; Park, U.H.; Kim, E.J.; Hwang, J.T.; Jeong, J.C.; Um, S.J. Tumor antigen PRAME is up-regulated by MZF1 in cooperation with DNA hypomethylation in melanoma cells. *Cancer Lett.* **2017**, *403*, 144–151. [CrossRef] [PubMed]
72. Lee, J.H.; Kim, S.S.; Lee, H.S.; Hong, S.; Rajasekaran, N.; Wang, L.H.; Choi, J.S.; Shin, Y.K. Upregulation of SMAD4 by MZF1 inhibits migration of human gastric cancer cells. *Int. J. Oncol.* **2017**, *50*, 272–282. [CrossRef] [PubMed]
73. Driver, J.; Weber, C.E.; Callaci, J.J.; Kothari, A.N.; Zapf, M.A.; Roper, P.M.; Borys, D.; Franzen, C.A.; Gupta, G.N.; Wai, P.Y.; et al. Alcohol inhibits osteopontin-dependent transforming growth factor-beta1 expression in human mesenchymal stem cells. *J. Biol. Chem.* **2015**, *290*, 9959–9973. [CrossRef] [PubMed]
74. Horinaka, M.; Yoshida, T.; Tomosugi, M.; Yasuda, S.; Sowa, Y.; Sakai, T. Myeloid zinc finger 1 mediates sulindac sulfide-induced upregulation of death receptor 5 of human colon cancer cells. *Sci. Rep.* **2014**, *4*, 6000. [CrossRef]
75. Verma, N.K.; Gadi, A.; Maurizi, G.; Roy, U.B.; Mansukhani, A.; Basilico, C. Myeloid Zinc Finger 1 and GA Binding Protein Co-Operate with Sox2 in Regulating the Expression of Yes-Associated Protein 1 in Cancer Cells. *Stem Cells* **2017**, *35*, 2340–2350. [CrossRef] [PubMed]
76. Hromas, R.; Davis, B.; Rauscher, F.J., 3rd; Klemsz, M.; Tenen, D.; Hoffman, S.; Xu, D.; Morris, J.F. Hematopoietic transcriptional regulation by the myeloid zinc finger gene, MZF-1. *Curr. Top. Microbiol. Immunol.* **1996**, *211*, 159–164. [CrossRef]
77. Tvingsholm, S.A.; Hansen, M.B.; Clemmensen, K.K.B.; Brix, D.M.; Rafn, B.; Frankel, L.B.; Louhimo, R.; Moreira, J.; Hautaniemi, S.; Gromova, I.; et al. Let-7 microRNA controls invasion-promoting lysosomal changes via the oncogenic transcription factor myeloid zinc finger-1. *Oncogenesis* **2018**, *7*, 14. [CrossRef]

78. Nana-Sinkam, S.P.; Croce, C.M. MicroRNAs as therapeutic targets in cancer. *Transl. Res.* **2011**, *157*, 216–225. [CrossRef]
79. Yu, F.; Yao, H.; Zhu, P.; Zhang, X.; Pan, Q.; Gong, C.; Huang, Y.; Hu, X.; Su, F.; Lieberman, J.; et al. let-7 regulates self renewal and tumorigenicity of breast cancer cells. *Cell* **2007**, *131*, 1109–1123. [CrossRef]
80. Noll, L.; Peterson, F.C.; Hayes, P.L.; Volkman, B.F.; Sander, T. Heterodimer formation of the myeloid zinc finger 1 SCAN domain and association with promyelocytic leukemia nuclear bodies. *Leuk. Res.* **2008**, *32*, 1582–1592. [CrossRef]
81. Nygaard, M.; Terkelsen, T.; Vidas Olsen, A.; Sora, V.; Salamanca Viloria, J.; Rizza, F.; Bergstrand-Poulsen, S.; Di Marco, M.; Vistesen, M.; Tiberti, M.; et al. The Mutational Landscape of the Oncogenic MZF1 SCAN Domain in Cancer. *Front. Mol. Biosci.* **2016**, *3*, 78. [CrossRef] [PubMed]
82. Raman, N.; Nayak, A.; Muller, S. The SUMO system: A master organizer of nuclear protein assemblies. *Chromosoma* **2013**, *122*, 475–485. [CrossRef] [PubMed]
83. Hay, R.T. SUMO: A history of modification. *Mol. Cell* **2005**, *18*, 1–12. [CrossRef]
84. Zhong, S.; Salomoni, P.; Pandolfi, P.P. The transcriptional role of PML and the nuclear body. *Nat. Cell Biol.* **2000**, *2*, E85–E90. [CrossRef] [PubMed]
85. Bernardi, R.; Pandolfi, P.P. Structure, dynamics and functions of promyelocytic leukaemia nuclear bodies. *Nat. Rev. Mol. Cell Biol.* **2007**, *8*, 1006–1016. [CrossRef] [PubMed]
86. Lallemand-Breitenbach, V.; de The, H. PML nuclear bodies: From architecture to function. *Curr. Opin. Cell Biol.* **2018**, *52*, 154–161. [CrossRef] [PubMed]
87. Mertins, P.; Mani, D.R.; Ruggles, K.V.; Gillette, M.A.; Clauser, K.R.; Wang, P.; Wang, X.; Qiao, J.W.; Cao, S.; Petralia, F.; et al. Proteogenomics connects somatic mutations to signalling in breast cancer. *Nature* **2016**, *534*, 55–62. [CrossRef] [PubMed]
88. Melton, C.; Reuter, J.A.; Spacek, D.V.; Snyder, M. Recurrent somatic mutations in regulatory regions of human cancer genomes. *Nat. Genet.* **2015**, *47*, 710–716. [CrossRef]
89. Tian, E.; Borset, M.; Sawyer, J.R.; Brede, G.; Vatsveen, T.K.; Hov, H.; Waage, A.; Barlogie, B.; Shaughnessy, J.D., Jr.; Epstein, J.; et al. Allelic mutations in noncoding genomic sequences construct novel transcription factor binding sites that promote gene overexpression. *Genes Chromosomes Cancer* **2015**, *54*, 692–701. [CrossRef]
90. Rafn, B.; Kallunki, T. A way to invade: A story of ErbB2 and lysosomes. *Cell Cycle* **2012**, *11*, 2415–2416. [CrossRef]
91. Brix, D.M.; Rafn, B.; Bundgaard Clemmensen, K.; Andersen, S.H.; Ambartsumian, N.; Jaattela, M.; Kallunki, T. Screening and identification of small molecule inhibitors of ErbB2-induced invasion. *Mol. Oncol.* **2014**, *8*, 1703–1718. [CrossRef] [PubMed]
92. Olson, O.C.; Joyce, J.A. Cysteine cathepsin proteases: Regulators of cancer progression and therapeutic response. *Nat. Rev. Cancer* **2015**, *15*, 712–729. [CrossRef] [PubMed]
93. Bawa-Khalfe, T.; Yeh, E.T. SUMO Losing Balance: SUMO Proteases Disrupt SUMO Homeostasis to Facilitate Cancer Development and Progression. *Genes Cancer* **2010**, *1*, 748–752. [CrossRef] [PubMed]
94. Kim, K.I.; Baek, S.H. SUMOylation code in cancer development and metastasis. *Mol. Cells* **2006**, *22*, 247–253.
95. Yang, Y.; Xia, Z.; Wang, X.; Zhao, X.; Sheng, Z.; Ye, Y.; He, G.; Zhou, L.; Zhu, H.; Xu, N.; et al. Small-Molecule Inhibitors Targeting Protein SUMOylation as Novel Anticancer Compounds. *Mol. Pharmacol.* **2018**, *94*, 885–894. [CrossRef]
96. P21-Activated Kinase 4 (PAK4) Inhibitors as Potential Cancer Therapy. Available online: https://pubs.acs.org/doi/pdf/10.1021/ml500445c (accessed on 13 January 2020).
97. This Is the First Study Using Escalating Doses of PF-03758309, an Oral Compound, in Patients with Advanced Solid Tumors. Available online: https://clinicaltrials.gov/ct2/show/NCT00932126 (accessed on 13 January 2020).
98. PAK4 and NAMPT in Patients with Solid Malignancies or NHL (PANAMA) (PANAMA). Available online: https://clinicaltrials.gov/ct2/show/NCT02702492 (accessed on 13 January 2020).

6

Mutations that Confer Drug-Resistance, Oncogenicity and Intrinsic Activity on the ERK MAP Kinases—Current State of the Art

Karina Smorodinsky-Atias [1,†], Nadine Soudah [1,†] and David Engelberg [1,2,3,*]

1 Department of Biological Chemistry, The Institute of Life Science, The Hebrew University of Jerusalem, Jerusalem 91904, Israel; karinasun@gmail.com (K.S.-A.); nadine.soudah@mail.huji.ac.il (N.S.)
2 CREATE-NUS-HUJ, Molecular Mechanisms Underlying Inflammatory Diseases (MMID), National University of Singapore, 1 CREATE WAY, Innovation Wing, Singapore 138602, Singapore
3 Department of Microbiology, Yong Loo Lin School of Medicine, National University of Singapore, Singapore 117456, Singapore
* Correspondence: engelber@mail.huji.ac.il or MICDE@nus.edu.sg
† These authors contributed equally to this work.

Abstract: Unique characteristics distinguish extracellular signal-regulated kinases (Erks) from other eukaryotic protein kinases (ePKs). Unlike most ePKs, Erks do not autoactivate and they manifest no basal activity; they become catalysts only when dually phosphorylated on neighboring Thr and Tyr residues and they possess unique structural motifs. Erks function as the sole targets of the receptor tyrosine kinases (RTKs)-Ras-Raf-MEK signaling cascade, which controls numerous physiological processes and is mutated in most cancers. Erks are therefore the executers of the pathway's biology and pathology. As oncogenic mutations have not been identified in Erks themselves, combined with the tight regulation of their activity, Erks have been considered immune against mutations that would render them intrinsically active. Nevertheless, several such mutations have been generated on the basis of structure-function analysis, understanding of ePK evolution and, mostly, via genetic screens in lower eukaryotes. One of the mutations conferred oncogenic properties on Erk1. The number of interesting mutations in Erks has dramatically increased following the development of Erk-specific pharmacological inhibitors and identification of mutations that cause resistance to these compounds. Several mutations have been recently identified in cancer patients. Here we summarize the mutations identified in Erks so far, describe their properties and discuss their possible mechanism of action.

Keywords: MAPK kinase; ERK1; ERK2; CD domain; Rolled; SCH772984; VRT-11E; *sevenmaker*

---

1. Introduction

The unusual biochemical properties of the extracellular signal-regulated Kinases (Erks), their numerous biological functions and their critical roles in essentially all types of cancer, make these enzymes important subjects for research, and attractive targets for therapeutic purposes. Indeed, more than 50,000 studies have addressed aspects of the biochemistry, biology and pathology of Erks. Nevertheless, serious obstacles, which seem to be related to the unusual characteristics of the Erk enzymes, have been hindering the research. One of the hurdles has been the lack of key reagents, such as intrinsically/constitutively active mutants of Erks, and another is the absence of specific pharmacological inhibitors, not to mention clinically relevant inhibitors. The unavailability of these tools was unexpected, because useful inhibitors and a variety of active mutants were readily developed for most other protein kinases, including those that function upstream and downstream of Erk and those that are similar to Erks, such as p38s and JNKs [1–16].

This situation has been changing dramatically in the last decade. An arsenal of over a dozen useful inhibitors was finally developed, and, soon after, numerous mutations that render Erks resistant to these drugs were identified. Other mutations in ERKs were found in screens for cells in culture that acquired resistance to inhibitors of Raf and MEK. The mutations that cause drug resistance joined a small number of mutations that had been generated on the basis of gain-of-function mutations in lower organisms, or via structural studies. Finally, sequencing of genomes of tens of thousands of cancer patients led to the discovery of a few more mutations in ERKs.

Thus, a large number of interesting mutations in ERKs has been finally gathered (Table 1). The effects of many of these mutations on the structure, biochemistry, biology, or pathology of Erks have not yet been fully characterized, but some notions are emerging. This review summarizes our current knowledge of ERK mutations and describes their effect on the catalytic, physiological, pharmacological and pathological properties of Erks.

1.1. The Erk MAP Kinases

1.1.1. The Erk MAP Kinases Are Conserved in All Eukaryotes and Carry Out a Plethora of Functions

Erk proteins form a small subgroup within the family of MAP kinases. In mammals this group is encoded by two genes, ERK1 and ERK2, and by several splicing variants thereof. Erk1 and Erk2 are expressed in all cells of the organism and are critical for the functionality of all tissues and body systems. An indication of the remarkable competency of Erks is the large number of substrates they phosphorylate—497 have been identified so far [17]. For comprehensive reviews on the Erks, see [18].

Erks are highly conserved in evolution structurally and functionally, so that many discoveries with Erks' orthologs of *S. cerevisiae* (Fus3, Kss1 and Slt2/Mpk1; [19–22]) or of *D. melanogaster* (Rolled; [23,24]) are directly relevant to the mammalian molecules.

Mammalian Erk1 and Erk2 share 83% sequence identity and 88% similarity (alignment of the human proteins) and seem to be equally activated in response to relevant signals, suggesting that many of their activities are redundant. Observations that raised the possibility of distinct functions for each isoform were made primarily with knockout mice [25–34]. The most significant finding in this regard was that knocking out *ERK2* resulted in embryonic lethality, whereas knocking out *ERK1* had only mild effects [35]. Yet, overexpression of Erk1 in mice knocked-out for *ERK2*, restores viability and the mice are normal and fertile [36]. It seems, therefore, that the physiological functions of Erk1 and Erk2 are almost fully redundant and the dramatic difference in the phenotype between ERK1$^{-/-}$ and ERK2$^{-/-}$ mice stems solely from the fact that in most tissues Erk2 is expressed at much higher levels than Erk1 [36]. Also pointing to similarity in structure-function relationships are the observations that the majority (but not all) of the mutations identified recently and discussed in this review confer similar effects on the Erk1 and Erk2 proteins. Finally, the newly developed pharmacological inhibitors manifest similar (but not identical) efficacy towards the two isoforms, although it should be noted that some of those inhibitors have not yet been tested against both isoforms. These observations combined suggest minor differences in functionality between Erk1 and Erk2 native proteins.

1.1.2. Erks Are Targets of the Proto-Oncogenic RTK-Ras-Raf-MEK Pathway

Erks function as the downstream targets of the receptor tyrosine kinase (RTK)-Ras-Raf-MEK pathway, which regulates a large number of biological processes in all cell types and in all developmental stages (for reviews on the RTK-Ras-Raf-MEK pathways see [37–41]). Although in particular cell-types and under some conditions Raf and MEK may phosphorylate various substrates [17], in response to most signals Erks seem to be the only targets of this cascade and therefore mediate most, if not all, of the effects of the pathway [42]. Erks are activated by all 20 subfamilies of RTKs [43], including the clinically important epidermal growth factor receptors (EGFRs), nerve growth factor receptors (NGFRs), vascular endothelial growth factor receptors (VEGFRs), platelet-derived growth factor receptors (PDGFRs), fibroblast growth factor receptors (FGFRs) and insulin receptors (InsRs) [43].

A series of consecutive reactions leads from ligand-bound receptor to Erk activation. Briefly, upon association with its ligand, the RTK dimerizes and trans-autophosphorylates on several tyrosine residues at its cellular domain [44]. The phosphorylated tyrosines serve as scaffolds for SH2- and PTB-containing cytoplasmic enzymes [38]. One of the protein complexes that bind to a phosphotyrosine on the RTK is Grb2-Sos, which in turn activates the small GTPase Ras. Active, GTP-bound, Ras recruits Raf proteins (A-Raf; B-Raf and c-Raf/Raf1) [45], the MAP3Ks of the Erk pathway. Raf kinases phosphorylate the MAP2Ks Mek1 and Mek2. Phosphorylated Meks dually phosphorylate Erk1/2 on neighboring Thr and Tyr residues, part of a TEY motif located at the activation loop. Several additional MAP3Ks may activate Mek, depending on the context of the cell and the type of stimulus (i.e., MOS [46], TPL2/Cot [47] and MLTK [48]). With only a few exceptions, Meks are the only known activators of Erk1/2. Without MEK-mediated dual phosphorylation, Erks are catalytically inactive. Erks can also be activated by GPCRs involving different subunits of G-proteins or β-arrestin, in a ligand-independent mechanism [49–52]. Thus, a variety of ligands, which activate either RTKs or GPCRs, as well as various environmental changes, lead to Erk activation. In addition to the interaction with the direct upstream activators, Erks interact with scaffold proteins such as KSR [53] and Mek partner-1 (MP-1) [54], which facilitate the association of the various cascade components thereby increasing the efficiency of their activation [55]. Activated Erks phosphorylate their substrates on Ser or Thr residues, in all cellular compartments. Cytoplasmic substrates include protein kinases, such as Rsk1/2, Mnk1/2 and Msk1 [56–58]. Nuclear targets include transcription factors of the Fos, Myc and Ets families [59]. Erks also phosphorylate upstream pathway components, such as Raf-1, B-Raf and Mek, as part of positive and negative feedback mechanisms [60–64]. Another manner of negative feedback is the Erk-induced expression of its own deactivating phosphatases [65]. For review on Erk substrates and downstream targets see [17].

1.1.3. Erk Activation Is Achieved by Dual Phosphorylation of a TEY Motif within the Activation Loop

The difficulty in obtaining mutations that render Erks intrinsically active may stem in part from its tight regulation, supported by unique structure-function properties that distinguish them from most other eukaryotic protein kinases (ePKs). Almost all ePKs share a common kinase domain, which includes a highly conserved ATP binding site, a catalytic site and an activation loop. ePKs reside in equilibrium between active and inactive conformations, so that these catalytically-relevant sites are functional only in the active conformation. The kinase domain of all ePKs, including Erks, consists of a small N-lobe and a larger C-lobe (Figure 1A). The N-lobe contains 5 β-strands and a single helix (αC-helix), which is dynamic and occupies the space between the lobes. The αC-helix contains a conserved Glu, which, in the active conformation, forms a salt bridge with a Lys residue located within the AXK motif in β3 strand. This bridge is important and conserved in all ePKs and ensures anchoring and proper orientation of the ATP molecule. The C-lobe, which is mainly α-helical, binds and brings substrates adjacent to the ATP. A short (20–30 amino acids long) fragment located between the N- and C-lobes, known as the activation segment, contains some important elements, such as the DFG and APE motifs, the P+1 site, the catalytic and the activation loops (Figure 1A; [66]). The DFG motif is important for proper positioning of the ATP for phosphate transfer. While the Asp in the DFG is critical for recognizing the Mg^{+2} ions, the Phe forms hydrophobic interactions with the αC-helix and also with the catalytic Asp of the Y/HRD motif. The Y/HRD motif belongs to the catalytic loop responsible for catalysis. The conserved catalytic Asp of the Y/HRD motif functions by orienting the phosphate accepting hydroxyl as well as a proton-transfer acceptor. The Tyr/His residue of this motif, which is also conserved, is part of the R-spine and forms hydrophobic interactions with the DFG. An important conserved moiety is a phosphoacceptor (commonly a threonine) within the activation loop. In most ePKs, phosphorylation of this Thr is a pre-requisite for activity, as it is essential for shifting the equilibrium towards the active conformation. This phosphorylation induces several structural changes, including a conformational change of the DFG motif (to DFG 'in'), rotation of the αC-helix, which enables the formation of a Glu–Lys salt bridge, and a domain closure between the N- and C-lobes, which ultimately stabilize the regulatory and the catalytic spines of the enzyme [67,68].

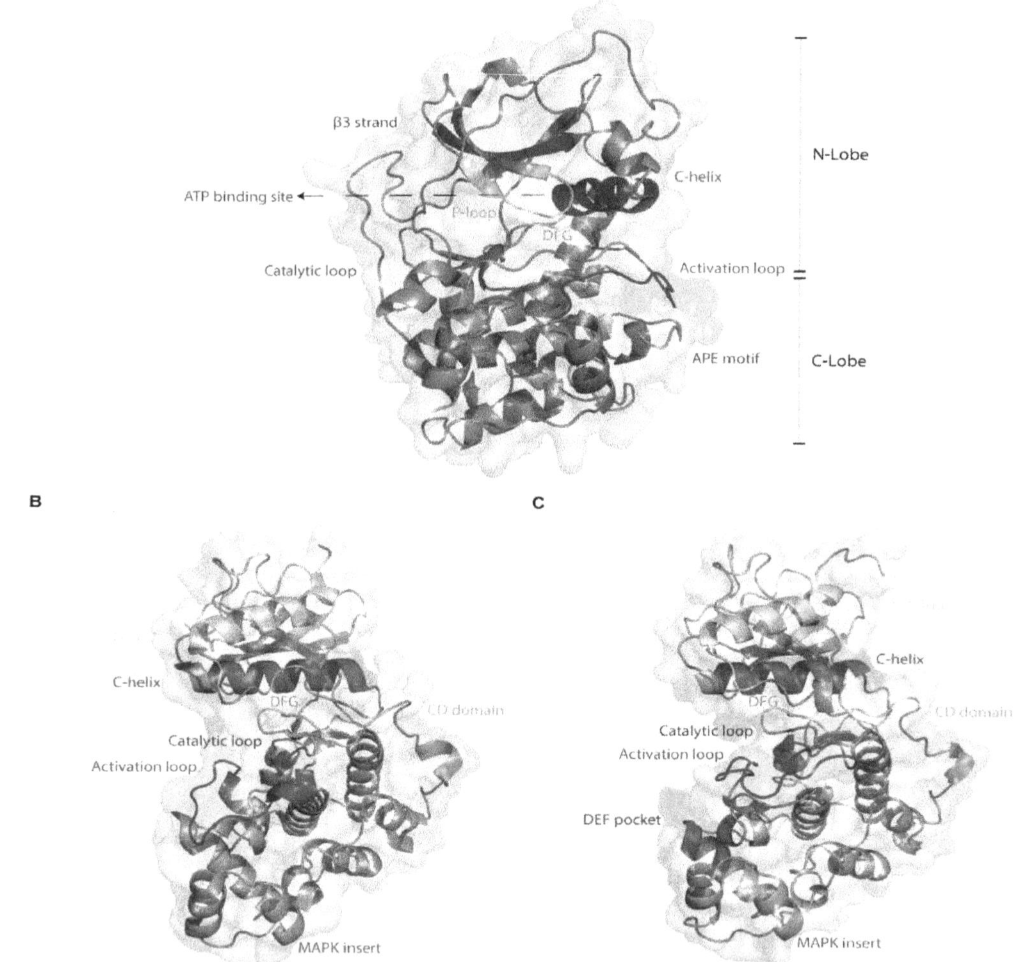

Figure 1. The kinase fold of Erks is highly similar to that of other ePKs, but they possess additional, specific domains. Shown are the crystal structures of (**A**) PKA (PDB 1FMO), (**B**) unphosphorylated Erk2 (PDB 4S31) and (**C**) dually phosphorylated Erk2 (PDB 2ERK). All panels show a cartoon representation covered with a transparent molecular surface with important regions presented and colored accordingly. Note the L16 helix and MAPK insert, not present in PKA, and the DEF pocket that forms only in phosphorylated Erk2.

As this dramatic shift from the non-active to active conformation is a result of the single phosphorylation event, the activation-loop phosphoacceptor Thr is an obvious target for regulation and for mutagenesis aimed at generating activating variants. In several ePKs, converting this Thr to Glu resulted in a constitutive activation of the kinase. However, for most ePKs, genetic manipulations are not required to achieve constant activity, because these enzymes are capable of autoactivating in a mechanism that probably involves dimerization, which enforces a 'prone-to-autophosphorylate' conformation [69–71]. The rate of this spontaneous autophosphorylation is different in each ePK, but in the majority of cases it is sufficient to give rise to a significant activity [69]. In Erks, autoactivation is extremely inefficient and almost non-measurable [72,73]. Erks are fully dependent, therefore, on MAP2Ks for activation loop phosphorylation and induction of catalysis. The lack of autophosphorylation/autoactivation capability in Erk molecules makes overexpression a non-useful experimental approach for studying their biological and pathological effects. As the overall structure of the kinase domain of Erk is very similar to that of the other eEPKs (Figure 1), the explanation for the lack of autophosphorylation and basal catalytic activity of Erks is not trivial [69]. Not only that Erks are incapable of autophosphorylation as opposed to most ePKs, several other structural features also distinguish them from common ePKs. For example, although, like most ePKs, Erks seem to reside in equilibrium between two conformations (termed L and R; [74]) these conformations differ from the classical active and inactive conformations of ePKs. For example, no conformational change in the DFG motif (from 'out' to 'in') is apparent in the structure.

The differences in the biochemical properties between MAPKs and other ePKs may be associated with structural motifs, not part of the kinase domain, which are not present in other ePKs. Two such prominent motifs are the MAPK insert and the C-terminal extension, which includes a domain termed the L16 helix (Figure 1B). However, a bioinformatics-based evolutionary study suggests that the inability to autophosphorylate and the dependence on MEK may stem from minor structural differences, and not necessarily involving the MAPK insert, or the C-terminal extension [75]. This study reconstituted an inferred common ancestor of Erk1, Erk2 and Erk5 that is able to autophosphorylate and an ancestor of Erk1 and Erk2 that cannot. Analysis of the two ancestors suggested that a single amino acid deletion in the linker loop connecting the αC-helix and the β3 strand (position 74 in modern Erk1) and a mutation in the gatekeeper residue (Gln122 in modern Erk1) account for the loss of autophosphorylation and dependence of modern Erk on its upstream activator. Indeed, inserting these two modifications into modern Erk1 was sufficient to generate Erk1 molecules that, when tested in kinase assays in vitro, showed high autophosphorylation ability and consequently catalytic capabilities similar to those of Mek-phosphorylated Erk1 [75]. This study clearly points at residues and domains that could be manipulated in an effort to generate intrinsically active, Mek-independent, Erks. These same residues were identified, in fact, as candidates for mutagenesis by other approaches as well [76].

Other unique Erk domains are the substrate binding motifs. Erks possess two distinct sites through which substrates, activators and deactivators can bind. The first is the common docking (CD) site, which is located about 10Å from the active site of Erk2 (Figure 1B) and is composed of amino acids such as Asp316 and Asp319. The second docking site of Erk2 is the hydrophobic DEF pocket, which is composed of residues Met197, Leu198, Tyr231, Leu232, Leu235 and Tyr261, and exists only in dually phosphorylated Erk adjacent to the catalytic site (Figure 1C). Important mutations, discussed here, occurred in these two domains [73,77,78].

1.1.4. ERK Molecules Are Highly Active in Most Cancers, but Oncogenic Mutations in ERK Themselves Are Very Rare

All upstream components of the Erk signaling cascade are frequently mutated in cancer [79], and it is believed, therefore, that Erks are abnormally overactive in essentially all cancer cases [80]. Accordingly, the Ras-Raf-MEK-Erk cascade has become a major target for anti-cancer therapy [81]. Oncogenic mutations or other genetic alterations (e.g., gene amplification) have been found in RTKs, Ras, Raf and MEKs, but no activating mutations or genetic alterations in Erk molecules themselves have been reported as oncogenic in tumor viruses or in patients. However, as the only known substrates of Rafs are the MEKs, and the only known substrates of MEKs are the Erks, it implies that the biological and pathological/oncogenic effects of the pathway are mediated exclusively via the Erk proteins (note some reports on deviations from the linearity of the RTK-Ras-Raf-MEK-Erk tier: [41,49–51], reviewed in [17]). It is not clear, therefore, why mutations in Erks are rarely found in cancer patients. This situation could be taken as another indication for the unusual tight regulation bestowed on Erks by the specific structural motifs, immunizing them against mutations that render them spontaneously active and oncogenic. Indeed, although some mutations that render Erks intrinsically active and even oncogenic (one mutation) have been discovered in the laboratory, they do not activate Erk to the maximal levels possible (that of Mek-activated Erk), and their oncogenic effect is markedly weaker than that of active, oncogenic, Ras or Raf [82,83].

Nevertheless, mutations in ERKs have been identified in a small number of patients (Table 1) and at least one of those, E320K in ERK2, seems to appear in a few dozen patients suffering from cervical and head and neck carcinoma (Table 1B). Perhaps activating mutations in ERKs are not fully oncogenic and do not have a causative effect, but may promote the disease.

1.1.5. Erk Inhibitors Have Been Recently Developed

Not only that Erks are obvious targets for anti-cancer therapy because they are the downstream components of the RTK-Ras-Raf-MEK pathway, in the majority of cases of tumors resistant to EGFR, B-Raf and MEK inhibitors, re-activation of Erk is observed [84]. These findings reinforce the need for direct Erk inhibitors. Specific inhibition of Erks should also be a powerful tool for research. For unknown reasons, developing pharmacological Erk inhibitors has lagged behind the development of inhibitors against the other MAP kinases, JNK and p38 and has required unusual efforts. Morris et al., for example, screened approximately five million compounds and performed multiple improvement steps in order to discover SCH772984, a small molecule that inhibits both Erk isoforms with an IC_{50} at the nano-molar range [85]. Further development of this inhibitor provided an orally administered analog, MK-8353 [86], which is being tested in phase-I clinical trials. Yet another potent Erk inhibitor is BVD-523 (Ulixertinib), a selective and reversible Erk1 and Erk2 ATP competitive molecule [87], which is currently in phase II clinical trials. GDC-0994 (Ravoxertinib) [88], a pyrazolylpyrrole-based inhibitor that was optimized specifically towards Erk by using structure-guided methods [89], is also undergoing clinical testing. Additional compounds that exhibit selectivity towards Erk are LY3214996 [90], FR180204 [91], VRT-11E [92] and the Erk dimerization inhibitor DEL22379 [93]. For a comprehensive description of Erk inhibitors, see [94].

In parallel to the biochemical and pharmacological characterization of the inhibitors, a large number of mutations that render Erk proteins resistant to them have been reported [95–97] (Table 1).

2. Identification of Various Mutations in ERKs and Study of Their Properties

2.1. Almost All Known Mutations in ERKs Have Been Identified Experimentally

Unlike the many mutations known in RTKs, Ras, Raf and MEK, mostly identified in tumors, almost all mutations known in ERKs have been identified in laboratory setups. Only a few have been identified in cancer patients, and even for those, it is not clear whether they are associated with the disease. Experimental systems were initially designed for identification of intrinsically active Erks. Later, following the development of Erk inhibitors, genetic screens were developed for identification of mutations that would cause drug resistance. The mutations identified in patients, in screens for drug-resistant molecules and for intrinsically active Erks are summarized in Table 1. It should be noted that numeration of the mutations in ERK1 (in text and in Table 1A) refer to the sequence of the human protein and numeration of mutations in ERK2 (in text and in Table 1B) refer to the sequence of rat protein. Notably, mutations that had been discovered (until 2006) in ERK orthologs in lower organisms were summarized in [98] and will not be discussed here.

2.2. Mutations Produced on the Basis of Structure-Function Studies

Original attempts to develop intrinsically active Erk molecules took the conventional approach of trying to mimic the activatory phosphorylation of the activation loop. As no phosphomimetic residue is available for tyrosine, this approach was limited to modifying the Thr of the TEY motif and turned out to be ineffective [99,100]. In fact, not only was changing this Thr to Glu unsuccessful, but the resulting $Erk2^{T183E}$ enzyme showed lower activity than $Erk2^{WT}$, even when phosphorylated by MEK [98,101,102]. Furthermore, even when mutations that render Erk2 intrinsically active were discovered, combining them with the T183E mutation did not create a more active molecule [103].

Other mutations devised on the basis of structure-function understanding, however, did lead to the development of interesting mutants. For example, mutating the gatekeeper residue of Erk2 resulted in an intrinsically active variant (Q103G and Q103A) [76]. Furthermore, mutating residues that interact with Gln103 provided even more active variants (when tested as purified recombinant proteins), primarily Erk2^{I82A} and Erk2^{I84A} [76]. As described above, the gatekeeper residue was also discovered as a site that distinguishes between an inferred ancestor kinase, which is capable of autophosphorylation, and the modern Erk1 and Erk2. Mutating the gatekeeper residue in Erk1 on the basis of comparison to the inferred ancestor (inserting the Q122M mutation) rendered the mutant intrinsically active [75].

The mechanism that renders all these mutants intrinsically active was shown to be the acquisition of an autophosphorylation capability. Namely, the mutations did not impose adoption of the native conformation, but rather unleashed an obstructed autophosphorylation capability and allowed autoactivation. These observations suggest that Erks are similar to most other ePKs that possess the autophosphorylation machinery, but this activity in Erks is not spontaneous. Structural blockers of autophosphorylation in Erks are not known implying that activating mutations could reveal them. An interesting mechanism of action for how substitutions at Gln103 or Ile84 unblock autophosphorylation was suggested by Emrick et al. It was proposed that the mutations induce a pathway of intramolecular interactions leading to flexibility in the activation lip, thereby enabling the phosphoacceptors to reach the catalytic Asp (D147 in Erk2). In the inactive form of Erk2, the intramolecular pathway includes hydrophobic interaction between Leu73, Gln103 or Ile84 and phe166 of the DFG motif, which in turn is linked to L168 through the backbone. The latter forms side-chain interactions with Val186 from the activation lip. Emrick et al. further suggested that T188 forms hydrogen bond with Asp147 and Lys149. These interactions together impede autoactivation by holding the activation lip in a stable conformation. It is therefore not surprising that mutating Leu73, Gln103 or Ile84 would lead to the movement of Phe166 and thus affect the hydrophobic interaction between Leu168 and Val186 and the hydrogen bond between Thr188 and Asp147/Lys149. This would cause an increase in flexibility of the activation loop and eventually autophosphorylation.

Although, when tested in vitro as recombinant proteins, these mutations render the Erk molecules intrinsically active, the significance of the mutants in the gatekeeper and nearby residues in living cells is not clear. While Erk2^{I84A} seems to be spontaneously active when expressed in HEK293 cells, it is not spontaneously active in NIH3T3 cells. The equivalent Erk1 mutant, Erk1^{I103A} is not spontaneously active in either cell line [82]. None of the mutants can oncogenically transform NIH3T3 cells [82], but, intriguingly, several mutations in the gatekeeper of Erk2 (Q103) were identified in screens for drug-resistant Erk2 molecules (Table 1B) and a mutation in I82 (I82T) was found in one cancer patient (Table 1B). Perhaps conversion of these residues to particular amino acids (e.g., Thr), other than those tested so far (i.e., Ala) would render them more active in cells and possibly even oncogenic.

Another mutation that was generated in Erk2 on the basis of structural studies is S151D. This mutation was designed following an alignment of the conserved sequence DLKPSN in MKK1 with the sequence DLKPEN in cAMP-dependent protein kinase. This mutant resulted in a 15-fold enhancement of MKK1 activity [99] and was therefore attempted in Erk2 [103]. Erk2^{S151D} manifested MEK-independent activity that was about 15-fold higher than that of Erk2^{WT}, but was just 1.5% of that of MEK-phosphorylated Erk2^{WT} [73,103].

2.3. Only a Few of the Mutations Identified via Genetic Screens in ERK Orthologs of Evolutionarily Low Organisms Are Relevant to Mammalian Erks

High throughput screens in *S. cerevisiae* and *D. melanogaster*, provided a variety of gain-of-function mutants of Erk orthologs in these organisms [73,77,104,105] (Reviewed in [98]). These mutations allowed important insights into the modes of regulation of the given Erk ortholog in each case and to interesting cross talks between yeast MAPK pathways. The relevance of most of those to mammalian Erks is, however, unclear, because some of the mutations occurred in residues that are not conserved in the mammalian enzymes, and of the conserved residues only a handful were tested [73,103,106]. Overall, very few of the mutations turned out to be relevant to mammalian Erks, but these are of significant importance.

For example, insertion of the L73P mutation to Erk2 (equivalent to the L63P mutation in Fus3 [107]) rendered Erk2 intrinsically active, as tested by an in vitro kinase assay with purified recombinant proteins, but to an activity level of approximately 1% of the activity displayed by Mek-activated Erk2 [103]. Combining L73P with other mutations, such as S151D and D319N, created a more active enzyme [103]. It required a combination of three mutations, L73P+S151D+D319N to create an Erk2 protein with a MEK-independent activity that was 100-fold higher than that of wild type Erk2 in vitro. Notably however, this activity is just about 6% of the MEK-phosphorylated Erk2 activity [103]. Thus, these mutants are *bona fide* intrinsically active, but their activity is not very high. Interestingly Leu73 is part of the hydrophobic cluster affected by the "gatekeeper mutations". It seems that mutations in Ser151 also interfere with the contacts of the catalytic base Asp147 with Thr188, resulting in increased activation lip flexibility and activation of the phosphoacceptors Tyr185 and Thr183.

The only Erk mutant that has been shown so far to oncogenically transform cells in cultures, Erk1^{R84S}, was generated on the basis of a mutation in the yeast ortholog Mpk1/Slt2. The mutation in Mpk1/Slt2, R68S, was identified in a screen that looked for Mpk1 mutants that rescue the phenotype of cells lacking the relevant MEKs [73]. Six Mpk1 mutants were isolated, but only the R68S mutation was found relevant to Erks of higher eukaryotes, including of *Drosophila* and mammals [73]. *Drosophila* and mammalian Erks carrying the equivalent mutation (R80S in *Drosophila's* ERK/Rolled; R84S in mammalian Erk1; R65S in mammalian Erk2) displayed high spontaneous intrinsic catalytic activity (>30% of the activity of Mek-activated Erk), independent of Mek activation in in vitro assays [73,82], in cell cultures [82] and in vivo, in transgenic mice and flies [83,108]. Furthermore, Erk1^{R84S} and Rolled^{R80S} were shown to function as oncogenes, capable of transforming NIH3T3 cells and to give rise to tumors in the fly, respectively [82,83]. Erk1^{R84S} was also shown to cause mild cardiac hypertrophy, when expressed as a transgene in the heart of mice [108]. The basic mechanism of action of the R80S/R84S/R65S mutation is similar to that of the other intrinsically active variants described above, namely, it bestowed upon the Rolled and Erk proteins an efficient autophosphorylation capability [73,82,83]. The structural basis for this capability is not clear, in part due to the extreme flexibility of Arg65 within the Erk2 structure. In many Erk2 structures it accommodates a different conformation (Figure 2).

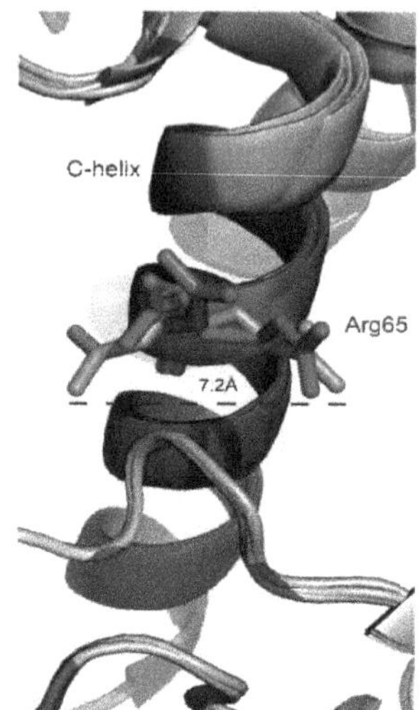

Figure 2. Unusual flexibility of the Arg65 residue at the αC-helix of different Erk2 crystal structures. 5 different crystal structures of Erk2 (PDB 1ERK, 4ERK, 4S31, 4GT3 and 5UMO) were superimposed and a zoom in into the αC-helix (colored in red) is presented. Arg65 is shown in sticks and the distance between the two extreme orientations is calculated.

Arg65 is located at a pivotal position in the αC-helix, the conserved helix within the N lobe, and interacts with the L16 domain, which is flexible and unstructured in the inactive form. Interestingly, in spite of the different conformation adopted by Arg65 in the various crystal structures of Erk2 (Figure 2), in many of them Arg65 is in association with amino acids of the conserved DFG motif

(D165, F166, G167). In the structure of Erk2^{WT}, PDB 1ERK, or 5UMO, Arg65 seems to have two possible conformations so that it forms a hydrogen bond with either the side chain of Asp165 or the backbone of Gly167. In the structure of Erk2^{R65S} (determined at a high resolution of 1.48Å (PDB 4SZ2)) the substituted serine is smaller than arginine and is not in association with the DFG motif. Instead, a new hydrogen bond is formed between Ser65 and Tyr34 of the P-loop (see Figure 8 in reference [82]). In addition, Ser65 stabilizes Thr183 from the activation loop and it is hypothesized that the Asp165 of the DFG motif can interact with ATP. It is noteworthy that in the crystal structure of dually phosphorylated Erk2 (PDB 2ERK), Thr183 interacts with the αC-helix, particularly with Arg65 via a water molecule [109].

Interestingly, similar to the case of Erk2^{R65S}, in the crystal structure of the intrinsically active Erk2^{I84A} (PDB code 4S30), a mutant that also autophosphorylates efficiently, the interaction of Arg65 with the DFG is also abolished, although the mutated residue is located in a distance from the αC-helix. As discussed above, the I84A mutation affects a hydrophobic cluster, involving, amongst other residues, Leu73 of the αC-helix, which may in turn divert Arg65. Also, in the Erk2^{I84A} structure in complex with AMP-PNP (PDB 4S34), a shift of Tyr34, causes it to form a hydrogen bond with Thr66 in addition to the Pi-Pi interactions with Tyr62 of the αC-helix observed in Erk2^{WT}. Tyr34 in Erk2 plays a pivotal role in catalysis and the DFG, especially Asp165, is involved in ATP binding by interacting with the gamma phosphate of ATP. Erk2 bearing mutations in Tyr34 (Y34H/N, in ERK1: Y53H) or Tyr62 (Y62N, in ERK1: Y81C) were shown to acquire resistance to the Erk inhibitors SCH77984 and VRT-11E in both ERK1 and ERK2 in two different screens (see below [95,96]). Finally, the association between Arg65 of Erk2 and the DFG is also abolished in other intrinsically active mutants, including mutations found in the CD site (PDB 6OT6) [110].

It is thus conceivable that the association of Arg65 with the DFG motif is crucial for blocking autophosphorylation activity by acting as a barrier between the ATP binding pocket, DFG motif and the activation loop. Tyr34 and Tyr62 of the P loop, which slightly change their conformation in several active mutants, may also play some role in suppressing spontaneous activity. Notably, mutations in Arg84 of Erk1, equivalent to Arg65 in Erk2, were identified in two cancer patients (Table 1A).

Intriguingly, another gain-of-function mutation, Y268C [73], was identified in the same genetic screen in yeast that provided the R68S mutation in Mpk1/Slt2. It was later shown that Y268A is also a gain-of-function mutation in Mpk1 [78]. Tyr268 is located at the heart of the DEF pocket, and in mammalian Erk2 a mutation in the equivalent Tyr, Y261A, is a partial loss-of-function mutation because Erk2^{Y261A} cannot bind and phosphorylate some of its substrates and cannot execute some of its biological functions [29,111,112]. As the mechanism through which Mpk1$^{Y268A/C}$ function as gain-of-function mutants is unknown, it is also unexplained why the equivalent mutations in Erk2 cause a loss of function [78].

Similar to the mammalian Erks, Rolled, the Erk ortholog in *Drosophila melanogaster*, is involved in numerous processes in the fly, including the development of the eye [23,24]. A screen aimed at isolation of mutants that facilitate proper eye development even in the absence of the ligand that activates the Erk pathway in the eye, identified a mutant fly that was termed *sevenmaker*. The mutation it carried was found to be D334N in the *Drosophila's* ERK/Rolled [77]. An equivalent mutation was isolated in another screen in yeast designed for identifying Fus3 molecules that are not inhibited by Hog1 [107], in a large-scale screen performed in mammalian cells for gain-of-function and inhibitor-resistant Erk2 mutants (D319 in Erk2) [95], and in cancer patients. As the *sevenmaker* mutation occurs at the CD site, its proposed mechanism of action is an elevated resistance to MAPK phosphatases resulting in increased sensitivity to low levels of MEK's activity [106]. This notion was based on the observation that the Erk2^{D319N} protein was less susceptible to inactivation by the MAPK phosphatase CL100 than the Erk2^{WT} recombinant protein, while both undergo inactivation in a dose-dependent manner [106]. Inserting this mutation into mammalian Erk2 showed minimal effect on catalytic activity in in vitro experiments and in cell culture [73,103,106]. It is not clear how the *sevenmaker* mutation affects Erk's association with phosphatases, but not with activators and substrates that also utilize the CD site.

Misiura et al. have shown, quantitatively, that the *sevenmaker* mutation increases the catalytic activity of Erk by changing the interaction energies. It specifically modifies the enzyme's susceptibility to deactivation by phosphatases, while not affecting the activation process by the MAPK kinase [113]. Nonetheless, the *sevenmaker* mutation may also affect catalysis *per se*. Indeed, recombinant Erk2^{D319N} does not manifest unusual catalytic properties, but when combining the D319N mutation with an activating mutation there is a dramatic elevation of catalysis [73,83,103]. Since Erk phosphatases do not exist in in vitro assays, the effect of the *sevenmaker* mutation should be explained by other mechanisms. Probably, in addition to reducing the affinity to phosphatases, the *sevenmaker* mutation also confers a conformational change that further stabilizes the "prone-to-autophosphorylate" conformation [69] induced by another mutation on the same protein. Supporting the role of the *sevenmaker* residue not only in substrate binding, but also in activation of catalysis, Molecular Dynamic simulations suggest that stabilization of the active conformation of Erk2, following phosphorylation of Thr183, is associated with disruption of several hydrogen bonding involving Asp334 [114]. Furthermore, in the structure of Erk2^{D319N} the interaction of Arg65 with the DFG is lost, a property of several of the autophosphorylating Erk mutants. Aside from this disruption, the crystal structure of Erk2^{D319N} is, essentially, indistinguishable from that of Erk2^{WT} [110].

The *sevenmaker* site seems to be a hot spot for mutations as it is being re-discovered in different screens. Mutations in Asp319 of Erk2 (D319N, D319V) or mutations in the neighboring residue (E320K and E320V), as well as in Glu79, which associates with D319, (E79K), were identified in a comprehensive screen that searched for gain-of-function and drug-resistant mutations, using A375 cells (see below; [95]). The *sevenmaker* mutation, itself, D319N, was also reported in four cases of carcinoma (COSMIC ID: D319N in ERK2—COSM98175) and three other patients carried another substitution in the 319 position (Table 1B). Interestingly, the ERK1 *sevenmaker* site was not found to be mutated in any screen, or in cancer patients.

2.4. Mutations in ERKs Are Very Rare in Cancer Patients, but Some Are Similar to Those Identified in Laboratory Models

Although several dozens of mutations in ERK1 and ERK2 have been identified in cancer patients (Table 1) the rate of mutations in ERK in patients is very low and most of the mutations appeared in only one of the samples tested. Mutations in ERK2 were observed in 179 out of 60,712 unique samples, approximately 0.3%. The COSMIC database lists 148 reported ERK1 mutations, out of 47,784 tumor samples tested (also approximately 0.3%). It is not clear whether these mutations have any causative effect on the malady. An exception is the E320K mutation, which was observed in 27 patients of squamous cell carcinoma (COSMIC ID: E320K in ERK2—COSM461148). Mutations in Glu320 were also identified in a screen for drug resistant Erk molecules. Notably Glu320 is neighboring Asp319 (the location of the *sevenmaker* mutation) within the CD site. Just like the *sevenmaker* mutation, the E320K does not affect the enzyme's intrinsic catalytic properties as tested in vitro with recombinant Erk2^{E320K}, and in transient transfections of HEK293 and NIH3T3 cells ([110]; Smorodinsky-Atias and Engelberg, unpublished observation). It may function, therefore, similar to the mutations in Asp319 by reducing the protein association with phosphatases (also supported by Brenan et al. [95]). Yet, unlike D319N, the E320K mutation enforces significant structural changes on the crystal structure of Erk2 and on its biophysical properties. Also, when equivalent mutations were inserted to the *Drosophila ERK/Rolled* they conferred different properties on the protein, suggesting that D319N and E320K function via different mechanisms [110,115]. More mutations of note identified in patients occurred in Glu79 (COSMIC ID: in ERK2—COSM444794), Ser140 (COSMIC ID: in ERK2—COSM3552430) and Pro56 (COSMIC ID: in ERK2—COSM4471756) residues. These substitutions were subsequently discovered as gain-of-function mutations in the screen that tested all possible missense mutations of ERK2 [95] (see below).

Nearly all of the ERK1 mutations recorded in patients, appeared only once. Only 18 mutations occurred in two or three independent samples. Notably, two patients carried the R84H mutation in

ERK1. As discussed above, another mutation at the same location, R84S, was shown to render Erk1 capable to oncogenically transform cells in culture [82]. This finding calls for testing the oncogenic potential of Erk1^{R84H} and perhaps of more Erk1 molecules in which Arg84 was substituted.

2.5. A Large Number of Mutations Can Render Erks Resistant to Pharmacological Inhibitors

The development of specific inhibitors towards Erks was the impetus for a series of studies that searched for mutations that cause drug resistance. Goetz et al., constructed a library of randomly mutagenized ERK1 and ERK2 cDNAs and induced its expression in A375 melanoma cells (harboring the BRAF^{V660E} oncogene) in the presence of either the Erk inhibitor VRT-11E, the MEK inhibitor trametinib, or with a combination of trametinib and the Raf inhibitor dabrafenib [96]. Overall, sequencing the ERK1 or ERK2 molecules in cell populations that survived the treatment identified 33 mutations in ERK1 (in 28 amino acids) and 24 in ERK2 (in 20 amino acids). In a separate screen for A375 colonies resistant to VRT-11E, another five mutations in ERK2 were discovered. All mutations are presented in Table 1. Only five of the mutations that caused resistance to VRT-11E were identified in both isoforms. These were (in ERK1/ERK2 order) Y53H/Y34H/N, G54A/G35S, P75L/P56L, Y81C/Y62N and C82Y/C63Y. A mutation at only one of the residues that caused resistance to the MEK inhibitor was also common in the two isoforms, Y148H/Y129N/H/F/C/S. Importantly, some of the residues that were found mutated in this screen were also reported to be mutated in patients, including Arg84 and Gly186 in Erk1 and Asp319 and Glu320 in Erk2. Another important finding of this study, with significant implications to therapeutic strategies, is that Erk variants that are resistant to RAF/MEK inhibitors are sensitive to Erk inhibition and vice versa [96].

As the mutations were not tested on purified Erk proteins it is not known how they affect the intrinsic biochemical and structural properties of the enzymes leaving the detailed mechanism of the acquired drug resistance open for future studies. It is possible however that mutations identified in the Erk-inhibitor screen interfere with drug binding as they cluster in proximity to the ATP/drug binding pocket. These mutations are located in the glycine-rich loop and the loop between β3 and αC-helix (in ERK1: I48N, Y53H, G54A, S74G, P75L. In ERK2: Y34H, G71S, P56L). Mutations residing in the αC-helix itself (ERK1: Y81C, C82Y, ERK2: Y62N, C63Y) may function similarly. ERK1 mutants that were identified in the Raf/MEK inhibitors screen probably function via a different mechanism. They are distributed along the molecule, but seem to cluster in domains important for catalysis and may render the kinase catalytically active. A206V/A187V and S219P/S200P (of ERK1/ERK2), for example, reside in the activation lip, R84H, C82Y and Q90R of Erk1 map to the αC-helix and Y148H of Erk1 and Y129F, D319G and E320K of Erk2 are located in the CD site. Mutations in the *sevenmaker* residue were already discussed above and probably function by reducing affinity to phosphatases in combination with some effect on catalysis. Another mutation, R84H in Erk1, occurred at the same residue in which the only oncogenic mutation identified so far in Erks, R84S, also occurred [82]. As Erk1^{R84S} was shown to be intrinsically catalytically active and spontaneously active when expressed in culture cells and in transgenic mice [82,108], it could be that Erk1^{R84H} also acquired similar properties and is independent of upstream activation, making it resistant to Raf and MEK inhibitors. Indeed, kinase assays using the various mutants, expressed in and immunoprecipitated from A375 cells, showed that the mutants maintained activity in the presence of either VRT-11E or SCH772984, another Erk inhibitor [96]. On the basis of the immunoprecipitation kinase assay it could be suggested that the mutants arising from the screen in the presence of RAF/MEK inhibitors acquired the capability to maintain sufficient kinase activity, even under these conditions, thereby rescuing the transformed cells from the inhibitors. As some of these mutations are found in patients, this conclusion is therapeutically relevant and may suggest that RAF and MEK inhibitors should be contraindicated for patients that harbor these mutants in the tumor.

Intriguingly, the mechanisms of action of the various mutants in vivo may be different for Erk1 and Erk2 as some of the mutations seem to be isoform-specific. Mutations in αC-helix were found only in ERK1 (C82Y, R84H and Q90R), while mutations in the CD site, such as D319G and E320K were only found in Erk2. Although the differences in the occurrence of the mutations could be a result of an unsaturated screen, the notion that the mutations are isoform-specific is supported by the situations observed in patients. The E320K mutation of Erk2 was found in 27 cancer patients while the equivalent mutation in Erk1 was not reported. Similarly, the *sevenmaker* site of Erk2, D319, which was mutated in seven patients, was not found so far to be mutated in ERK1 in patients. In line with these observations Goetz et al. inserted the equivalents of the D319G and E320K mutations into ERK1, and observed that the resulting proteins, $Erk1^{D338N}$ and $Erk1^{E339K}$ were not resistant to inhibitors, at least in the cell assay [96]. It is reasonable to conclude that different mutations may render Erk1 and Erk2 resistant to drugs. Given that the biological functions of the two isoforms is almost fully redundant [36] and that the inhibitors affect both isoforms similarly *in vitro*, it is currently difficult to explain the dichotomy in the mutations that cause resistance of each isoform.

A mutation that renders Erks resistant to SCH772984 was identified when cells of the colorectal cancer cell line HCT-116 (harboring a mutated KRAS) were serially passaged in the presence of increasing concentration of the inhibitor for 4 months [97]. Sequencing the ERK1/2 genes isolated from resistant clones, revealed a reoccurring point mutation, G186D, in ERK1 [97]. Gly186 resides in the DFG motif of the activation segment. The mutant displayed a several-fold reduction in binding affinity to the inhibitor, compared to the wild-type protein. Crystal structure of SCH772984-associated Erk2 suggests that this reduction is a direct result of a steric clash imposed by the aspartic acid in the active site, which destabilized the binding of the inhibitor. The same $Erk1^{G186D}$ mutant did not provide resistance to another ATP-competitive Erk inhibitor (VRT-11E), an observation that is explained by the structural difference between the two inhibitors, significantly altering the interactions with the binding pocket, predominantly the distance of the molecule from the new aspartic acid [97]. Notably, the orthologous residue in Erk2, Gly167 was found mutated to Asp in a screen for Erk2 mutants that are resistant to SCH772984 and VRT-11E in A375 cells. In this screen Gly167 was mutated to many other residues, but only the $Erk2^{G167D}$ was selected as rendering the kinase drug-resistance [95]. The interference of Asp at position 169 for drug binding seems very particular.

$Erk2^{G167D}$ was in fact isolated in a large-scale screen that led to the discovery of many more mutants. In this effort, Brenan et al. employed saturation mutagenesis and were able to screen a library of 6810 variants of ERK2, out of 6821 possible, each carrying a point mutation. They searched for gain-of-function, loss-of-function, as well as for drug-resistant mutants. The ERK2 mutants library was introduced into A375 cells and inducibly expressed, under the premise that cells expressing gain-of-function mutants will proliferate slower, while cells expressing loss-of-function mutants will proliferate faster, than cells expressing $Erk2^{WT}$ [95]. The relative abundance of Erk2 molecules that were expressed in the cells after 96 h was determined by parallel sequencing.

Indeed, mutants considered to be carrying GOF mutations on the basis of previous screens or appearance in tumors, such as Glu320 and Asp319, were depleted from the proliferative culture. Mutations in an additional 19 residues caused the Erk2 molecules to be depleted to a degree equivalent to or greater than that of $Erk2^{Glu320}$ and $Erk2^{Asp319}$. The 19 residues were Glu79, Gly83, Gly8, Leu333, Pro56, Val47, Ser358, Val16, Pro354, Arg13, Glu320, Glu58, Ala3, Ala350, Ala7, Ser140, Thr24, Gln15, Asp319, Gly20 and Phe346 (from the most depleted to the least). Many of the mutants considered to have acquired gain-of-function mutations were shown to be catalytically active when immunoprecipitated from cells treated with the RAF inhibitor trametinib. As the mutants were not tested as recombinant purified proteins it is not clear whether they possess any unusual catalytic properties, and, specifically, if they are intrinsically active.

The mutants library was also inducibly expressed in A375 cells exposed to sublethal doses of VRT-11E, or SCH772984 in order to discover Erk2 mutants that are resistant to these inhibitors. The relative enrichment of the Erk2 mutants was quantified after 12 days of exposure to inhibitors. The rationale in this experiment was that cells harboring an Erk2 mutant insensitive to an inhibitor would allow proliferation in its presence. Mutations in 12 residues rendered Erk2 resistant to VRT-11E (Arg13, Ile29, Gly30, Ala33, Met36, Val37, Arg65, Gln95, Met96, Asp98, Thr108, Leu154), mutations in

9 residues confer resistance to SCH772984 (Glu31, Tyr41, Val47, Lys53, Glu68, Leu67, Ile101, Asp122, Asp125) and mutations in 18 residues render Erk2 resistant to both inhibitors (Tyr34, Gly35, Cys38, Asp42, Val49, Ile54, Ser55, Pro56, Phe57, Gln60, Tyr62, Cys63, Thr66, Glu69, Leu73, Gln103, Gly167, Ile345). Curiously, half of the mutations that cause resistant to VRT-11E occurred in residues that make direct contacts with the inhibitor, but none of the mutants that confer specific resistance to SCH772984 are mutated in residues that contact the inhibitor. Projection of the mutations identified in this study into cancer associated mutations showed that within the top 20 residues harboring GOF mutations, five were reported to be mutated in patients (E320K/V, D319N/V, E79K, P56L and S140L). Erk2 mutants carrying any of these GOF mutations were found to rescue A375 cells from the anti-proliferative effect of Raf/MEK inhibitors, but only one, $Erk2^{P56L/G}$ was able to rescue the cells from SCH772984. All GOF mutations clustered within the CD site, whereas LOF mutations altered the DEF pocket. The LOF mutations in the DEF pocket seem dominant since when combined, on a single Erk2 molecule, with a GOF mutation in the CD site the resulting protein was not able to rescue cells and promote the downstream signaling. It seems that the mechanism of action of the GOF mutants residing in the CD site is similar to that of the *sevenmaker* mutation. This hypothesis was validated by co-expressing Erk2 mutants with $BRAF^{V600E}$ and dual specificity phosphatase (DUSP) in 293T cells and monitoring Erk2 phosphorylation. Erk2 molecules mutated at the CD site (E320K/V; D319N/V E79K) exhibited sustained phosphorylation levels relative to $Erk2^{WT}$ [95]. It is worth noting that the GOF mutant P56L showed a reduced level of phosphorylation, suggesting that constant phosphorylation in the presence of DUSP is not a general property of all GOF mutations. Most mutants identified in this comprehensive study await further biochemical, structural and pharmacological analysis.

3. Discussion

Table 1 lists an impressive number of mutations in Erk1 and Erk2, many of them discovered in screens for drug-resistant mutants. The mutations that confer drug resistance outscore the very few mutations that render Erks intrinsically active and the single mutant that was shown so far to possess oncogenic properties. The mutations causing drug-resistant occur throughout the protein so that various mechanisms are involved. It is not clear whether the list in Table 1 reflects all relevant mutations possible in Erks. Indeed, most of the screens that provided the currently known mutations were high throughput, but they were performed in a particular context of a given cell line, or against specific pharmacological inhibitors. Also, it is not clear if these screens themselves were saturated. It is a plausible assumption therefore that further screening, particularly in novel experimental setups, would result in yet unidentified mutations. Also, once Erk inhibitors reach the clinic, patients may develop resistance by acquiring mutations other than those discovered in the laboratory. As the research of Erk mutations is relatively young many properties of the known mutation are still elusive. For most of the mutations that cause resistant to inhibitors the mechanism of action is not known and for many of them even the effects on Erks' conformation and catalytic properties are yet to be revealed. Finally, it may take a long time to reveal the role (if any) of the rare mutations identified in cancer patients, in disease etiology. Most mutations that were identified in a single patient, may be bystanders with no role in the disease, while others may contribute to disease development or even disease onset. Prime suspects for a causative role are the R84H mutation in Erk1, because an equivalent mutation, R84S, was shown to be oncogenic in cells in culture, and E320K in Erk2 that is found in patients in a higher rate than all other mutations.

3.1. Mutations Identified in Erks Could Not Have Been Predicted by Structural or Mechanistic Analysis

It is not currently possible to predict the location and type of more Erk mutations. Although Erk proteins have been the subject of comprehensive structural studies, including via X-ray crystallography, NMR and HX-MS approaches, and although critical features of their structure-function properties have been revealed, it is not clear how to translate this knowledge into predicting specific mutations that will modify Erks' biochemical or pharmacological properties or biological functions. Also, modifying Erks' biological effects requires understanding of additional mechanisms, responsible for sub-cellular localization and interaction with partners and scaffold proteins. Some of these mechanisms could be isoform-specific and, consequently, mutations that affect these processes may be different in Erk1 and Erk2, similar to the case of the CD site mutations that seem relevant only to Erk2 and mutation in the αC-helix, which are more relevant to Erk1. As a result of our inability to translate structural and mechanistic knowledge into mutation design, most mutations identified so far were discovered via unbiased screens, and even following their isolation, their mechanism of action is not understood.

3.2. Mutations Identified in Erks Disclose 3 Hotspots for Mutagenesis, Perhaps Reflecting Some Prevailing Mechanisms

Although mutations discussed in this review are spread along the Erk molecules, some hotspots re-appear in several laboratory screens as well as in cancer patients. The *sevenmaker* residue and its neighbor at the CD site, Glu320, are prominent examples, relevant for Erk2. αC-helix, mainly Arg84/Arg65 (in ERK1/ERK2), is another hotspot, which seems relevant primarily to Erk1. Yet another important residue is the gatekeeper that was discovered as a target for mutagenesis by studying the evolution of Erks and by structural approaches. Mutations that occur in the CD site affect protein-protein interactions, primarily with phosphatases, while mutations in the gatekeeper, in the residues that are in proximity to it and in residues of the αC-helix, significantly increase the commonly negligible intrinsic catalytic activity of the kinases. All mutations that caused elevation of the basal catalytic activity did so via identical mechanism, increasing the autocatalytic capability of the proteins. So far, no mutation was discovered that allows Erks to bypass the requirement of activation loop phosphorylation and enforces by itself adoption of the active conformation. Rather, the mutations discovered so far caused the Erk molecule to acquire a 'prone to autophosphorylate' conformation. Erks may be immune against mutations that induce the active conformation by themselves.

4. Conclusions

Clinical and Biochemical Lessons from the Erk Mutant

Most of the mutations described in this review seem to be directly relevant to understanding cancer etiology and patients response to drugs. An important lesson is that Erks, at least Erk1, could become oncogenic. This finding strongly suggests that the oncogenicity of the RTK-Ras-Raf-MEK pathway is mediated primarily via Erks, reinforcing the effort to inhibit Erk as a powerful anti-cancer approach. The analysis of the mutants may further suggest that isoform-specific inhibitors should be developed with higher priority to Erk1-specific inhibitors. This would be a difficult challenge for drug developers. The mutations that cause drug resistance could be already taken into consideration when a therapeutic strategy is planned. Namely, drugs should be applied according to the mutation that appears in the tumor. This requires deep understanding of the effect of each of the many mutations discovered so far (Table 1) on Erks' biochemistry, biology and pathology.

Table 1. (**A**) Mutations identified in ERK1 (MAPK3; mutations numeration is according to the sequence of the human ERK1). (**B**) Mutations identified in ERK2 (MAPK1) (numeration of the mutants is according to the sequence of rat ERK2).

Mutation	Mode of Identification	Reference
	(A)	
A6_Q7insA	In cancer patients	COSMIC, cBioPortal
A6dup	In cancer patients	COSMIC
Q7R	In cancer patients	COSMIC
Q7H	In cancer patients	COSMIC, cBioPortal
G10R	In cancer patients	COSMIC
G11V	In cancer patients	COSMIC
G11_Splice	In cancer patients	COSMIC, cBioPortal
G12E	In cancer patients	COSMIC
E13K	In cancer patients	COSMIC, cBioPortal
E13*	In cancer patients	COSMIC, cBioPortal
R15G	In cancer patients	COSMIC, cBioPortal
R16I	In cancer patients	COSMIC, cBioPortal
E18Q	In cancer patients	COSMIC, cBioPortal, TumorPortal
V20V	In cancer patients	COSMIC
G23G	In cancer patients, and in a screen for mutants resistant to Erk inhibitors	COSMIC, [96]
V24F	In cancer patients	COSMIC, cBioPortal
V24S	In cancer patients	cBioPortal
V24fs*8	In cancer patients	cBioPortal
P25S	In cancer patients	COSMIC, cBioPortal
E27fs*35	In cancer patients	COSMIC, cBioPortal
E27G	In cancer patients	COSMIC
M30I	In cancer patients	COSMIC, cBioPortal

Table 1. *Cont.*

Mutation	Mode of Identification	Reference
G33W	In cancer patients	cBioPortal
P35S	In cancer patients	COSMIC
D37D	In cancer patients	COSMIC, TumorPortal
Q46H	In cancer patients	cBioPortal
I48N	In a screen for mutants resistant to VRT-11E	[96]
G51S	In a screen for mutants resistant to RAF/MEK inhibitors	[96]
A52P	In cancer patients	COSMIC, cBioPortal
Y53Y	In cancer patients	COSMIC
Y53H	In a screen for mutants resistant to VRT-11E and SCH772984	[96]
Y53C	In a screen for mutants resistant to Erk inhibitors	[96]
G54S	In a screen for mutants resistant to VRT-11E and SCH772984	[96]
G54C	In cancer patients	cBioPortal
G54A	In a screen for mutants resistant to Erk inhibitors	[96]
S57G	In a screen for mutants resistant to RAF/MEK inhibitors	[96]
X57_splice	In cancer patients	cBioPortal
S58L	In cancer patients	cBioPortal, TumorPortal
Y60C	In a screen for mutants resistant to Erk inhibitors	[96]
D61E	In cancer patients	COSMIC, cBioPortal
H62_S74>R	In cancer patients	COSMIC, cBioPortal
V63M	In cancer patients	COSMIC
R64C	In cancer patients	COSMIC, cBioPortal
R64L	In cancer patients	cBioPortal
K65R	In a screen for mutants resistant to Erk and RAF/MEK inhibitors	[96]
R67C	In cancer patients	COSMIC

Table 1. *Cont.*

Mutation	Mode of Identification	Reference
V68L	In cancer patients	cBioPortal
K72N	In cancer patients	COSMIC, cBioPortal
K72R	In a screen for mutants resistant to Erk inhibitors	[96]
I73S	In a screen for mutants resistant to Erk inhibitors	[96]
I73M	In Cancer patients	COSMIC, cBioPortal
S74G	In a screen for mutants resistant to VRT-11E	[96]
Insertion 74N	An activating mutation. On the basis of inferred ancestor	[75]
P75P	In Cancer patients	TumorPortal
P75L	In a screen for mutants resistant to VRT-11E and SCH772984	[96]
P75S	In a screen for mutants resistant to VRT-11E and SCH772984	[96]
E77E	In cancer patients, and in a screen for mutants resistant to Erk inhibitors	COSMIC, cBioPortal, TumorPortal, [96]
Q79H	In cancer patients	cBioPortal
Q79*	In cancer patients	COSMIC, cBioPortal, TumorPortal
Y81C	In a screen for mutants resistant to VRT-11E	[96]
C82Y	In cancer patients	cBioPortal, [96]
R84H	In cancer patients, and in a screen for mutants resistant to trametinib and dabrafenib	COSMIC, cBioPortal,[96]
R84S	In a screen for mutants resistant to RAF/MEK inhibitors, and in a screen for MEK-independent mutants	[73,96]
T85T	In cancer patients	COSMIC
L86L	In cancer patients	COSMIC
L86R	In a screen for mutants resistant to RAF/MEK inhibitors	[96]
L86P	In a screen for mutants resistant to RAF/MEK inhibitors	[96]
R87W	In cancer patients	COSMIC, cBioPortal

Table 1. *Cont.*

Mutation	Mode of Identification	Reference
Q90R	In a screen for mutants resistant to trametinib and dabrafenib	[96]
R94C	In cancer patients	COSMIC, cBioPortal, TumorPortal
R96H	In cancer patients	COSMIC, cBioPortal
R96C	In cancer patients	cBioPortal
R96R	In cancer patients	COSMIC
H97H	In cancer patients	COSMIC
E98K	In cancer patients	COSMIC, cBioPortal
E98D	In cancer patients	COSMIC, cBioPortal
I101I	In cancer patients	COSMIC
G102D	In cancer patients	COSMIC, cBioPortal
I103A	On the basis of structural considerations	[76]
R104Q	In cancer patients	cBioPortal
L107L	In cancer patients	TumorPortal
R108W	In cancer patients	COSMIC, cBioPortal
A109P	In cancer patients	COSMIC
Q122M	An activating mutation. On the basis of inferred ancestor	[75]
L124L	In cancer patients	COSMIC
E126*	In cancer patients	COSMIC, cBioPortal, TumorPortal
S135N	In a screen for mutants resistant to RAF/MEK inhibitors	[96]
Q136fs*4	In cancer patients	cBioPortal
Q136*	In cancer patients	cBioPortal
Q136H	In cancer patients	cBioPortal
L138L	In cancer patients	COSMIC

Table 1. *Cont.*

Mutation	Mode of Identification	Reference
H142H	In cancer patients	COSMIC
Y145*	In cancer patients	COSMIC
Y148H	In a screen for mutants resistant to trametinib and dabrafenib	[96]
Y148C	In cancer patients	COSMIC, cBioPortal
R152L	In cancer patients	TumorPortal
R152W	In cancer patients	COSMIC, cBioPortal, TumorPortal
G153S	In cancer patients	COSMIC, cBioPortal
G153G	In cancer patients	COSMIC
H158L	In cancer patients	COSMIC
S159S	In cancer patients	COSMIC, TumorPortal
A160T	In cancer patients	COSMIC, cBioPortal
A160A	In cancer patients	COSMIC
L163L	In cancer patients	COSMIC
R165L	In cancer patients	COSMIC
P169L	In cancer patients	cBioPortal
N171D	In cancer patients	COSMIC, cBioPortal
T177I	In cancer patients	COSMIC, cBioPortal
C178R	In cancer patients	COSMIC
C178Y	In cancer patients	COSMIC
C178C	In cancer patients	COSMIC
D179N	In cancer patients	COSMIC
I182N	In cancer patients	cBioPortal
I182-splice	In cancer patients	TumorPortal
F185F	In cancer patients	COSMIC

Table 1. *Cont.*

Mutation	Mode of Identification	Reference
F185I	In cancer patients	cBioPortal
G186R	In cancer patients	COSMIC, cBioPortal, TumorPortal
G186D	In a screen for mutants resistant to VRT-1E and SCH772984	[96,97]
R189W	In cancer patients	COSMIC, cBioPortal
R189Q	In cancer patients	COSMIC
R189R	In cancer patients	COSMIC
I190T	In cancer patients	COSMIC, cBioPortal
P193T	In cancer patients	COSMIC, cBioPortal
P193H	In cancer patients	COSMIC, cBioPortal
P193S	In cancer patients	cBioPortal, TumorPortal
E194Q	In cancer patients	COSMIC, cBioPortal
T198T	In cancer patients	COSMIC
G199D	In cancer patients	COSMIC, cBioPortal
T202M	In cancer patients	COSMIC, cBioPortal
E203K	In cancer patients	cBioPortal
A206V	In a screen for mutants resistant to trametinib and dabrafenib	[96]
T207T	In cancer patients	COSMIC, TumorPortal
R211Q	In cancer patients	COSMIC, cBioPortal
R211P	In cancer patients	COSMIC, cBioPortal
R211W	In cancer patients	cBioPortal
E214D	In cancer patients	cBioPortal
M216I	In cancer patients, and in a screen for mutants resistant to RAF/MEK inhibitors	COSMIC, cBioPortal,[96]
N218N	In cancer patients	COSMIC

Table 1. *Cont.*

Mutation	Mode of Identification	Reference
S219F	In cancer patients	COSMIC, cBioPortal
S219P	In a screen for mutants resistant to trametinib and dabrafenib	[96]
X221_splice	In cancer patients	cBioPortal
D227N	In cancer patients	cBioPortal
V231L	In cancer patients	COSMIC
A236T	In cancer patients	COSMIC
S240C	In cancer patients	COSMIC
R242R	In cancer patients	TumorPortal
L251L	In cancer patients	COSMIC
Q253P	In cancer patients	COSMIC, cBioPortal
I257V	In cancer patients	COSMIC, cBioPortal
I260H	In cancer patients	COSMIC, cBioPortal
Q266*	In cancer patients	COSMIC, cBioPortal
L269P	In cancer patients	COSMIC, cBioPortal, TumorPortal
I273M	In Cancer patients	cBioPortal
R278*	In cancer patients, and in a screen for mutants resistant to RAF/MEK inhibitors	cBioPortal, [96]
L281I	In cancer patients	cBioPortal
V290A	In cancer patients	COSMIC, cBioPortal, TumorPortal
F296F	In cancer patients	COSMIC
D300E	In cancer patients	COSMIC, cBioPortal
A303V	In cancer patients, and in a screen for mutants resistant to RAF/MEK inhibitors	COSMIC, cBioPortal, [96]
L304P	In Cancer patients	cBioPortal
L306L	In Cancer patients, and in a screen for mutants resistant to Erk inhibitors	cBioPortal, [96]
T312S	In cancer patients	cBioPortal

Table 1. *Cont.*

Mutation	Mode of Identification	Reference
N314I	In cancer patients	COSMIC, cBioPortal, TumorPortal
N314N	In cancer patients	COSMIC
P315H	In cancer patients	COSMIC
R318W	In cancer patients	COSMIC, cBioPortal
R318R	In cancer patients	COSMIC
V321fs*40	In cancer patients	cBioPortal
V321W	In cancer patients	cBioPortal
P328L	In cancer patients	COSMIC, cBioPortal
E331E	In cancer patients	COSMIC
Q332H	In cancer patients	COSMIC
D335N	In cancer patients	COSMIC, cBioPortal
P336Q	In cancer patients	COSMIC
T337T	In cancer patients	COSMIC
E339V	In cancer patients	COSMIC, cBioPortal
E343K	In cancer patients	cBioPortal
P345T	In cancer patients	COSMIC
F346I	In cancer patients	COSMIC, cBioPortal
F346F	In cancer patients	COSMIC
F348F	In cancer patients	COSMIC
A349T	In cancer patients	cBioPortal
R359W	In cancer patients	COSMIC, cBioPortal, TumorPortal
R359Q	In cancer patients	COSMIC
R359L	In cancer patients	COSMIC, cBioPortal

Table 1. *Cont.*

Mutation	Mode of Identification	Reference
E362K	In cancer patients	COSMIC, cBioPortal
E362*	In cancer patients	COSMIC, TumorPortal
F365C	In cancer patients	cBioPortal
Q366H	In cancer patients	cBioPortal
E367D	In cancer patients	COSMIC
P373P	In cancer patients	COSMIC, TumorPortal
G374*	In cancer patients	COSMIC
G374K	In cancer patients	COSMIC, cBioPortal
L376R	In cancer patients	COSMIC, cBioPortal
A378G	In cancer patients	COSMIC, cBioPortal
	(B)	
A2V	In cancer patients	COSMIC, cBioPortal
A6_A7delAA	In cancer patients	COSMIC
A5delA	In cancer patients	COSMIC
A7T	In cancer patients	COSMIC, cBioPortal
G8S	In cancer patients	COSMIC, cBioPortal
R13P	In a screen for mutants that are resistant to VRT-11E and SCH772984	[95]
Q15Q	In cancer patients	COSMIC
P21S	In cancer patients	COSMIC, cBioPortal
I29M	In Cancer patients, and in a screen for mutants that are resistant to VRT-11E	COSMIC, cBioPortal,[95]
I29Q	In a screen for mutants that are resistant to VRT-11E	[95]
I29R	In a screen for mutants that are resistant to VRT-11E	[95]
I29L	In a screen for mutants that are resistant to VRT-11E	[95]
I29E	In a screen for mutants that are resistant to VRT-11E	[95]

Table 1. *Cont.*

Mutation	Mode of Identification	Reference
I29K	In a screen for mutants that are resistant to VRT-11E	[95]
I29H	In a screen for mutants that are resistant to VRT-11E	[95]
I29Y	In a screen for mutants that are resistant to VRT-11E	[95]
I29D	In a screen for mutants that are resistant to VRT-11E	[95]
I29C	In a screen for mutants that are resistant to VRT-11E	[95]
I29W	In a screen for mutants that are resistant too VRT-11E	[95]
I29N	In a screen for mutants that are resistant to VRT-11E	[95]
G30P	In a screen for mutants that are resistant to VRT-11E	[95]
E31P	In a screen for mutants that are resistant to SCH772984	[95]
E31Q	In cancer patients	COSMIC, cBioPortal
G32D	In cancer patients	COSMIC, cBioPortal
G32C	In cancer patients	cBioPortal
A33N	In a screen for mutants that are resistant to VRT-11E	[95]
Y34Y	In cancer patients	COSMIC
Y34H	In a screen for mutants that are resistant to VRT-11E and SCH772984	[95,96]
Y34V	In a screen for mutants that are resistant to VRT-11E and SCH772984	[95]
Y34T	In a screen for mutants that are resistant to VRT-11E and SCH772984	[95]
Y34Q	In a screen for mutants that are resistant to VRT-11E and SCH772984	[95]
Y34G	In a screen for mutants that are resistant to VRT-11E and SCH772984	[95]
Y34S	In a screen for mutants that are resistant to VRT-11E and SCH772984	[95]
Y34C	In a screen for mutants that are resistant to VRT-11E and SCH772984	[95]
Y34I	In a screen for mutants that are resistant to VRT-11E and SCH772984	[95]
Y34D	In a screen for mutants that are resistant to VRT-11E and SCH772984	[95]
Y34R	In a screen for mutants that are resistant to VRT-11E and SCH772984	[95]

Table 1. *Cont.*

Mutation	Mode of Identification	Reference
Y34N	In a screen for mutants that are resistant to VRT-11E and SCH772984	[95,96]
Y34L	In a screen for mutants that are resistant to VRT-11E and SCH772984	[95]
Y34M	In a screen for mutants that are resistant to VRT-11E and SCH772984	[95]
G35D	In a screen for mutants that are resistant to VRT-11E and SCH772984	[95]
G35T	In a screen for mutants that are resistant to VRT-11E and SCH772984	[95]
G35K	In a screen for mutants that are resistant to VRT-11E and SCH772984	[95]
G35S	In a screen for mutants that are resistant to VRT-11E and SCH772984	[95,96]
G35A	In a screen for mutants that are resistant to VRT-11E and SCH772984	[95]
G35N	In a screen for mutants that are resistant to VRT-11E	[95]
G35P	In a screen for mutants that are resistant to VRT-11E	[95]
G35C	In a screen for mutants that are resistant to VRT-11E and SCH772984	[95]
M36P	In a screen for mutants that are resistant to VRT-11E	[95]
V37A	In a screen for mutants that are resistant to VRT-11E	[95]
C38P	In a screen for mutants that are resistant to VRT-11E and SCH772984	[95]
C38R	In a screen for mutants that are resistant to SCH772984	[95]
Y41W	In a screen for mutants that are resistant to SCH772984	[95]
Y41E	In a screen for mutants that are resistant to SCH772984	[95]
D42H	In a screen for mutants that are resistant to VRT-11E and SCH772984	[95]
V44F	In cancer patients	cBioPortal
V47A	In a screen for mutants that are resistant to SCH772984	[95]
R48*	In cancer patients	COSMIC, cBioPortal
V49K	Causes resistance to SCH772984	[95]
V49H	In a screen for mutants that are resistant to VRT-11E and SCH772984	[95]
A50S	In Cancer patients	COSMIC, TumorPortal

Table 1. *Cont.*

Mutation	Mode of Identification	Reference
K53G	In a screen for mutants that are resistant to SCH772984	[95]
I54H	In a screen for mutants that are resistant to SCH772984	[95]
I54D	In a screen for mutants that are resistant to SCH772984	[95]
54W	In a screen for mutants that are resistant to SCH772984	[95]
I54K	In a screen for mutants that are resistant to SCH772984	[95]
I54Y	In a screen for mutants that are resistant to SCH772984	[95]
I54E	In a screen for mutants that are resistant to SCH772984	[95]
I54Q	In a screen for mutants that are resistant to VRT-11E and SCH772984	[95]
I54S	In a screen for mutants that are resistant to VRT-11E and SCH772984	[95]
I54G	In a screen for mutants that are resistant to VRT-11E and SCH772984	[95]
I54P	In a screen for mutants that are resistant to VRT-11E	[95]
S55P	In a screen for mutants that are resistant to VRT-11E	[95]
S55G	In a screen for mutants that are resistant to VRT-11E	[95]
S55F	In a screen for mutants that are resistant to VRT-11E and SCH772984	[95]
P56L	In cancer patients, In a screen for mutants that are resistant to VRT-11E and SCH772984	COSMIC, cBioPortal, [95,96]
P56S	In a screen for mutants that are resistant to VRT-11E and SCH772984	[95,96]
P56W	In a screen for mutants that are resistant to VRT-11E and SCH772984	[95]
P56R	In a screen for mutants that are resistant to VRT-11E and SCH772984	[95]
P56K	In a screen for mutants that are resistant to VRT-11E and SCH772984	[95]
P56A	In a screen for mutants that are resistant to VRT-11E and SCH772984	[95]
P56M	In a screen for mutants that are resistant to VRT-11E and SCH772984	[95]
P56N	In a screen for mutants that are resistant to VRT-11E and SCH772984	[95]

Table 1. *Cont.*

Mutation	Mode of Identification	Reference
P56G	In a screen for mutants that are resistant to VRT-11E and SCH772984	[95]
P56Y	In a screen for mutants that are resistant to VRT-11E and SCH772984	[95]
P56F	In a screen for mutants that are resistant to VRT-11E and SCH772984	[95]
P56Q	In a screen for mutants that are resistant to VRT-11E	[95]
P56V	In a screen for mutants that are resistant to VRT-11E	[95]
P56T	In a screen for mutants that are resistant to VRT-11E	[95,96]
P56I	In a screen for mutants that are resistant to VRT-11E	[95]
F57G	In a screen for mutants that are resistant to VRT-11E	[95]
F57P	In a screen for mutants that are resistant to VRT-11E	[95]
F57S	In a screen for mutants that are resistant to VRT-11E and SCH772984	[95]
F57R	In a screen for mutants that are resistant to VRT-11E and SCH772984	[95]
E58Q	In a screen for mutants that are resistant to SCH772984	[95]
E58S	In a screen for mutants that are resistant to SCH772984	[95]
Q60P	In a screen for mutants that are resistant to VRT-11E and SCH772984	[95]
T61T	In cancer patients	COSMIC
T61I	In cancer patients	COSMIC
Y62G	In a screen for mutants that are resistant to VRT-11E	[95]
Y62E	In a screen for mutants that are resistant to VRT-11E	[95]
Y62D	In a screen for mutants that are resistant to VRT-11E	[95]
Y62S	In a screen for mutants that are resistant to VRT-11E	[95]
Y62C	In a screen for mutants that are resistant to VRT-11E	[95]
Y62T	In a screen for mutants that are resistant to VRT-11E	[95]
Y62Q	In a screen for mutants that are resistant to VRT-11E	[95]
Y62A	In a screen for mutants that are resistant to VRT-11E	[95]

Table 1. *Cont.*

Mutation	Mode of Identification	Reference
Y62P	In a screen for mutants that are resistant to VRT-11E	[95]
Y62V	In a screen for mutants that are resistant to VRT-11E and SCH772984	[95]
Y62M	In a screen for mutants that are resistant to VRT-11E and SCH772984	[95]
Y62K	In a screen for mutants that are resistant to VRT-11E and SCH772984	[95]
Y62I	In a screen for mutants that are resistance to VRT-11E and SCH772984	[95]
Y62L	In a screen for mutants that are resistance to VRT-11E and SCH772984	[95]
Y62R	In a screen for mutants that are resistant to VRT-11E and SCH772984	[95]
Y62N	In a screen for mutants that are resistant to VRT-11E	[95,96]
C63F	In a screen for mutants that are resistant to VRT-11E	[95]
C63W	In a screen for mutants that are resistant to VRT-11E	[95]
C63fs*3	In Cancer patients	COSMIC, cBioPortal
C63Y	In a screen for mutants that are resistant to VRT-11E and SCH772984	[95,96]
R65I	In cancer patients, and in a screen for mutants that are resistant to VRT-11E	COSMIC, cBioPortal,[95]
R65K	In a screen for mutants that are resistant to Erk inhibitors and RAF/MEK inhibitors	[96]
R65S	Genetic screen for Mpk1 intrinsically active mutants	[73]
T66T	In Cancer patients	COSMIC
T66M	In a screen for mutants that are resistant to VRT-11E	[95,96]
T66Q	In a screen for mutants that are resistant to VRT-11E	[95,96]
T66F	In a screen for mutants that are resistant to VRT-11E	[95,96]
T66I	In a screen for mutants that are resistant to VRT-11E	[95,96]
T66L	In a screen for mutants that are resistant to VRT-11E	[95,96]
T66P	In a screen for mutants that are resistant to VRT-11E	[95,96]

Table 1. *Cont.*

Mutation	Mode of Identification	Reference
T66D	In a screen for mutants that are resistant to VRT-11E and SCH772984	[95,96]
T66Y	In a screen for mutants that are resistant to VRT-11E and SCH772984	[95,96]
T66H	In a screen for mutants that are resistant to VRT-11E	[95,96]
T66N	In a screen for mutants that are resistant to VRT-11E and SCH772984	[95,96]
L67L	In cancer patients	COSMIC
R68R	In cancer patients	COSMIC
E69P	In a screen for mutants that are resistant to VRT-11E	[95,96]
E69C	In a screen for mutants that are resistant to VRT-11E	[95,96]
E69G	In a screen for mutants that are resistant to VRT-11E	[95,96]
E69K	In a screen for mutants that are resistant to VRT-11E and SCH772984	[95,96]
E69A	In a screen for mutants that are resistant to VRT-11E and SCH772984	[95,96]
I72fs*8	In cancer patients	COSMIC
L73E	In a screen for mutants that are resistant to VRT-11E	[95,96]
L73H	In a screen for mutants that are resistant to VRT-11E	[95,96]
L73R	In a screen for mutants that are resistant to VRT-11E	[95,96]
L73W	In a screen for mutants that are resistant to VRT-11E and SCH772984	[95]
L73P	In a screen for mutants that are resistant to VRT-11E, and on the basis of genetic screen for intrinsically active FUS3	[95,103]
R75C	In cancer patients	COSMIC, cBioPortal
R77S	In cancer patients	cBioPortal
R77K	In cancer patients	COSMIC, cBioPortal
E79K	In cancer patients	COSMIC, cBioPortal, TumorPortal
N80fs*18	In cancer patients	COSMIC, cBioPortal
I82T	In cancer patients	COSMIC, cBioPortal
I82A	Activating mutation. On the basis of structural considerations	[76]

Table 1. *Cont.*

Mutation	Mode of Identification	Reference
I84A	Activating mutation. On the basis of structural considerations	[76]
D86-del	In cancer patients	cBioPortal
I88F	In cancer patients	COSMIC
I93I	In cancer patients	COSMIC, TumorPortal
Q95R	In a screen for mutants that are resistant to VRT-11E	[95]
M96W	In a screen for mutants that are resistant to VRT-11E	[95]
M96I	In cancer patients	cBioPortal
D98N	In cancer patients	cBioPortal
D98M	In a screen for mutants that are resistant to VRT-11E	[95]
I101Q	In a screen for mutants that are resistant to SCH772984	[95]
I101W	In a screen for mutants that are resistant to SCH772984	[95]
I101Y	In a screen for mutants that are resistant to SCH772984	[95]
I101R	In cancer patients	COSMIC
V102V	In a screen for mutants that are resistant to Erk inhibitors and RAF/MEK inhibitors	[96]
Q103A	Generated in order to study the biological effect the gatekeeper residue	[76]
Q103G	Generated in order to study the biological effect the gatekeeper residue	[76]
Q103I	In a screen for mutants that are resistant to SCH772984	[95]
Q103F	In a screen for mutants that are resistant to SCH772984	[95]
Q103T	In a screen for mutants that are resistant to SCH772984	[95]
Q103W	In a screen for mutants that are resistant to VRT-11E and SCH772984	[95]
Q103V	In a screen for mutants that are resistant to VRT-11E and SCH772984	[95]
Q103N	In a screen for mutants that are resistant to VRT-11E	[95]
Q103Y	In a screen for mutants that are resistant to VRT-11E and SCH772984	[95]
D104D	In a screen for mutants that are resistant to Erk inhibitors	[96]

Table 1. *Cont.*

Mutation	Mode of Identification	Reference
D104H	In cancer patients	cBioPortal
T108P	In a screen for mutants that are resistant to VRT-11E	[95]
L110R	In cancer patients	cBioPortal
L114S	In cancer patients	cBioPortal
L119I	In cancer patients	COSMIC, cBioPortal, TumorPortal
D122T	In a screen for mutants that are resistant to VRT-11E and SCH772984	[95]
I124F	In cancer patients	COSMIC
C125I	In a screen for mutants that are resistant to VRT-11E and SCH772984	[95]
Y129N	In a screen for mutants that are resistant to RAF/MEK inhibitors	[96]
Y129H	In a screen for mutants that are resistant to RAF/MEK inhibitors	[96]
Y129F	In a screen for mutants that are resistant to trametinib and dabrafenib	[96]
Y129C	In Cancer patients, and In a screen for mutants that are resistant to trametinib and dabrafenib	COSMIC, cBioPortal, [96]
Y129S	In a screen for mutants that are resistant totrametinib and dabrafenib	[96]
Q130E	In cancer patients	COSMIC, cBioPortal
L132P	In cancer patients	COSMIC, cBioPortal
R133K	In cancer patients	COSMIC, cBioPortal
G134E	In cancer patients	COSMIC, cBioPortal
I138I	In cancer patients	COSMIC
H139Y	In cancer patients	COSMIC, cBioPortal, TumorPortal
H139R	In cancer patients	cBioPortal
S140L	In cancer patients	COSMIC, cBioPortal
A141A	In cancer patients	COSMIC, TumorPortal
N142K	In cancer patients	COSMIC, cBioPortal
N142N	In cancer patients	COSMIC

Table 1. *Cont.*

Mutation	Mode of Identification	Reference
H145Y	In cancer patients	COSMIC, cBioPortal
H145R	In cancer patients	cBioPortal
R146S	In cancer patients	COSMIC, cBioPortal
R146L	In cancer patients	cBioPortal, TumorPortal
R146C	In cancer patients	cBioPortal
R146H	In cancer patients	COSMIC, cBioPortal
D147Y	In cancer patients	cBioPortal
S151D	On the basis of alignment with MKK1	[103]
L154N	In a screen for mutants that are resistant to VRT-11E	[95]
L154G	In a screen for mutants that are resistant to VRT-11E	[95]
L155L	In cancer patients	COSMIC, TumorPortal
D160N	In cancer patients	COSMIC, cBioPortal, TumorPortal
D160G	In cancer patients	COSMIC, cBioPortal, TumorPortal
I163I	In cancer patients	cBioPortal
C164R	In cancer patients	COSMIC, cBioPortal
D165G	In cancer patients	COSMIC, cBioPortal
G167D	In a screen for mutants that are resistant to VRT-11E and SCH772984	[95,97]
L168L	In a screen for mutants that are resistant to Erk inhibitors	[96]
R170H	In cancer patients	COSMIC, cBioPortal, TumorPortal
V171I	In cancer patients	COSMIC
P174T	In cancer patients	COSMIC, cBioPortal
P174S	In cancer patients	COSMIC, cBioPortal
D177G	In cancer patients	cBioPortal
T179fs*29	In cancer patients	COSMIC, cBioPortal
F181S	In cancer patients	COSMIC

Table 1. *Cont.*

Mutation	Mode of Identification	Reference
E184*	In cancer patients	cBioPortal
A187V	In a screen for mutants that are resistant to trametinib and dabrafenib	[96]
R189C	In cancer patients	COSMIC, cBioPortal
R189H	In cancer patients	COSMIC, cBioPortal
W190L	In cancer patients	cBioPortal
E195*	In cancer patients	cBioPortal
L198F	In cancer patients	COSMIC
S200P	In a screen for mutants that are resistant to trametinib and dabrafenib	[96]
G202C	In cancer patients	COSMIC, cBioPortal,[96]
G202S	In cancer patients	cBioPortal,[96]
G202G	In cancer patients	COSMIC, [96]
Y203N	In a screen for mutants that are resistant to RAF/MEK inhibitors	[96]
T204I	In cancer patients	COSMIC, cBioPortal
I209V	In cancer patients	COSMIC, cBioPortal
V212A	In a screen for mutants that are resistant to RAF/MEK inhibitors	[96]
E218K	In cancer patients	COSMIC
S220Y	In cancer patients	COSMIC, cBioPortal
I225F	In cancer patients	COSMIC, cBioPortal
P227S	In cancer patients	COSMIC
P227L	In cancer patients	COSMIC, cBioPortal
G228E	In cancer patients	COSMIC, cBioPortal
D233E	In cancer patients	COSMIC, cBioPortal
D233G	In cancer patients	cBioPortal

Table 1. *Cont.*

Mutation	Mode of Identification	Reference
D233V	In cancer patients	COSMIC, cBioPortal
D233*	In cancer patients	TumorPortal
G240_splice	In cancer patients	cBioPortal
L242I	In cancer patients	COSMIC, cBioPortal
L242F	In cancer patients	COSMIC, cBioPortal, TumorPortal
S244F	In cancer patients	COSMIC, cBioPortal
S244S	In cancer patients	COSMIC
L250L	In a screen for mutants that are resistant to RAF/MEK inhibitors	[96]
N255S	In cancer patients	COSMIC, cBioPortal
R259G	In cancer patients	COSMIC, cBioPortal
N260T	In cancer patients	COSMIC, cBioPortal, TumorPortal
Y261C	In cancer patients	COSMIC, cBioPortal
L263F	In a screen for mutants that are resistant to Erk inhibitors	[96]
S264F	In cancer patients	COSMIC
L265P	In cancer patients	COSMIC
P266L	In cancer patients	COSMIC, cBioPortal
P272S	In cancer patients	COSMIC
L276L	In cancer patients	COSMIC, TumorPortal
L276M	In cancer patients	cBioPortal
F277F	In cancer patients	COSMIC
K283T	In cancer patients	cBioPortal
L285M	In a screen for mutants that are resistant to RAF/MEK inhibitors	[96]
L288L	In cancer patients	COSMIC
D289G	In cancer patients	COSMIC, cBioPortal, TumorPortal
D289H	In cancer patients	cBioPortal

Table 1. *Cont.*

Mutation	Mode of Identification	Reference
P296T	In cancer patients	COSMIC
E301K	In a screen for mutants that are resistant to RAF/MEK inhibitors	[96]
A305S	In cancer patients	cBioPortal
L311P	In cancer patients	COSMIC
Y314F	In cancer patients	COSMIC, cBioPortal, TumorPortal
Y314C	In cancer patients	cBioPortal
D316N	In cancer patients	COSMIC, cBioPortal
P317S	In cancer patients	COSMIC, cBioPortal
P317P	In cancer patients	COSMIC
S318C	In cancer patients	COSMIC
D319N	In cancer patients, and in a genetic screen in *Drosophila*	COSMIC, cBioPortal, [77]
D319A	In cancer patients	COSMIC
D319G	In a screen for mutants that are resistant to trametinib and dabrafenib	cBioPortal, [96]
D319V	In cancer patients	COSMIC, cBioPortal
D319E	In cancer patients	COSMIC, cBioPortal
E320K	In a screen for mutants that are resistant to trametinib and dabrafenib	CISMIC, cBioPortal, TumorPortal,[96]
E320*	In cancer patients	cBioPortal, TumorPortal
E320N	In cancer patients	cBioPortal
E320A	In cancer patients	COSMIC, cBioPortal
E320V	In cancer patients	COSMIC
P321P	In a screen for mutants that are resistant to Erk inhibitors	[96]
P321S	In a screen for mutants that are resistant to RAF/MEK inhibitors	[96]
P321L	In a screen for mutants that are resistant to RAF/MEK inhibitors	[96]
I322V	In cancer patients	cBioPortal

Table 1. *Cont.*

Mutation	Mode of Identification	Reference
A323T	In cancer patients	cBioPortal
A323S	In cancer patients	cBioPortal
A323V	In cancer patients	cBioPortal
E324*	In cancer patients	COSMIC, cBioPortal
F329F	In cancer patients	COSMIC
F329Y	In cancer patients	COSMIC
D330N	In cancer patients	COSMIC, cBioPortal
M331I	In cancer patients	COSMIC, cBioPortal
D335N	In a screen for mutants that are resistant to RAF/MEK inhibitors	[96]
E343*	In cancer patients	COSMIC
I345H	In a screen for mutants that are resistant to to VRT-11E	[95]
I345M	In a screen for mutants that are resistant to VRT-11E	[95]
I345F	In a screen for mutants that are resistant to VRT-11E	[95]
I345L	In a screen for mutants that are resistant to VRT-11E	COSMIC
I345Y	In a screen for mutants that are resistant to VRT-11E and SCH772984	[95]
I345W	In a screen for mutants that are resistant to VRT-11E and SCH772984	[95]
E347*	In cancer patients	COSMIC
E347K	In cancer patients, and in a screen for mutants that are resistant to RAF/MEK inhibitors	COSMIC, cBioPortal,[96]
T349T	In cancer patients	COSMIC
A350S	In cancer patients	COSMIC
A350V	In cancer patients	COSMIC
R351K	In a screen for mutants that are resistant to RAF/MEK inhibitors	[96]
Y356D	In cancer patients	COSMIC, cBioPortal
Y356Y	In cancer patients	COSMIC
R357T	In cancer patients	cBioPortal

References

1. Askari, N.; Diskin, R.; Avitzour, M.; Capone, R.; Livnah, O.; Engelberg, D. Hyperactive variants of p38α induce, whereas hyperactive variants of p38γ suppress, activating protein 1-mediated transcription. *J. Biol. Chem.* **2007**, *282*, 91–99. [CrossRef] [PubMed]
2. Avitzour, M.; Diskin, R.; Raboy, B.; Askari, N.; Engelberg, D.; Livnah, O. Intrinsically active variants of all human p38 isoforms. *FEBS J.* **2007**, *274*, 963–975. [CrossRef] [PubMed]
3. Fujimura, T. Current status and future perspective of robot-assisted radical cystectomy for invasive bladder cancer. *Int. J. Urol.* **2019**, *26*, 1033–1042. [CrossRef] [PubMed]
4. Roskoski, R., Jr. Targeting oncogenic Raf protein-serine/threonine kinases in human cancers. *Pharmacol. Res.* **2018**, *135*, 239–258. [CrossRef]
5. Keith, W.M.; Kenichi, N.; Sara, W. Recent advances of MEK inhibitors and their clinical progress. *Curr. Top. Med. Chem.* **2007**, *7*, 1364–1378.
6. Zhao, Y.; Adjei, A.A. The clinical development of MEK inhibitors. *Nat. Rev. Clin. Oncol.* **2014**, *11*, 385–400. [CrossRef]
7. Roskoski, R., Jr. Allosteric MEK1/2 inhibitors including cobimetanib and trametinib in the treatment of cutaneous melanomas. *Pharmacol. Res.* **2017**, *117*, 20–31. [CrossRef]
8. Dominguez, C.; Powers, D.A.; Tamayo, N. p38 MAP kinase inhibitors: Many are made, but few are chosen. *Curr. Opin. Drug Discov. Dev.* **2005**, *8*, 421–430.
9. Yong, H.Y.; Koh, M.S.; Moon, A. The p38 MAPK inhibitors for the treatment of inflammatory diseases and cancer. *Expert Opin. Investig. Drugs* **2009**, *18*, 1893–1905. [CrossRef]
10. Pettus, L.H.; Wurz, R.P. Small molecule p38 MAP kinase inhibitors for the treatment of inflammatory diseases: Novel structures and developments during 2006–2008. *Curr. Top. Med. Chem.* **2008**, *8*, 1452–1467. [CrossRef]
11. Messoussi, A.; Feneyrolles, C.; Bros, A.; Deroide, A.; Daydé-Cazals, B.; Chevé, G.; Van Hijfte, N.; Fauvel, B.; Bougrin, K.; Yasri, A. Recent progress in the design, study, and development of c-Jun N-terminal kinase inhibitors as anticancer agents. *Chem. Biol.* **2014**, *21*, 1433–1443. [CrossRef] [PubMed]
12. Mansour, S.J.; Matten, W.T.; Hermann, A.S.; Candia, J.M.; Rong, S.; Fukasawa, K.; Woude, G.V.; Ahn, N.G. Transformation of mammalian cells by constitutively active MAP kinase kinase. *Science* **1994**, *265*, 966–970. [CrossRef] [PubMed]
13. Kolibaba, K.S.; Druker, B.J. Protein tyrosine kinases and cancer. *Biochim. Biophys. Acta* **1997**, *1333*, F217–F248. [CrossRef]
14. Garnett, M.J.; Marais, R. Guilty as charged: B-RAF is a human oncogene. *Cancer Cell* **2004**, *6*, 313–319. [CrossRef] [PubMed]
15. Raingeaud, J.; Whitmarsh, A.J.; Barrett, T.; Derijard, B.; Davis, R.J. MKK3-and MKK6-regulated gene expression is mediated by the p38 mitogen-activated protein kinase signal transduction pathway. *Mol. Cell. Biol.* **1996**, *16*, 1247–1255. [CrossRef] [PubMed]
16. Wick, M.J.; Wick, K.R.; Chen, H.; He, H.; Dong, L.Q.; Quon, M.J.; Liu, F. Substitution of the autophosphorylation site Thr516 with a negatively charged residue confers constitutive activity to mouse 3-phosphoinositide-dependent protein kinase-1 in cells. *J. Biol. Chem.* **2002**, *277*, 16632–16638. [CrossRef]
17. Yang, L.; Zheng, L.; Chng, W.J.; Ding, J.L. Comprehensive Analysis of ERK1/2 Substrates for Potential Combination Immunotherapies. *Trends Pharmacol. Sci.* **2019**, *40*, 897–910. [CrossRef]
18. Kyriakis, J.M.; Avruch, J. Mammalian MAPK signal transduction pathways activated by stress and inflammation: A 10-year update. *Physiol. Rev.* **2012**, *92*, 689–737. [CrossRef]
19. Brewster, J.L.; Gustin, M.C. Hog1: 20 years of discovery and impact. *Sci. Signal* **2014**, *7*, re7. [CrossRef]
20. Engelberg, D.; Perlman, R.; Levitzki, A. Transmembrane signaling in Saccharomyces cerevisiae as a model for signaling in metazoans: State of the art after 25 years. *Cell. Signal.* **2014**, *26*, 2865–2878. [CrossRef]
21. Saito, H. Regulation of cross-talk in yeast MAPK signaling pathways. *Curr. Opin. Microbiol.* **2010**, *13*, 677–683. [CrossRef] [PubMed]
22. Chen, R.E.; Thorner, J. Function and regulation in MAPK signaling pathways: Lessons learned from the yeast Saccharomyces cerevisiae. *Biochim. Biophys. Acta* **2007**, *1773*, 1311–1340. [CrossRef] [PubMed]
23. Shilo, B.Z. The regulation and functions of MAPK pathways in Drosophila. *Methods* **2014**, *68*, 151–159. [CrossRef] [PubMed]

24. Ashton-Beaucage, D.; Therrien, M. *How Genetics Has Helped Piece Together the MAPK Signaling Pathway*; Humana Press: New York, NY, USA, 2017; Volume 1487, pp. 1–21.
25. Bost, F.; Aouadi, M.; Caron, L.; Even, P.; Belmonte, N.; Prot, M.; Dani, C.; Hofman, P.; Pagès, G.; Pouysségur, J.; et al. The extracellular signal-regulated kinase isoform ERK1 is specifically required for in vitro and in vivo adipogenesis. *Diabetes* **2005**, *54*, 402–411. [CrossRef] [PubMed]
26. Bourcier, C.; Jacquel, A.; Hess, J.; Peyrottes, I.; Angel, P.; Hofman, P.; Auberger, P.; Pouysségur, J.; Pagès, G. p44 mitogen-activated protein kinase (extracellular signal-regulated kinase 1)-dependent signaling contributes to epithelial skin carcinogenesis. *Cancer Res.* **2006**, *66*, 2700–2707. [CrossRef] [PubMed]
27. Guihard, S.; Clay, D.; Cocault, L.; Saulnier, N.; Opolon, P.; Souyri, M.; Pagès, G.; Pouysségur, J.; Porteu, F.; Gaudry, M. The MAPK ERK1 is a negative regulator of the adult steady-state splenic erythropoiesis. *Blood* **2010**, *115*, 3686–3694. [CrossRef]
28. Lefloch, R.; Pouysségur, J.; Lenormand, P. Single and combined silencing of ERK1 and ERK2 reveals their positive contribution to growth signaling depending on their expression levels. *Mol. Cell. Biol.* **2008**, *28*, 511–527. [CrossRef]
29. Shin, S.; Dimitri, C.A.; Yoon, S.O.; Dowdle, W.; Blenis, J. ERK2 but not ERK1 induces epithelial-to-mesenchymal transformation via DEF motif-dependent signaling events. *Mol. Cell* **2010**, *38*, 114–127. [CrossRef]
30. Voisin, L.; Saba-El-Leil, M.K.; Julien, C.; Frémin, C.; Meloche, S. Genetic demonstration of a redundant role of extracellular signal-regulated kinase 1 (ERK1) and ERK2 mitogen-activated protein kinases in promoting fibroblast proliferation. *Mol. Cell. Biol.* **2010**, *30*, 2918–2932. [CrossRef]
31. Frémin, C.; Ezan, F.; Boisselier, P.; Bessard, A.; Pagès, G.; Pouysségur, J.; Baffet, G. ERK2 but not ERK1 plays a key role in hepatocyte replication: An RNAi-mediated ERK2 knockdown approach in wild-type and ERK1 null hepatocytes. *Hepatology* **2007**, *45*, 1035–1045. [CrossRef]
32. Radtke, S.; Milanovic, M.; Rossé, C.; De Rycker, M.; Lachmann, S.; Hibbert, A.; Kermorgant, S.; Parker, P.J. ERK2 but not ERK1 mediates HGF-induced motility in non-small cell lung carcinoma cell lines. *J. Cell Sci.* **2013**, *126 Pt 11*, 2381–2391. [CrossRef]
33. Chang, S.F.; Lin, S.S.; Yang, H.C.; Chou, Y.Y.; Gao, J.I.; Lu, S.C. LPS-Induced G-CSF Expression in Macrophages Is Mediated by ERK2, but Not ERK1. *PLoS ONE* **2015**, *10*, e0129685. [CrossRef] [PubMed]
34. Samuels, I.S.; Karlo, J.C.; Faruzzi, A.N.; Pickering, K.; Herrup, K.; Sweatt, J.D.; Saitta, S.C.; Landreth, G.E. Deletion of ERK2 mitogen-activated protein kinase identifies its key roles in cortical neurogenesis and cognitive function. *J. Neurosci.* **2008**, *28*, 6983–6995. [CrossRef] [PubMed]
35. Hatano, N.; Mori, Y.; Oh-hora, M.; Kosugi, A.; Fujikawa, T.; Nakai, N.; Niwa, H.; Miyazaki, J.I.; Hamaoka, T.; Ogata, M. Essential role for ERK2 mitogen-activated protein kinase in placental development. *Genes Cells* **2003**, *8*, 847–856. [CrossRef] [PubMed]
36. Frémin, C.; Saba-El-Leil, M.K.; Lévesque, K.; Ang, S.L.; Meloche, S. Functional Redundancy of ERK1 and ERK2 MAP Kinases during Development. *Cell Rep.* **2015**, *12*, 913–921. [CrossRef]
37. Marshall, C.J. Specificity of receptor tyrosine kinase signaling: Transient versus sustained extracellular signal-regulated kinase activation. *Cell* **1995**, *80*, 179–185. [CrossRef]
38. McKay, M.M.; Morrison, D.K. Integrating signals from RTKs to ERK/MAPK. *Oncogene* **2007**, *26*, 3113–3121. [CrossRef]
39. Wee, P.; Wang, Z. Epidermal Growth Factor Receptor Cell Proliferation Signaling Pathways. *Cancers* **2017**, *9*, 52.
40. Katz, M.; Amit, I.; Yarden, Y. Regulation of MAPKs by growth factors and receptor tyrosine kinases. *Biochim. Biophys. Acta* **2007**, *1773*, 1161–1176. [CrossRef]
41. Schlessinger, J. Receptor tyrosine kinases: Legacy of the first two decades. *Cold Spring Harb. Perspect. Biol.* **2014**, *6*, a008912. [CrossRef]
42. Liu, F.; Yang, X.; Geng, M.; Huang, M. Targeting ERK, an Achilles' Heel of the MAPK pathway, in cancer therapy. *Acta Pharm. Sin. B* **2018**, *8*, 552–562. [CrossRef] [PubMed]

43. Lemmon, M.A.; Schlessinger, J. Cell signaling by receptor tyrosine kinases. *Cell* **2010**, *141*, 1117–1134. [CrossRef] [PubMed]
44. van der Geer, P.; Hunter, T.; Lindberg, R.A. Receptor Protein-Tyrosine Kinases and Their Signal-Transduction Pathways. *Annu. Rev. Cell Biol.* **1994**, *10*, 251–337. [CrossRef] [PubMed]
45. Wellbrock, C.; Karasarides, M.; Marais, R. The RAF proteins take centre stage. *Nat. Rev. Mol. Cell Biol.* **2004**, *5*, 875–885. [CrossRef] [PubMed]
46. Okazaki, K.; Sagata, N. The Mos/MAP kinase pathway stabilizes c-Fos by phosphorylation and augments its transforming activity in NIH 3T3 cells. *EMBO J.* **1995**, *14*, 5048–5059. [CrossRef]
47. Das, S.; Cho, J.; Lambertz, I.; Kelliher, M.A.; Eliopoulos, A.G.; Du, K.; Tsichlis, P.N. Tpl2/cot signals activate ERK, JNK, and NF-kappaB in a cell-type and stimulus-specific manner. *J. Biol. Chem.* **2005**, *280*, 23748–23757. [CrossRef]
48. Gotoh, I.; Adachi, M.; Nishida, E. Identification and characterization of a novel MAP kinase kinase kinase, MLTK. *J. Biol. Chem.* **2001**, *276*, 4276–4286. [CrossRef]
49. Shenoy, S.K.; Drake, M.T.; Nelson, C.D.; Houtz, D.A.; Xiao, K.; Madabushi, S.; Reiter, E.; Premont, R.T.; Lichtarge, O.; Lefkowitz, R.J. beta-arrestin-dependent, G protein-independent ERK1/2 activation by the beta2 adrenergic receptor. *J. Biol. Chem.* **2006**, *281*, 1261–1273. [CrossRef]
50. Choi, M.; Staus, D.P.; Wingler, L.M.; Ahn, S.; Pani, B.; Capel, W.D.; Lefkowitz, R.J. G protein-coupled receptor kinases (GRKs) orchestrate biased agonism at the beta2-adrenergic receptor. *Sci. Signal* **2018**, *11*, eaar7084. [CrossRef]
51. Jain, R.; Watson, U.; Vasudevan, L.; Saini, D.K. ERK Activation Pathways Downstream of GPCRs. *Int. Rev. Cell Mol. Biol.* **2018**, *338*, 79–109.
52. Watson, U.; Jain, R.; Asthana, S.; Saini, D.K. Spatiotemporal Modulation of ERK Activation by GPCRs. *Int. Rev. Cell Mol. Biol.* **2018**, *338*, 111–140. [PubMed]
53. Morrison, D.K. KSR: A MAPK scaffold of the Ras pathway? *J. Cell Sci.* **2001**, *114*, 1609–1612. [PubMed]
54. Sharma, C.; Vomastek, T.; Tarcsafalvi, A.; Catling, A.D.; Schaeffer, H.J.; Eblen, S.T.; Weber, M.J. MEK partner 1 (MP1): Regulation of oligomerization in MAP kinase signaling. *J. Cell. Biochem.* **2005**, *94*, 708–719. [CrossRef] [PubMed]
55. Morrison, D.K.; Davis, R.J. Regulation of MAP kinase signaling modules by scaffold proteins in mammals. *Annu. Rev. Cell Dev. Biol.* **2003**, *19*, 91–118. [CrossRef] [PubMed]
56. Frodin, M.; Gammeltoft, S. Role and regulation of 90 kDa ribosomal S6 kinase (RSK) in signal transduction. *Mol. Cell. Endocrinol.* **1999**, *151*, 65–77. [CrossRef]
57. Reyskens, K.M.; Arthur, J.S.C. Emerging Roles of the Mitogen and Stress Activated Kinases MSK1 and MSK2. *Front. Cell Dev. Biol.* **2016**, *4*, 56. [CrossRef]
58. Gaestel, M. Specificity of signaling from MAPKs to MAPKAPKs: kinases' tango nuevo. *Front. Biosci.* **2008**, *13*, 6050–6059. [CrossRef]
59. Cruzalegui, F.H.; Cano, E.; Treisman, R. ERK activation induces phosphorylation of Elk-1 at multiple S/T-P motifs to high stoichiometry. *Oncogene* **1999**, *18*, 7948–7957. [CrossRef]
60. Dougherty, M.K.; Müller, J.; Ritt, D.A.; Zhou, M.; Zhou, X.Z.; Copeland, T.D.; Conrads, T.P.; Veenstra, T.D.; Lu, K.P.; Morrison, D.K. Regulation of Raf-1 by direct feedback phosphorylation. *Mol. Cell* **2005**, *17*, 215–224. [CrossRef]
61. Fritsche-Guenther, R.; Witzel, F.; Sieber, A.; Herr, R.; Schmidt, N.; Braun, S.; Brummer, T.; Sers, C.; Blüthgen, N. Strong negative feedback from Erk to Raf confers robustness to MAPK signalling. *Mol. Syst. Biol.* **2011**, *7*, 489. [CrossRef]
62. Shin, S.Y.; Rath, O.; Choo, S.M.; Fee, F.; McFerran, B.; Kolch, W.; Cho, K.H. Positive- and negative-feedback regulations coordinate the dynamic behavior of the Ras-Raf-MEK-ERK signal transduction pathway. *J. Cell Sci.* **2009**, *122 Pt 3*, 425–435. [CrossRef]
63. Dong, C.; Waters, S.B.; Holt, K.H.; Pessin, J.E. SOS phosphorylation and disassociation of the Grb2-SOS complex by the ERK and JNK signaling pathways. *J. Biol. Chem.* **1996**, *271*, 6328–6332.
64. Xu, B.E.; Wilsbacher, J.L.; Collisson, T.; Cobb, M.H. The N-terminal ERK-binding site of MEK1 is required for efficient feedback phosphorylation by ERK2 in vitro and ERK activation in vivo. *J. Biol. Chem.* **1999**, *274*, 34029–34035. [CrossRef] [PubMed]

65. Ekerot, M.; Stavridis, M.P.; Delavaine, L.; Mitchell, M.P.; Staples, C.; Owens, D.M.; Keenan, I.D.; Dickinson, R.J.; Storey, K.G.; Keyse, S.M. Negative-feedback regulation of FGF signalling by DUSP6/MKP-3 is driven by ERK1/2 and mediated by Ets factor binding to a conserved site within the DUSP6/MKP-3 gene promoter. *Biochem. J.* **2008**, *412*, 287–298. [CrossRef] [PubMed]
66. Nolen, B.; Taylor, S.; Ghosh, G. Regulation of protein kinases; controlling activity through activation segment conformation. *Mol. Cell* **2004**, *15*, 661–675. [CrossRef] [PubMed]
67. Kornev, A.P.; Haste, N.M.; Taylor, S.S.; Eyck, L.F. Surface comparison of active and inactive protein kinases identifies a conserved activation mechanism. *Proc. Natl. Acad. Sci. USA* **2006**, *103*, 17783–17788. [CrossRef]
68. Kornev, A.P.; Taylor, S.S. Dynamics-Driven Allostery in Protein Kinases. *Trends Biochem. Sci.* **2015**, *40*, 628–647. [CrossRef]
69. Beenstock, J.; Mooshayef, N.; Engelberg, D. How Do Protein Kinases Take a Selfie (Autophosphorylate)? *Trends Biochem. Sci.* **2016**, *41*, 938–953. [CrossRef]
70. Shi, F.; Telesco, S.E.; Liu, Y.; Radhakrishnan, R.; Lemmon, M.A. ErbB3/HER3 intracellular domain is competent to bind ATP and catalyze autophosphorylation. *Proc. Natl. Acad. Sci. USA* **2010**, *107*, 7692–7697. [CrossRef]
71. Pike, A.C.; Rellos, P.; Niesen, F.H.; Turnbull, A.; Oliver, A.W.; Parker, S.A.; Turk, B.E.; Pearl, L.H.; Knapp, S. Activation segment dimerization: A mechanism for kinase autophosphorylation of non-consensus sites. *EMBO J.* **2008**, *27*, 704–714. [CrossRef]
72. Seger, R.; Ahn, N.G.; Boulton, T.G.; Yancopoulos, G.D.; Panayotatos, N.; Radziejewska, E.; Ericsson, L.; Bratlien, R.L.; Cobb, M.H.; Krebs, E.G. Microtubule-associated protein 2 kinases, ERK1 and ERK2, undergo autophosphorylation on both tyrosine and threonine residues: Implications for their mechanism of activation. *Proc. Natl. Acad. Sci. USA* **1991**, *88*, 6142–6146. [CrossRef] [PubMed]
73. Levin-Salomon, V.; Kogan, K.; Ahn, N.G.; Livnah, O.; Engelberg, D. Isolation of intrinsically active (MEK-independent) variants of the ERK family of mitogen-activated protein (MAP) kinases. *J. Biol. Chem.* **2008**, *283*, 34500–34510. [CrossRef] [PubMed]
74. Pegram, L.M.; Liddle, J.C.; Xiao, Y.; Hoh, M.; Rudolph, J.; Iverson, D.B.; Vigers, G.P.; Smith, D.; Zhang, H.; Wang, W.; et al. Activation loop dynamics are controlled by conformation-selective inhibitors of ERK2. *Proc. Natl. Acad. Sci. USA* **2019**, *116*, 15463–15468. [CrossRef] [PubMed]
75. Sang, D.; Pinglay, S.; Wiewiora, R.P.; Selvan, M.E.; Lou, H.J.; Chodera, J.D.; Turk, B.E.; Gumus, Z.H.; Holt, L.J. Ancestral reconstruction reveals mechanisms of ERK regulatory evolution. *eLife* **2019**, *8*, e38805. [CrossRef] [PubMed]
76. Emrick, M.A.; Lee, T.; Starkey, P.J.; Mumby, M.C.; Resing, K.A.; Ahn, N.G. The gatekeeper residue controls autoactivation of ERK2 via a pathway of intramolecular connectivity. *Proc. Natl. Acad. Sci. USA* **2006**, *103*, 18101–18106. [CrossRef] [PubMed]
77. Brunner, D.; Oellers, N.; Szabad, J.; Biggs, W.H.; Zipursky, S.L.; Hafen, E. A gain-of-function mutation in Drosophila MAP kinase activates multiple receptor tyrosine kinase signaling pathways. *Cell* **1994**, *76*, 875–888. [CrossRef]
78. Goshen-Lago, T.; Goldberg-Carp, A.; Melamed, D.; Darlyuk-Saadon, I.; Bai, C.; Ahn, N.G.; Admon, A.; Engelberg, D. Variants of the yeast MAPK Mpk1 are fully functional independently of activation loop phosphorylation. *Mol. Biol. Cell* **2016**, *27*, 2771–2783. [CrossRef]
79. Dhillon, A.S.; Hagan, S.; Rath, O.; Kolch, W. MAP kinase signalling pathways in cancer. *Oncogene* **2007**, *26*, 3279–3290. [CrossRef]
80. Hanahan, D.; Weinberg, R.A. Hallmarks of cancer: The next generation. *Cell* **2011**, *144*, 646–674. [CrossRef]
81. Samatar, A.A.; Poulikakos, P.I. Targeting RAS-ERK signalling in cancer: Promises and challenges. *Nat. Rev. Drug Discov.* **2014**, *13*, 928–942. [CrossRef]
82. Smorodinsky-Atias, K.; Goshen-Lago, T.; Goldberg-Carp, A.; Melamed, D.; Shir, A.; Mooshayef, N.; Beenstock, J.; Karamansha, Y.; DArlyuk-Saadon, I.; Livnah, O.; et al. Intrinsically active variants of Erk oncogenically transform cells and disclose unexpected autophosphorylation capability that is independent of TEY phosphorylation. *Mol. Biol. Cell* **2016**, *27*, 1026–1039. [CrossRef] [PubMed]
83. Kushnir, T.; Bar-Cohen, S.; Mooshayef, N.; Lange, R.; Bar-Sinai, A.; Rozen, H.; Salzberg, A.; Engelberg, D.; Paroush, Z. An Activating Mutation in ERK Causes Hyperplastic Tumors in a scribble Mutant Tissue in Drosophila. *Genetics* **2019**. [CrossRef] [PubMed]
84. Groenendijk, F.H.; Bernards, R. Drug resistance to targeted therapies: Deja vu all over again. *Mol. Oncol.* **2014**, *8*, 1067–1083. [CrossRef] [PubMed]

85. Morris, E.J.; Jha, S.; Restaino, C.R.; Dayananth, P.; Zhu, H.; Cooper, A.; Carr, D.; Deng, Y.; Jin, W.; Black, S.; et al. Discovery of a novel ERK inhibitor with activity in models of acquired resistance to BRAF and MEK inhibitors. *Cancer Discov.* **2013**, *3*, 742–750. [CrossRef]
86. Moschos, S.J.; Sullivan, R.J.; Hwu, W.J.; Ramanathan, R.K.; Adjei, A.A.; Fong, P.C.; Shapira-Frommer, R.; Tawbi, H.A.; Rubino, J.; Rush, T.S.; et al. Development of MK-8353, an orally administered ERK1/2 inhibitor, in patients with advanced solid tumors. *JCI Insight* **2018**, *3*, e92352. [CrossRef]
87. Germann, U.A.; Furey, B.F.; Markland, W.; Hoover, R.R.; Aronov, A.M.; Roix, J.J.; Hale, M.; Boucher, D.M.; Sorrell, D.A.; Martinez-Botella, G.; et al. Targeting the MAPK Signaling Pathway in Cancer: Promising Preclinical Activity with the Novel Selective ERK1/2 Inhibitor BVD-523 (Ulixertinib). *Mol. Cancer Ther.* **2017**, *16*, 2351–2363. [CrossRef]
88. Blake, J.F.; Burkard, M.; Chan, J.; Chen, H.; Chou, K.J.; Diaz, D.; Dudley, D.A.; Gaudino, J.J.; Gould, S.E.; Grina, J.; et al. Discovery of (S)-1-(1-(4-Chloro-3-fluorophenyl)-2-hydroxyethyl)-4-(2-((1-methyl-1H-pyrazol-5-yl)amino)pyrimidin-4-yl)pyridin-2(1H)-one (GDC-0994), an Extracellular Signal-Regulated Kinase 1/2 (ERK1/2) Inhibitor in Early Clinical Development. *J. Med. Chem.* **2016**, *59*, 5650–5660. [CrossRef]
89. Aronov, A.M.; Baker, C.; Bemis, G.W.; Cao, J.; Chen, G.; Ford, P.J.; Germann, U.A.; Green, J.; Hale, M.R.; Jacobs, M.; et al. Flipped out: Structure-guided design of selective pyrazolylpyrrole ERK inhibitors. *J. Med. Chem.* **2007**, *50*, 1280–1287. [CrossRef]
90. Bhagwat, S.V.; McMillen, W.T.; Cai, S.; Zhao, B.; Whitesell, M.; Kindler, L.; Flack, R.S.; Wu, W.; Huss, K.; Anderson, B.; et al. Discovery of LY3214996, a selective and novel ERK1/2 inhibitor with potent antitumor activities in cancer models with MAPK pathway alterations. *Cancer Res.* **2017**, *77*. [CrossRef]
91. Ohori, M.; Kinoshita, T.; Okubo, M.; Sato, K.; Yamazaki, A.; Arakawa, H.; Nishimura, S.; Inamura, N.; Nakajima, H.; Neya, M.; et al. Identification of a selective ERK inhibitor and structural determination of the inhibitor-ERK2 complex. *Biochem. Biophys. Res. Commun.* **2005**, *336*, 357–363. [CrossRef]
92. Aronov, A.M.; Tang, Q.; Martinez-Botella, G.; Bemis, G.W.; Cao, J.; Chen, G.; Ewing, N.P.; Ford, P.J.; Germann, U.A.; Green, J.; et al. Structure-guided design of potent and selective pyrimidylpyrrole inhibitors of extracellular signal-regulated kinase (ERK) using conformational control. *J. Med. Chem.* **2009**, *52*, 6362–6368. [CrossRef] [PubMed]
93. Herrero, A.; Pinto, A.; Colon-Bolea, P.; Casar, B.; Jones, M.; Agudo-Ibanez, L.; Vidal, R.; Tenbaum, S.P.; Nuciforo, P.; Valdizan, E.M.; et al. Small Molecule Inhibition of ERK Dimerization Prevents Tumorigenesis by RAS-ERK Pathway Oncogenes. *Cancer Cell* **2015**, *28*, 170–182. [CrossRef] [PubMed]
94. Ryan, M.B.; Corcoran, R.B. Therapeutic strategies to target RAS-mutant cancers. *Nat. Rev. Clin. Oncol.* **2018**, *15*, 709–720. [CrossRef] [PubMed]
95. Brenan, L.; Andreev, A.; Cohen, O.; Pantel, S.; Kamburov, A.; Cacchiarelli, D.; Persky, N.S.; Zhu, C.; Bagul, M.; Goettz, E.M.; et al. Phenotypic Characterization of a Comprehensive Set of MAPK1/ERK2 Missense Mutants. *Cell Rep.* **2016**, *17*, 1171–1183. [CrossRef]
96. Goetz, E.M.; Ghandi, M.; Treacy, D.J.; Wagle, N.; Garraway, L.A. ERK mutations confer resistance to mitogen-activated protein kinase pathway inhibitors. *Cancer Res.* **2014**, *74*, 7079–7089. [CrossRef]
97. Jha, S.; Morris, E.J.; Hruza, A.; Mansueto, M.S.; Schroeder, G.K.; Arbanas, J.; McMasters, D.; Restaino, C.R.; Dayanath, P.; Black, S.; et al. *Dissecting* Therapeutic Resistance to ERK Inhibition. *Mol. Cancer Ther.* **2016**, *15*, 548–559. [CrossRef]
98. Askari, N.; Diskin, R.; Avitzour, M.; Yaakov, G.; Livnah, O.; Engelberg, D. MAP-quest: Could we produce constitutively active variants of MAP kinases? *Mol. Cell. Endocrinol.* **2006**, *252*, 231–240. [CrossRef]
99. Cowley, S.; Paterson, H.; Kemp, P.; Marshall, C.J. Activation of Map Kinase Kinase Is Necessary and Sufficient for Pc12 Differentiation and for Transformation of Nih 3t3 Cells. *Cell* **1994**, *77*, 841–852. [CrossRef]
100. Huang, S.; Jiang, Y.; Li, Z.; Nishida, E.; Mathias, P.; Lin, S.; Ulevitch, R.J.; Nemerow, G.R.; Hanj, J. Apoptosis signaling pathway in T cells is composed of ICE/Ced-3 family proteases and MAP kinase kinase 6b. *Immunity* **1997**, *6*, 739–749. [CrossRef]
101. Prowse, C.N.; Deal, M.S.; Lew, J. The complete pathway for catalytic activation of the mitogen-activated protein kinase, ERK2. *J. Biol. Chem.* **2001**, *276*, 40817–40823. [CrossRef]
102. Robbins, D.J.; Zhen, E.; Owaki, H.; Vanderblit, C.A.; Ebert, D.; Geppert, T.D.; Cobb, M.H. Regulation and properties of extracellular signal-regulated protein kinases 1 and 2 in vitro. *J. Biol. Chem.* **1993**, *268*, 5097–5106. [PubMed]

103. Emrick, M.A.; Hoofnagle, A.N.; Miller, A.S.; Ten Eyck, L.F.; Ahn, N.G. Constitutive activation of extracellular signal-regulated kinase 2 by synergistic point mutations. *J. Biol. Chem.* **2001**, *276*, 46469–46479. [CrossRef] [PubMed]
104. Brill, J.A.; Elion, E.A.; Fink, G.R. A role for autophosphorylation revealed by activated alleles of FUS3, the yeast MAP kinase homolog. *Mol. Biol. Cell* **1994**, *5*, 297–312. [CrossRef] [PubMed]
105. Madhani, H.D.; Styles, C.A.; Fink, G.R. MAP kinases with distinct inhibitory functions impart signaling specificity during yeast differentiation. *Cell* **1997**, *91*, 673–684. [CrossRef]
106. Bott, C.M.; Thorneycroft, S.G.; Marshall, C.J. The sevenmaker gain-of-function mutation in p42 MAP kinase leads to enhanced signalling and reduced sensitivity to dual specificity phosphatase action. *FEBS Lett.* **1994**, *352*, 201–205. [CrossRef]
107. Hall, J.P.; Cherkasova, V.; Elion, E.; Gustin, M.C.; Winter, E. The osmoregulatory pathway represses mating pathway activity in Saccharomyces cerevisiae: Isolation of a FUS3 mutant that is insensitive to the repression mechanism. *Mol. Cell. Biol.* **1996**, *16*, 6715–6723. [CrossRef]
108. Mutlak, M.; Schlesinger-Laufer, M.; Haas, T.; Shofti, R.; Ballan, N.; Lewis, Y.E.; Zuler, M.; Zohar, Y.; Caspi, L.H.; Kehat, I. Extracellular signal-regulated kinase (ERK) activation preserves cardiac function in pressure overload induced hypertrophy. *Int. J. Cardiol.* **2018**, *270*, 204–213. [CrossRef]
109. Canagarajah, B.J.; Khokhlatchev, A.; Cobb, M.H.; Golsdmisth, E.J. Activation mechanism of the MAP kinase ERK2 by dual phosphorylation. *Cell* **1997**, *90*, 859–869. [CrossRef]
110. Taylor, C.A.; Cormier, K.W.; Keenan, S.E.; Earnest, S.; Stippec, S.; Wichaidit, C.; Juang, Y.C.; Wang, J.; Shvartsman, S.Y.; Goldsmith, E.J.; et al. Functional divergence caused by mutations in an energetic hotspot in ERK2. *Proc. Natl. Acad. Sci. USA* **2019**, *116*, 15514–15523. [CrossRef]
111. Lee, T.; Hoofnagle, A.N.; Kabuyama, Y.; Stoud, J.; Min, X.; Goldsmith, E.J.; Chen, L.; Resing, K.A.; Ahn, N.G. Docking motif interactions in MAP kinases revealed by hydrogen exchange mass spectrometry. *Mol. Cell* **2004**, *14*, 43–55. [CrossRef]
112. Dimitri, C.A.; Dowdle, W.; MacKeiga, J.P.; Blenis, J.; Murphy, L.O. Spatially separate docking sites on ERK2 regulate distinct signaling events in vivo. *Curr. Biol.* **2005**, *15*, 1319–1324. [CrossRef]
113. Misiura, M.; Kolomeisky, A.B. Kinetic network model to explain gain-of-function mutations in ERK2 enzyme. *J. Chem. Phys.* **2019**, *150*, 155101. [CrossRef] [PubMed]
114. Barr, D.; Oashi, T.; Burkhard, K.; Lucius, S.; Samadani, R.; Zhang, J.; Shapiro, P.; MacKerell, A.D.; van der Vaart, A. Importance of domain closure for the autoactivation of ERK2. *Biochemistry* **2011**, *50*, 8038–8048. [CrossRef] [PubMed]
115. Mahalingam, M.; Arvind, R.; Ida, H.; Murugan, A.K.; Yamaguchi, M.; Tsuchida, N. ERK2 CD domain mutation from a human cancer cell line enhanced anchorage-independent cell growth and abnormality in Drosophila. *Oncol. Rep.* **2008**, *20*, 957–962. [PubMed]

7

Disruption of the NF-κB/IL-8 Signaling Axis by Sulconazole Inhibits Human Breast Cancer Stem Cell Formation

Hack Sun Choi [1,2,†], Ji-Hyang Kim [3,†], Su-Lim Kim [1,3] and Dong-Sun Lee [1,2,3,*]

1 School of Biomaterials Sciences and Technology, College of Applied Life Science, Jeju National University, Jeju 63243, Korea
2 Subtropical/tropical Organism Gene Bank, Jeju National University, Jeju 63243, Korea
3 Interdisciplinary Graduate Program in Advanced Convergence Technology & Science, Jeju National University, Jeju 63243, Korea
* Correspondence: dongsunlee@jejunu.ac.kr
† These authors contributed equally to this work.

Abstract: Breast cancer stem cells (BCSCs) are tumor-initiating cells that possess the capacity for self-renewal. Cancer stem cells (CSCs) are responsible for poor outcomes caused by therapeutic resistance. In our study, we found that sulconazole—an antifungal medicine in the imidazole class—inhibited cell proliferation, tumor growth, and CSC formation. This compound also reduced the frequency of cells expressing CSC markers ($CD44^{high}/CD24^{low}$) as well as the expression of another CSC marker, aldehyde dehydrogenase (ALDH), and other self-renewal-related genes. Sulconazole inhibited mammosphere formation, reduced the protein level of nuclear NF-κB, and reduced extracellular IL-8 levels in mammospheres. Knocking down NF-κB expression using a p65-specific siRNA reduced CSC formation and secreted IL-8 levels in mammospheres. Sulconazole reduced nuclear NF-κB protein levels and secreted IL-8 levels in mammospheres. These new findings show that sulconazole blocks the NF-κB/IL-8 signaling pathway and CSC formation. NF-κB/IL-8 signaling is important for CSC formation and may be an important therapeutic target for BCSC treatment.

Keywords: sulconazole; NF-κB; IL-8; mammosphere; breast cancer stem cells

1. Introduction

Breast cancer is a cancer that develops from common breast tissue and a major fatal health problem among females [1]. Patients treated with different therapeutics suffer from cancer relapse and metastasis because of cancer stem cells (CSCs), a subpopulation of tumor cells. CSCs are heterogeneous bulk tumor cells that differentiate into cancer cells. CSCs are resistant to chemotherapies and contribute to tumor heterogeneity [2]. CSCs were first identified in leukemia and found to show properties similar to those of stem cells by Bonnet and Dick [3]. Markers of breast cancer stem cells (BCSCs) include CD44, CD133, and ALDH1. CD44 expression is upregulated in the microenvironment that promotes cancer progression and metastasis [4]. Additionally, CD44 isoforms are reliable markers of CSCs. The CD44 isoform CD44v-xCT regulates redox in cancer stem cells [5]. The signaling pathways regulating CSC stemness and differentiation are the Wnt, Hedgehog, Hippo, and Notch signaling pathways. Molecular targeting of these pathways to inhibit BCSCs may be a useful tool for cancer treatment [6]. Sox2, Nanog, Oct4, and c-Myc are crucial for CSC formation and potential targets for cancer therapy. One report showed that NF-κB was involved in CSCs from primary acute myeloid leukemia (AML) samples [7]. Additionally, BCSCs overexpress NF-κB signaling pathway components and induce NF-κB activity. BCSCs have high protein expression of NF-κB [8]. Inhibiting NF-κB signaling with BMS-345541 in lung cancer reduces the stemness and self-renewal capacity of lung CSCs [9]. The cytokines IL-6 and IL-8 regulate links between CSCs and the microenvironment. The Stat3 and NF-κB pathways regulate the gene expression of IL-6 and IL-8 in breast cancer. Microenvironmental IL-6 and IL-8 regulate BCSC populations [10]. In lung cancer patients, high extracellular IL-6 levels are associated with a poor prognosis [11,12]. IL-6 regulates BCSC formation through the IL-6/IL-6 receptor interaction [13]. The protein expression level of IL-8 is higher in breast cancer cells than in normal breast tissue cells, and IL-8 promotes cancer progression. IL-8 promotes BCSC activity through the CXCR1/IL8 interaction. IL-8/CXCR1 signaling is an important pathway for targeting BCSCs [14]. Azole compounds used as antifungal drugs inhibit the ergosterol biosynthesis pathway through suppression of the enzyme lanosterol 14-α-demethylase, a cytochrome P450 (CYP) enzyme. Azole antifungal drugs consist of an imidazole (clotrimazole and ketoconazole) and a triazole (fluconazole and itraconazole). Recently, antifungal imidazole drugs have well-established pharmacokinetic profiles and known toxicity, which can make these generic drugs strong candidates for repositioning as antitumor therapies [15]. Sulconazole is an antifungal medicine in the imidazole class and has broad-spectrum activity against dermatophytes [16]. We demonstrated that sulconazole had antiproliferative properties in breast cancer and inhibited BCSC formation through a reduction in IL-8 expression induced by disrupting the NF-κB pathway.

2. Materials and Methods

2.1. Cell Lines and Media

MCF-7 and MDA-MB-231 cells were grown in Dulbecco's modified Eagle's medium (DMEM; Gibco, Thermo Fisher Scientific, Waltham, CA, USA) supplemented with 10% (v/v) fetal bovine serum (FBS; Thermo Fisher Scientific, Waltham, CA, USA), 1% penicillin and streptomycin in a humidified 5% CO_2 incubator at 37 °C. Breast cancer cells were cultured at a concentration of 3.5×10^4 or 0.5×10^4 cells/well in an Ultralow Adherent plate containing MammoCult™ medium (STEMCELL Technologies, Vancouver, BC, Canada) supplemented with heparin and hydrocortisone in a humidified 5% CO_2 incubator at 37 °C. A 6-well plate was scanned, and mammosphere counting was performed using the NICE program [17]. A mammosphere formation assay was determined by evaluating mammosphere formation efficiency (MFE) (%) as previously described [18].

2.2. Antibodies, siRNAs, and Plasmids

Anti-pStat3 (Y705) (rabbit monoclonal) antibodies were obtained from Cell Signaling Technology. Anti-p65 (mouse polyclonal), anti-pp65, anti-Stat3 (rabbit monoclonal), anti-β-actin (mouse polyclonal), and anti-Lamin b antibodies were purchased from Santa Cruz Biotechnology. Anti-CD44 FITC-conjugated and anti-CD24 PE-conjugated antibodies were obtained from BD Pharmingen. A human p65-specific siRNA and scrambled siRNA were purchased from Bioneer (Daejeon, Korea).

2.3. Cell Proliferation

We used a previously reported method [19]. Breast cancer cells were incubated in a 96-well plate with sulconazole for 24 h. We followed the manufacturer's protocol for a CellTiter 96® Aqueous One Solution cell kit (Promega), and the optical density at 490 nm (OD_{490}) was determined using a plate reader (SpectraMax, Molecular Devices, San Jose, CA, USA).

2.4. Colony Formation and Migration Assays

MDA-MB-231 cells were cultured at 2×10^3 cells/well with different concentrations of sulconazole in DMEM/10% FBS. The cancer cells were incubated, and colonies were counted. The cancer cells were incubated in a 6-well plate, and a scratch was made using a microtip. After washing with

DMEM, the breast cancer cells were cultured with sulconazole. We followed a previously described method [20].

2.5. *Flow Cytometry Analysis of the Expression of CD24 and CD44 and an ALDEFLUOR Assay*

We used a previously described method [20]. In total, 1×10^6 cells were incubated with FITC-conjugated anti-CD44 and PE-conjugated anti-CD24 antibodies (BD, San Jose, CA, USA) and incubated on ice for 20 min. The breast cancer cells were washed two times with 1X PBS and assayed by using a flow cytometer (BD curi C6, San Jose, CA, USA). An ALDH1 assay was performed using an ALDEFUOR kit (STEMCELL Technologies, Vancouver, BC, Canada). We followed a previously described method [20]. Breast cancer cells were incubated in ALDH assay buffer at 37 °C for 20 min. ALDH-positive cells were determined by using a personal flow cytometer (BD Accuri C6).

2.6. *RNA Isolation and Real-Time RT-qPCR*

Total RNA was purified, and RT-qPCR was performed using a one-step RT-qPCR kit (Takara, Tokyo, Japan). We followed a previously described method [19]. The specific primers used can be found in Supplementary Table S1. The β-actin gene was used as an internal control for RT-qPCR.

2.7. *Immunoblot Analysis*

Proteins isolated from breast cancer cells and mammospheres were separated by 10% SDS-PAGE and transferred to a polyvinylidene fluoride (PVDF) membrane (EMD Millipore, Burlington, MA, USA). The blots were blocked in 5% skim milk in 1X PBS-Tween 20 at room temperature for 60 min and then incubated overnight at 4 °C with primary antibodies. The antibodies were anti-JAK2, anti-Stat3, anti-p65, anti-pp65, anti-lamin B, anti-phospho-Stat3 (Cell Signaling, Danvers, MA, USA), and anti-β-actin (Santa Cruz Biotechnology, Dallas, TA, USA) antibodies. After washing, the blots were detected with IRDye 680 RD and 800 CW secondary antibodies, and images were detected by using ODYSSEY CLx (LI-COR, Lincoln, NE, USA).

2.8. *Electrophoretic Mobility Shift Assays (EMSAs)*

Nuclear extracts were prepared as described previously [21]. An EMSA for NF-κB binding was performed using an IRDye 800-labeled NF-κB consequence oligonucleotide (LI-COR) for 30 min at room temperature. Samples were run on a nondenaturing 6% PAGE gel, and EMSA data were captured by ODYSSEY CLx (LI-COR). Supershifts were analyzed by incubating nuclear extracts for 30 min before the addition of the IRDye 800-labeled NF-κB consequence oligonucleotide.

2.9. *In Vivo Mouse Experiments*

Twelve female BALB/C nude mice were injected with MDA-MB-231 cells and treated with/without sulconazole (10 mg/kg). Tumor volume was measured after 1.5 months using a formula (Figure 2). Mouse experiments were performed as described previously [22]. Animal care and animal experiments were conducted in accordance with protocols approved by the Jeju National University Animal Care and Use Committee. Female BALB/C nude mice (5 weeks old) were obtained from OrientBio (Seoul, Korea) and kept in mouse facilities for 7 days. Twelve female BALB/C nude mice injected with MDA-MB-231 cells were monitored. Nude mice ($n = 6$) received sulconazole using mammary fat pad injection with an optimized dosage of 10 mg/kg. The dose of drug used was 10 mg/kg (200 μg/100 μL) once a week. The measurement was made every 3 to 4 days starting from day 10. The solvent used is DMSO. Tumor volumes were measured using the formula: $V = (\text{width}^2 \times \text{length})/2$.

2.10. Statistical Analysis

All data from three independent experiments are shown as the mean ± standard deviation (SD). Data were analyzed using one-way ANOVA. A p-value less than 0.05 was considered statistically significant.

3. Results

3.1. Sulconazole Inhibits the Proliferation of Breast Cancer Cells

We examined the antiproliferative effect of sulconazole on human breast cancer cells. Sulconazole inhibited proliferation (Figure 1A,B). Apoptosis in breast cancer cells was induced by sulconazole at a concentration of 20 μM (Figure 1C). Sulconazole induced caspase3/7 activity in breast cancer cells (Figure 1D). The breast cancer cells showed formation of apoptotic bodies in response to sulconazole treatment (Figure 1E). Sulconazole inhibited the migration of cancer cells and reduced the number of colonies (Figure 1F,G). Our data showed that sulconazole effectively inhibited proliferation, migration, and colony formation.

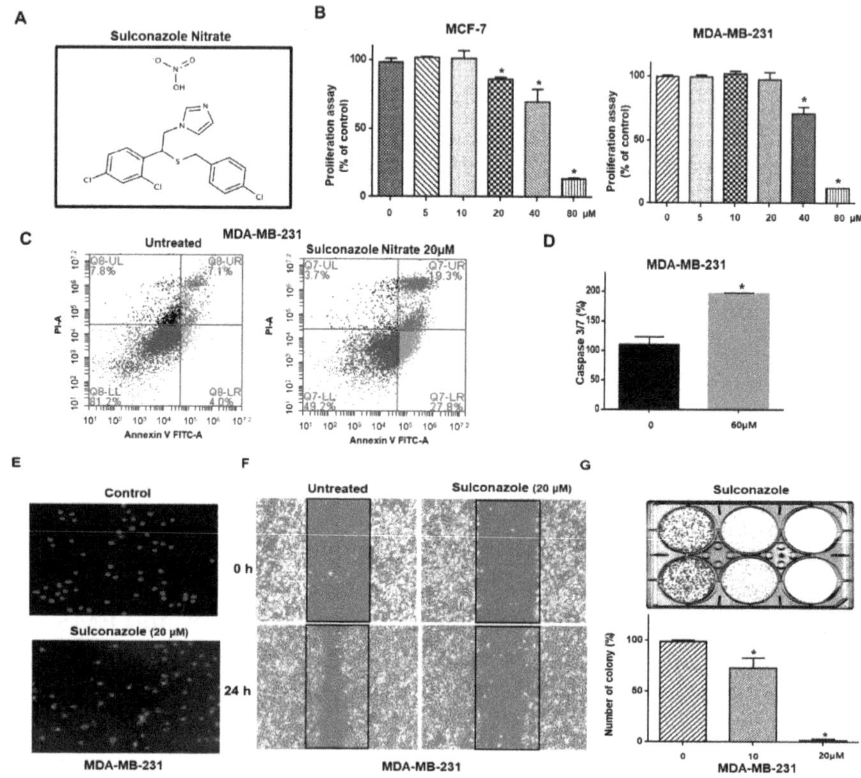

Figure 1. Sulconazole inhibits cell proliferation in breast cancer. (**A**) The molecular structure of sulconazole is shown. (**B**) Breast cancer cells were incubated in a 96-well plate with the indicated concentration of sulconazole. Cell proliferation was measured by an MTS assay. (**C**) Sulconazole induced apoptosis in cancer cells at the indicated concentration. Apoptotic cells were determined using Annexin V/PI staining. (**D**) The caspase3/7 activity of cancer cells was determined using a Caspase-Glo 3/7 assay kit (Promega). The data are presented as the mean ± SD; $n = 3$ independent experiments; * $p <$ 0.05 vs. the control (0.3% DMSO). (**E**) Apoptotic cells were analyzed by fluorescence nuclear staining using Hoechst 33,258 dye (magnification, 40×). (**F**) The effect of sulconazole on the migration of cancer cells was evaluated using a scratch assay. The scratch assay was performed with cancer cells treated with sulconazole. (**G**) The effect of sulconazole on colony formation is shown. 1000 cancer cells were incubated in 6-well plates with sulconazole (0.1% DMSO) and 0.1% DMSO. Representative images were recorded. The data are presented as the mean ± SD; $n = 3$ independent experiments; * $p < 0.05$ vs. the control.

3.2. Sulconazole Inhibits Tumor Growth

As sulconazole has cytotoxic activity in breast cancer, we tested whether sulconazole inhibits tumor growth in an in vivo mouse model. The tumor volume in sulconazole-injected mice was smaller than that in control mice (Figure 2A). The tumor weights in the sulconazole-injected mice were lower than those in the control mice (Figure 2B). The sulconazole-treated mice showed body weights similar to those of the control mice (data not shown). Our data showed that sulconazole effectively decreased tumor growth in the xenograft mouse model.

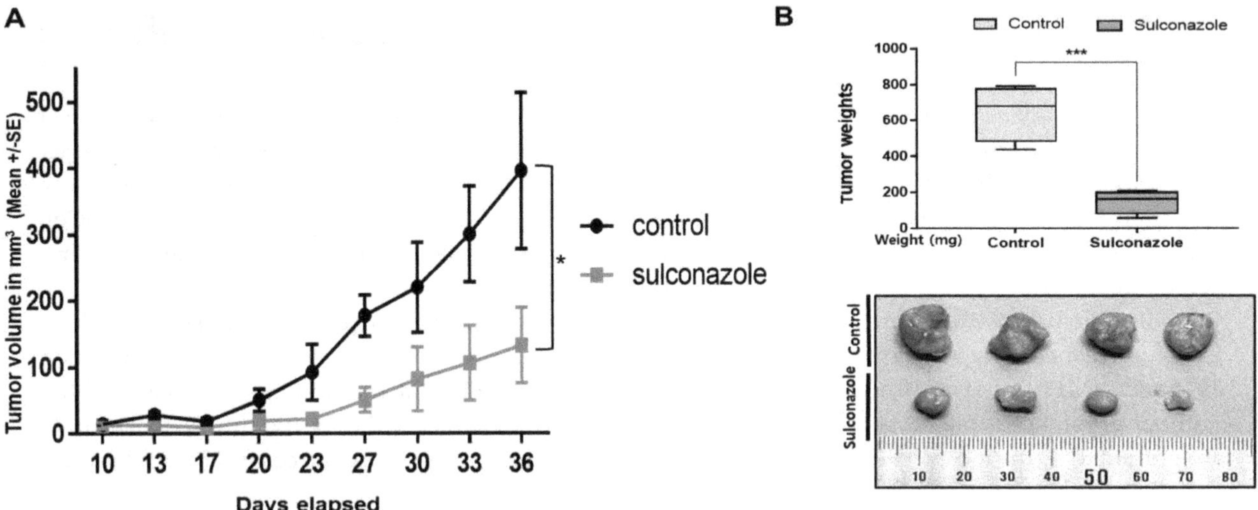

Figure 2. Effect of sulconazole on in vivo tumor growth. (**A**) NOD-SCID nude mice were inoculated with MDA-MB-231 cells and treated with sulconazole or vehicle. The dose of drug used was 10 mg/kg once a week. Tumor volume was measured at the indicated time points using a caliper and calculated as (width^2 × length)/2 and are reported (Mean ± SE). (**B**) The effect of sulconazole on tumor weights was evaluated. Tumor weights were assayed after sacrifice. Photographs were taken of isolated tumors from control or sulconazole-treated mice. * $p < 0.05$ and *** $p < 0.05$ vs. the control.

3.3. Effect of Sulconazole on the Properties of BCSCs

To examine whether sulconazole inhibits mammosphere formation, we treated mammospheres derived from breast cancer cells (MCF-7 and MDA-MB-231) with different concentrations of sulconazole. Sulconazole inhibited mammosphere formation. The number of mammospheres declined by 90%, and mammosphere size also decreased (Figure 3A,B). $CD44^+/CD24^-$ cancer cells were assessed under sulconazole treatment. Sulconazole reduced the percentage of $CD44^+/CD24^-$ cells from 14.23% to 3.53% (Figure 4A). Additionally, we performed an ALDEFLUOR assay to examine the effect of sulconazole on ALDH-positive cells. Sulconazole reduced the ALDH-positive cell percentage from 3.2% to 1.5% (Figure 4B). Our data show that sulconazole inhibits BCSCs.

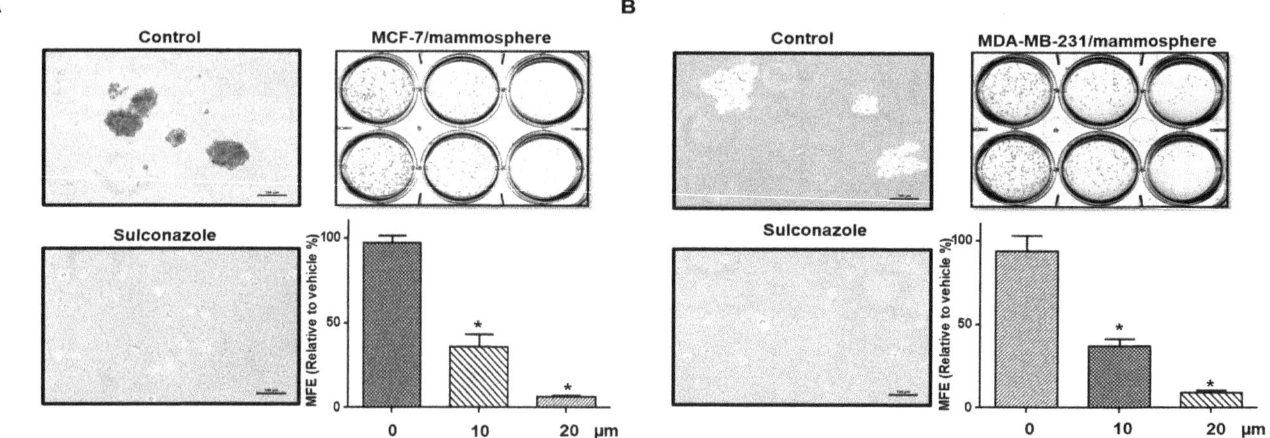

Figure 3. Effect of sulconazole on the mammosphere-forming ability of breast cancer cells. (**A, B**) Effect of sulconazole on the mammosphere formation of breast cancer cells. To establish mammospheres, MCF-7 and MDA-MB-231 cells were seeded at a density of 4×10^4 and 1×10^4 cells/well, respectively, in ultralow attachment 6-well plates containing 2 mL of complete MammoCult^{TM} medium (StemCell Technologies) which was supplemented with 4 μg/mL heparin, 0.48 μg/mL hydrocortisone, 100 U/mL penicillin, and 100 μg/mL streptomycin. Mammospheres were cultured with sulconazole (10 or 20 μM) solubilized in 0.05% DMSO or 0. 1% DMSO. The breast cancer cells were incubated with sulconazole in CSC culture medium for 7 days. A mammosphere formation assay evaluated mammosphere formation efficiency (MFE, % of control), which corresponds to the number of mammospheres per well/the number of total cells plated per well ×100 as previously described (scale bar = 100 μm) [22]. The data are presented as the mean ± SD; $n = 3$ independent experiments;* $p < 0.05$ vs. the control (0. 1% DMSO).

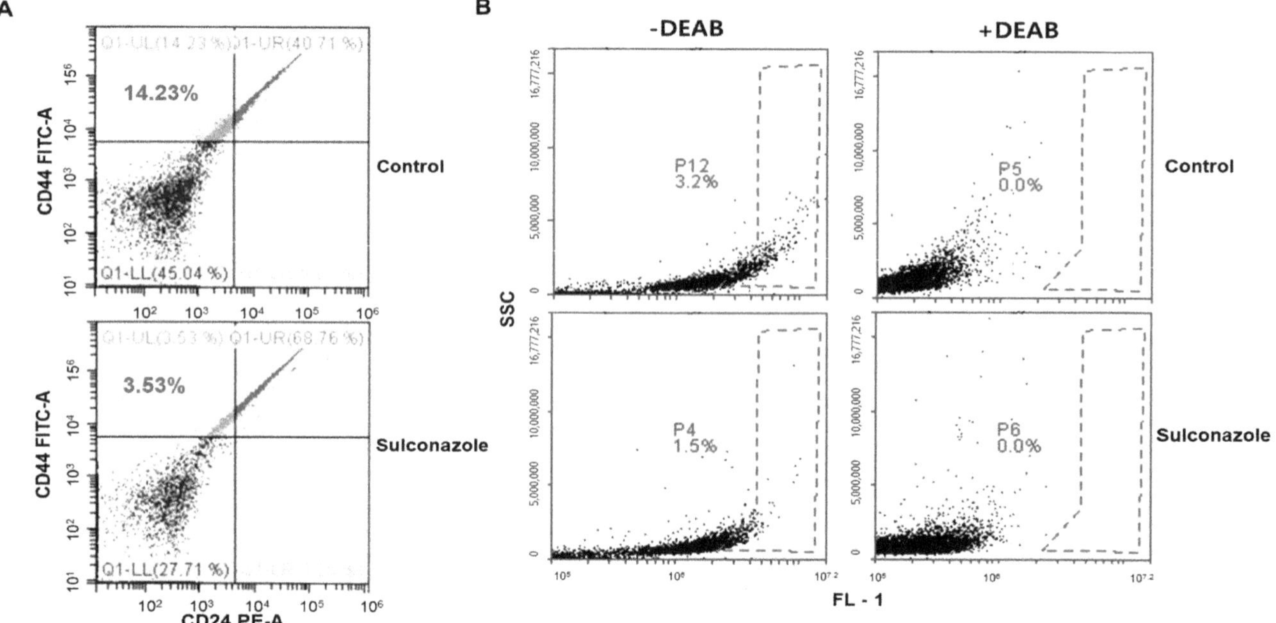

Figure 4. Effect of sulconazole on $CD44^+/CD24^-$-and ALDH-positive cell populations. (**A**) The $CD44^+/CD24^-$ cell population treated with sulconazole (20 μM) was assayed by flow cytometry. For FACS analysis, 10,000 cells were assayed. Gating was based on binding of the control antibody (Red cross). (**B**) ALDH-positive cells were detected by using an ALDEFLUOR kit. A representative flow cytometry dot plot is shown. The right panel indicates ALDH-positive cells treated with the ALDH inhibitor DEAB (7.5 μM), and the left panel shows ALDH-positive cells without DEAB treatment. The ALDH-positive population was gated in a box (red dot line box).

3.4. *Sulconazole Inhibits Mammosphere Formation Through the Inhibition of p65 Nuclear Translocation*

To understand the molecular mechanism of sulconazole in mammosphere formation, the nuclear translocation of p65 was evaluated in mammospheres. Our data showed that nuclear phosphor-p65 and p65 levels were reduced significantly in a dose-dependent manner under sulconazole treatment (Figure 5A). Because caffeic acid phenethyl ester (CAPE) inhibits the nuclear translocation of p65 and the activation of the NF-κB signaling pathway [23], we evaluated mammosphere formation after treatment with CAPE. CAPE inhibited mammosphere formation. As a result of the use of sulconazole and CAPE, we showed that the inhibition of p65 nuclear translocation blocked mammosphere formation (Figure 5C). To examine p65 function in BCSCs, we tested the effect of NF-kB using a p65-specific siRNA. siRNA-p65 inhibited mammosphere formation in breast cancer (Figure 5B). In conclusion, we show that NF-κB regulates CSC formation and a CSC survival factor (Figure 5).

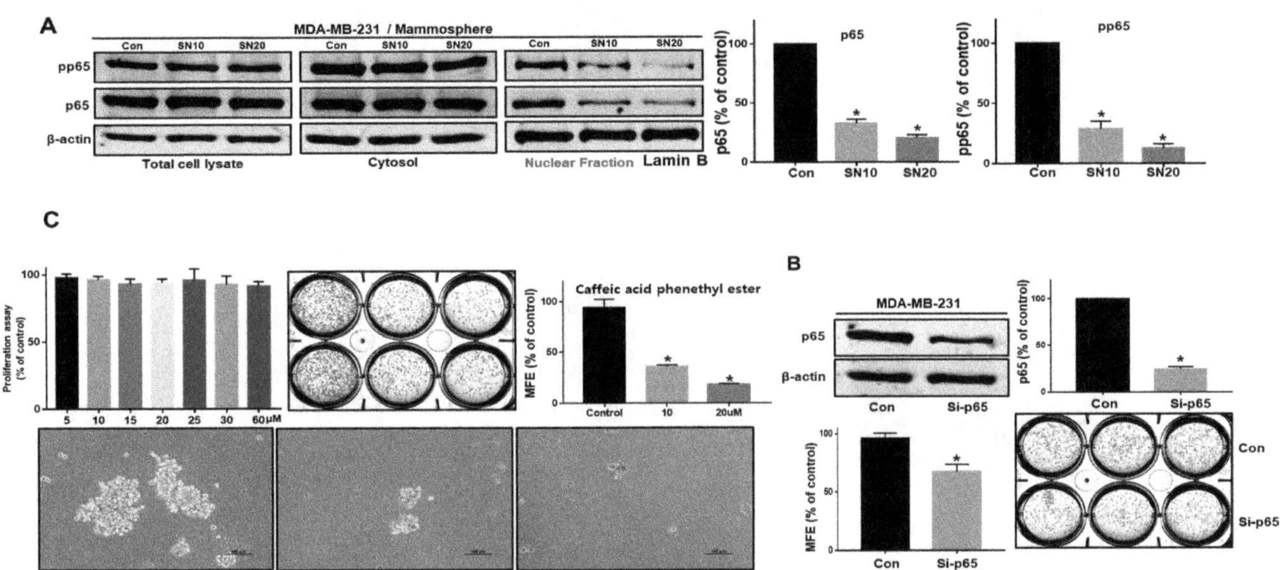

Figure 5. Sulconazole inhibits mammosphere formation through disruption of NF-κB activity. (**A**) Cancer cells were treated with sulconazole for 24 h. Nuclear and cytosolic proteins were run on a 10% SDS-PAGE gel, followed by immunoblotting with anti-p65 and anti-pp65 antibodies. (**B**) The effect of knocking down p65 expression using a siRNA specific for p65 on mammosphere formation was evaluated. The p65-knockdown effect was confirmed by immunoblotting using an anti-p65 antibody. (**C**) The effect of caffeic acid phenethyl ester, an NF-κB-specific inhibitor, on mammosphere formation was evaluated. A mammosphere formation assay evaluated mammosphere formation efficiency (MFE) (scale bar = 100 μm). The data are presented as the mean ± SD; $n = 3$ independent experiments;* $p < 0.05$ vs. the control.

3.5. *Sulconazole Inhibits the NF-κB Signaling Pathway and Production of Extracellular IL-8 in Mammospheres*

To analyze the biological function of sulconazole, we examined NF-κB signaling and the extracellular IL-8 level in mammospheres treated with sulconazole. Compared with a vehicle, sulconazole reduced nuclear p65 protein levels (Figure 6A). We checked NF-κB binding with sulconazole-treated nuclear proteins using an IRDye 800-NF-κB probe that binds an NF-κB oligonucleotide with high affinity. Sulconazole reduced the ability of p65 to bind to the IRDye 800-NF-κB probe (Figure 6B, lane 3). NF-κB/IRDye 800-NF-κB probe specificity was confirmed using a 10-fold increased concentration of self-competitor oligonucleotides (Figure 6B, lane 4). Sulconazole decreased the DNA-binding capacities of NF-κB. Extracellular IL-6 and IL-8 have essential functions in CSC formation [13]. NF-κB regulated the transcription of the IL-6 and IL-8 genes, binding to the promoter regions of the IL-6 and IL-8 genes. To assess the transcriptional levels of IL-6 and IL-8 under sulconazole treatment, we performed real-time RT-qPCR analysis of mammospheres using IL-6- and IL-8-specific primers. The transcript data showed that sulconazole reduced the transcript level of IL-8 but not that of IL-6 (Figure 6C). After using a siRNA targeting p65, the transcript data showed that sulconazole reduced the transcript level of IL-8 (Figure 6D). To test the level of extracellular IL-8, we performed cytokine profiling of the culture medium from mammospheres. After sulconazole treatment, the cytokine profiling data showed that sulconazole reduced the level of extracellular IL-8 but not that of IL-6 (Figure 6E).

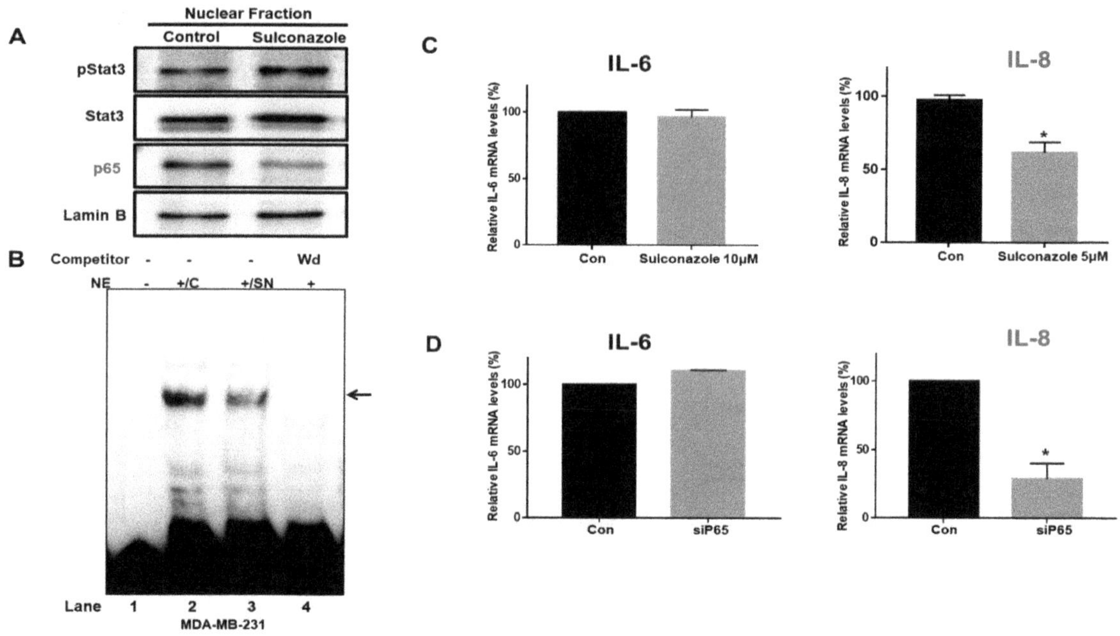

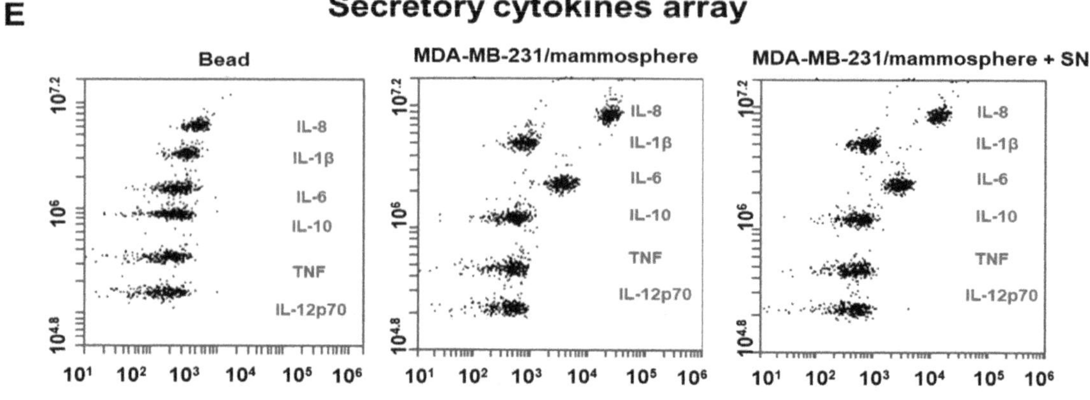

Figure 6. *Cont.*

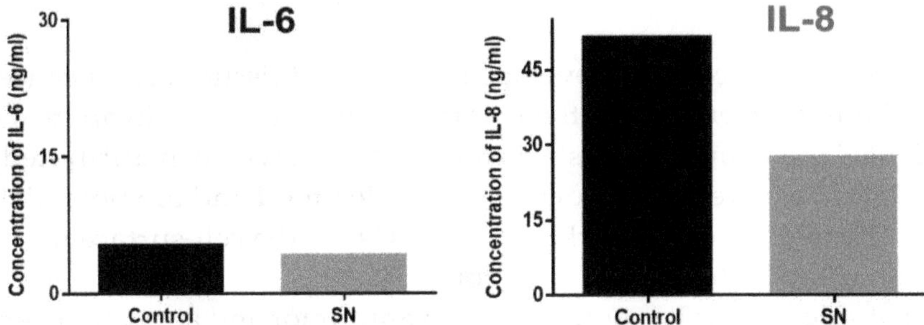

Figure 6. Effect of sulconazole on the NF-κB and IL-8 signaling pathways. (**A**) Cancer cells were treated with sulconazole for 24 h. Nuclear proteins were resolved on a 10% SDS-PAGE gel, followed by western blotting with anti-pStat3, anti-Stat3, anti-p65, and anti-Lamin B antibodies. (**B**) An electrophoretic mobility shift assay (EMSA) was used to assess nuclear lysates from mammospheres treated with sulconazole. The nuclear proteins were incubated with an IRDye 800-NF-κB probe and separated by 6% PAGE. Lane 1: probe only; lane 2: nuclear proteins with probe; lane 3: sulconazole-treated nuclear proteins with probe; lane 4: 10× self-competition. The arrow indicates the DNA/NF-κB interaction in the nuclear lysates. (**C**,**D**) Transcriptional levels of the IL-6 and IL-8 genes were determined in sulconazole-treated mammospheres and p65-knockout samples treated with a siRNA specific for p65. IL-6- and IL-8-specific primers were used for real-time RT-PCR. β-actin acted as an internal control. The data are presented as the mean ± SD; $n = 3$ independent experiments; * $p < 0.05$ vs. the control. (**E**) The cytokine profiles of conditioned media from mammosphere cultures were determined with cytokine-specific antibodies and cytokine beads. Sulconazole reduced extracellular IL-8 levels in the mammosphere cultures.

3.6. Sulconazole Inhibits Stem Cell Marker Gene Expression and Mammosphere Growth

To determine whether sulconazole regulates stem cell marker genes, we tested the transcription of stem cell marker genes. Sulconazole inhibited the expression of genes such as Nanog, c-Myc, and CD44 in BCSCs (Figure 7A). To verify that sulconazole reduces mammosphere growth, we added sulconazole to a mammosphere culture and counted the mammosphere cells. Sulconazole induced cell death in the mammospheres. These data showed that sulconazole led to a dramatic reduction in mammosphere growth (Figure 7B). These data showed that NF-κB signaling was essential for regulating mammosphere growth and that sulconazole inhibited mammosphere formation through deregulation of the NF-κB/IL-8 signaling pathway.

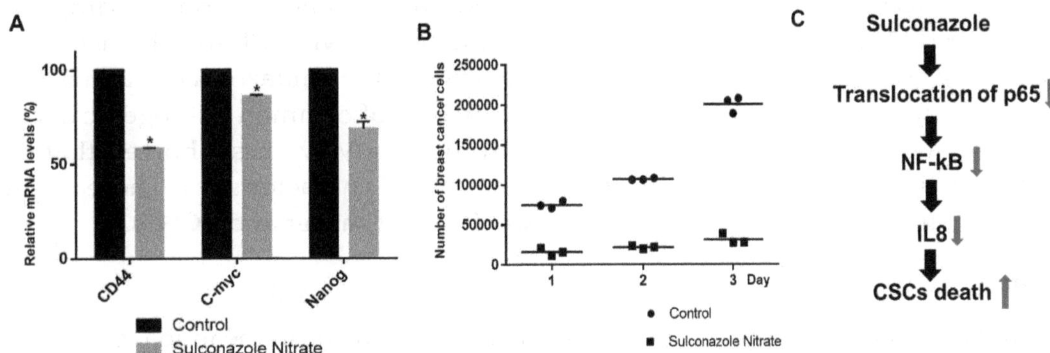

Figure 7. Effects of CSC loads on breast cancer. (**A**) The transcriptional levels of Nanog, C-myc, and CD44 were assayed in sulconazole- and 0.1% DMSO-treated mammospheres using specific primers. β-actin acted as an internal control. The data are presented as the mean ± SD; $n = 3$ independent experiments;* $p < 0.05$ vs. the control. (**B**) Sulconazole prevented mammosphere growth. Sulconazole-treated mammospheres were dissociated into single cells and plated in 6-well plates with equal numbers of cells. The cells were counted in triplicate 1, 2, and 3 days after plating and the mean value was plotted. The data shown represent the mean ± SD of three independent experiments. (**C**) The proposed model for CSC death induced by sulconazole is shown.

4. Discussion

Breast cancer is a female cancer that develops in the breast tissue. Breast cancer treatment using chemotherapy and radiotherapy eradicates the primary tumor, resulting in an increased survival rate in breast cancer patients [24]. Cancer metastasis and relapse have been attributed to CSC existence after chemotherapy [25]. BCSCs remain incompletely understood and are potential targets for breast cancer therapies [26]. The minimum biomarkers for BCSCs are the cell-surface markers CD44+/CD24- and CD44 upregulation is linked to tumor formation [27].

Our data show that sulconazole has potential as an antitumor and anti-CSC agent for breast cancer therapy. Sulconazole inhibits breast cancer hallmarks (Figure 1) and BCSC hallmarks (Figures 3 and 4). It is well known that the maintenance of BCSC properties is regulated by Stat3 [19,28,29]. We checked the Stat3 signaling pathway in the context of sulconazole treatment, but sulconazole did not regulate the Stat3 signaling pathway (Figure 6). The involvement of the NF-κB signaling pathway has been observed in primary AML samples, and elevated or constitutive NF-κB signaling activation is known to be present in many solid tumor types [30]. A high level of nuclear p65 is an essential feature of CSC formation [31]. As the NF-κB signaling pathway is important for BCSC survival, we examined the localization of the p65 subunit. Our results showed that sulconazole inhibited the translocation of p65. The inhibition of p65 translocation induced the inhibition of BCSC formation. CAPE is a strong specific inhibitor of NF-κB and prevents the nuclear translocation of p65 [32]. CAPE inhibited the translocation of p65 and pp65 and induced the inhibition of mammosphere formation. A siRNA specific for p65 inhibited mammosphere formation. Pyrrolidinedithiocarbamate (PDTC), another NF-κB pathway inhibitor, is known to inhibits CSC formation [33]. The imidazole-class drug BMS-345541 IKK inhibitor as an NF-kB inhibitor reduced their stem cell concentrations and self-renewal capacity in lung cancer cells. The nuclear levels of p65 and NF-κB signaling are important for BCSC survival.

Tumor progression and CSC survival can be regulated by the cytokines IL-6 and IL-8 in an autocrine or paracrine manner [10,34,35]. The JAK2/STAT3/IL-6 pathway is hyperactivated in several types of cancer and important to the growth of BCSCs [28]. This hyperactivation is related to a poor prognosis [36]. Extracellular IL-8 is overexpressed in triple-negative breast cancer (TNBC) and is an important therapeutic target in TNBC [37]. IL-8 signaling is an important key for targeting BCSCs [14]. We know that NF-κB can regulate the transcriptional regulation of the IL-6 and IL-8 genes in BCSCs. We assessed IL-6 and IL-8 gene transcripts in BCSCs treated with a p65 translocation inhibitor, sulconazole, and a siRNA specific for p65 that induced p65 downregulation. Both conditions showed that the RNA level of IL-8 was lower in treated samples than in control samples, but the RNA level of IL-6 was not changed between the treated samples and the control samples (Figure 6). Sulconazole reduced CSC formation through downregulation of NF-κB/IL-8 in breast cancer.

Sulconazole is an antifungal and antibacterial medicine in the imidazole class and is available as a cream to treat skin infection. Sulconazole inhibits the growth of common pathogenic dermatophytes by blocking sterol 14α-demethylase (CYP51) [38]. In this study, we first showed that sulconazole has cytotoxicity against breast cancer cells and reduces BCSC characteristics. These results support sulconazole as an important therapeutic agent to inhibit breast cancer and BCSCs.

5. Conclusions

In this study, we found that sulconazole—an antifungal medicine in the imidazole class—inhibited cell proliferation, tumor growth, and CSC formation. This compound also reduced the frequency of cells with the CSC marker phenotype of $CD44^{+}/CD24^{-}$ as well as the expression of ALDH and self-renewal-related genes. Sulconazole inhibited mammosphere formation and reduced the protein level of nuclear NF-κB. NF-κB knockdown using a p65-specific siRNA reduced CSC formation and secreted IL-8 levels in mammospheres. Sulconazole reduced nuclear NF-κB protein levels and extracellular IL-8 levels. These new findings showed that sulconazole blocked the NF-κB/IL-8 signaling pathway and CSC formation. NF-κB/IL-8 signaling is important for CSC formation and may be an important therapeutic target for BCSC treatment.

Author Contributions: H.S.C. and J.-H.K. designed and performed all the experiments; H.S.C. and D.-S.L. wrote the manuscript; S.-L.K. helped to design and perform the experiments; D.-S.L. supervised the study.

References

1. Torre, L.A.; Bray, F.; Siegel, R.L.; Ferlay, J.; Lortet-Tieulent, J.; Jemal, A. Global cancer statistics, 2012. *CA Cancer J. Clin.* **2015**, *65*, 87–108. [CrossRef] [PubMed]
2. Kusoglu, A.; Biray Avci, C. Cancer stem cells: A brief review of the current status. *Gene* **2019**, *681*, 80–85. [CrossRef] [PubMed]
3. Bonnet, D.; Dick, J.E. Human acute myeloid leukemia is organized as a hierarchy that originates from a primitive hematopoietic cell. *Nat. Med.* **1997**, *3*, 730–737. [CrossRef] [PubMed]
4. Gotte, M.; Yip, G.W. Heparanase, hyaluronan, and CD44 in cancers: A breast carcinoma perspective. *Cancer Res.* **2006**, *66*, 10233–10237. [CrossRef] [PubMed]
5. Nagano, O.; Okazaki, S.; Saya, H. Redox regulation in stem-like cancer cells by CD44 variant isoforms. *Oncogene* **2013**, *32*, 5191–5198. [CrossRef] [PubMed]
6. Koury, J.; Zhong, L.; Hao, J. Targeting Signaling Pathways in Cancer Stem Cells for Cancer Treatment. *Stem Cells Int.* **2017**, *2017*, 2925869. [CrossRef] [PubMed]
7. Guzman, M.L.; Neering, S.J.; Upchurch, D.; Grimes, B.; Howard, D.S.; Rizzieri, D.A.; Luger, S.M.; Jordan, C.T. Nuclear factor-kappaB is constitutively activated in primitive human acute myelogenous leukemia cells. *Blood* **2001**, *98*, 2301–2307. [CrossRef] [PubMed]
8. Vazquez-Santillan, K.; Melendez-Zajgla, J.; Jimenez-Hernandez, L.E.; Gaytan-Cervantes, J.; Munoz-Galindo, L.; Pina-Sanchez, P.; Martinez-Ruiz, G.; Torres, J.; Garcia-Lopez, P.; Gonzalez-Torres, C.; et al. NF-kappaBeta-inducing kinase regulates stem cell phenotype in breast cancer. *Sci. Rep.* **2016**, *6*, 37340. [CrossRef]
9. Zakaria, N.; Mohd Yusoff, N.; Zakaria, Z.; Widera, D.; Yahaya, B.H. Inhibition of NF-kappaB Signaling Reduces the Stemness Characteristics of Lung Cancer Stem Cells. *Front. Oncol.* **2018**, *8*, 166. [CrossRef]
10. Korkaya, H.; Liu, S.; Wicha, M.S. Regulation of cancer stem cells by cytokine networks: Attacking cancer's inflammatory roots. *Clin. Cancer Res.* **2011**, *17*, 6125–6129. [CrossRef]
11. Silva, E.M.; Mariano, V.S.; Pastrez, P.R.A.; Pinto, M.C.; Castro, A.G.; Syrjanen, K.J.; Longatto-Filho, A. High systemic IL-6 is associated with worse prognosis in patients with non-small cell lung cancer. *PLoS ONE* **2017**, *12*, e0181125. [CrossRef] [PubMed]
12. Lippitz, B.E.; Harris, R.A. Cytokine patterns in cancer patients: A review of the correlation between interleukin 6 and prognosis. *Oncoimmunology* **2016**, *5*, e1093722. [CrossRef] [PubMed]
13. Sansone, P.; Storci, G.; Tavolari, S.; Guarnieri, T.; Giovannini, C.; Taffurelli, M.; Ceccarelli, C.; Santini, D.; Paterini, P.; Marcu, K.B.; et al. IL-6 triggers malignant features in mammospheres from human ductal breast carcinoma and normal mammary gland. *J. Clin. Investig.* **2007**, *117*, 3988–4002. [CrossRef] [PubMed]
14. Singh, J.K.; Simoes, B.M.; Howell, S.J.; Farnie, G.; Clarke, R.B. Recent advances reveal IL-8 signaling as a potential key to targeting breast cancer stem cells. *Breast Cancer Res.* **2013**, *15*, 210. [CrossRef] [PubMed]
15. Bae, S.H.; Park, J.H.; Choi, H.G.; Kim, H.; Kim, S.H. Imidazole Antifungal Drugs Inhibit the Cell Proliferation and Invasion of Human Breast Cancer Cells. *Biomol. Ther.* **2018**, *26*, 494–502. [CrossRef] [PubMed]
16. Benfield, P.; Clissold, S.P. Sulconazole. A review of its antimicrobial activity and therapeutic use in superficial dermatomycoses. *Drugs* **1988**, *35*, 143–153. [CrossRef] [PubMed]
17. Clarke, M.L.; Burton, R.L.; Hill, A.N.; Litorja, M.; Nahm, M.H.; Hwang, J. Low-cost, high-throughput, automated counting of bacterial colonies. *Cytom. Part A* **2010**, *77*, 790–797. [CrossRef] [PubMed]
18. Choi, H.S.; Kim, D.A.; Chung, H.; Park, I.H.; Kim, B.H.; Oh, E.S.; Kang, D.H. Screening of breast cancer stem cell inhibitors using a protein kinase inhibitor library. *Cancer Cell Int.* **2017**, *17*, 25. [CrossRef] [PubMed]
19. Choi, H.S.; Kim, J.H.; Kim, S.L.; Deng, H.Y.; Lee, D.; Kim, C.S.; Yun, B.S.; Lee, D.S. Catechol derived from aronia juice through lactic acid bacteria fermentation inhibits breast cancer stem cell formation via modulation Stat3/IL-6 signaling pathway. *Mol. Carcinog.* **2018**, *57*, 1467–1479. [CrossRef] [PubMed]
20. Choi, H.S.; Kim, S.L.; Kim, J.H.; Deng, H.Y.; Yun, B.S.; Lee, D.S. Triterpene Acid (3-*O*-*p*-Coumaroyltormentic Acid) Isolated From Aronia Extracts Inhibits Breast Cancer Stem Cell Formation through Downregulation of c-Myc Protein. *Int. J. Mol. Sci.* **2018**, *19*, 2528. [CrossRef] [PubMed]

21. Choi, H.S.; Hwang, C.K.; Kim, C.S.; Song, K.Y.; Law, P.Y.; Wei, L.N.; Loh, H.H. Transcriptional regulation of mouse mu opioid receptor gene: Sp3 isoforms (M1, M2) function as repressors in neuronal cells to regulate the mu opioid receptor gene. *Mol. Pharmacol.* **2005**, *67*, 1674–1683. [CrossRef] [PubMed]
22. Kim, S.L.; Choi, H.S.; Kim, J.H.; Jeong, D.K.; Kim, K.S.; Lee, D.S. Dihydrotanshinone-Induced NOX5 Activation Inhibits Breast Cancer Stem Cell through the ROS/Stat3 Signaling Pathway. *Oxid. Med. Cell. Longev.* **2019**, *2019*, 9296439. [CrossRef] [PubMed]
23. Liang, Y.; Feng, G.; Wu, L.; Zhong, S.; Gao, X.; Tong, Y.; Cui, W.; Qin, Y.; Xu, W.; Xiao, X.; et al. Caffeic acid phenethyl ester suppressed growth and metastasis of nasopharyngeal carcinoma cells by inactivating the NF-kappaB pathway. *Drug Des. Dev. Ther.* **2019**, *13*, 1335–1345. [CrossRef] [PubMed]
24. Siegel, R.L.; Miller, K.D.; Jemal, A. Cancer statistics, 2016. *CA Cancer J. Clin.* **2016**, *66*, 7–30. [CrossRef] [PubMed]
25. Yu, Y.; Ramena, G.; Elble, R.C. The role of cancer stem cells in relapse of solid tumors. *Front. Biosci.* **2012**, *4*, 1528–1541. [CrossRef]
26. Saeg, F.; Anbalagan, M. Breast cancer stem cells and the challenges of eradication: A review of novel therapies. *Stem Cell Investig* **2018**, *5*, 39. [CrossRef] [PubMed]
27. Fillmore, C.; Kuperwasser, C. Human breast cancer stem cell markers CD44 and CD24: Enriching for cells with functional properties in mice or in man? *Breast Cancer Res.* **2007**, *9*, 303. [CrossRef] [PubMed]
28. Marotta, L.L.; Almendro, V.; Marusyk, A.; Shipitsin, M.; Schemme, J.; Walker, S.R.; Bloushtain-Qimron, N.; Kim, J.J.; Choudhury, S.A.; Maruyama, R.; et al. The JAK2/STAT3 signaling pathway is required for growth of CD44(+)CD24(−) stem cell-like breast cancer cells in human tumors. *J. Clin. Investig.* **2011**, *121*, 2723–2735. [CrossRef]
29. An, H.; Kim, J.Y.; Oh, E.; Lee, N.; Cho, Y.; Seo, J.H. Salinomycin Promotes Anoikis and Decreases the CD44+/CD24− Stem-Like Population via Inhibition of STAT3 Activation in MDA-MB-231 Cells. *PLoS ONE* **2015**, *10*, e0141919. [CrossRef]
30. Rinkenbaugh, A.L.; Baldwin, A.S. The NF-kappaB Pathway and Cancer Stem Cells. *Cells* **2016**, *5*, 16. [CrossRef]
31. Garner, J.M.; Fan, M.; Yang, C.H.; Du, Z.; Sims, M.; Davidoff, A.M.; Pfeffer, L.M. Constitutive activation of signal transducer and activator of transcription 3 (STAT3) and nuclear factor kappaB signaling in glioblastoma cancer stem cells regulates the Notch pathway. *J. Biol. Chem.* **2013**, *288*, 26167–26176. [CrossRef]
32. Natarajan, K.; Singh, S.; Burke, T.R., Jr.; Grunberger, D.; Aggarwal, B.B. Caffeic acid phenethyl ester is a potent and specific inhibitor of activation of nuclear transcription factor NF-kappa B. *Proc. Natl. Acad. Sci. USA* **1996**, *93*, 9090–9095. [CrossRef]
33. Zhou, J.; Zhang, H.; Gu, P.; Bai, J.; Margolick, J.B.; Zhang, Y. NF-kappaB pathway inhibitors preferentially inhibit breast cancer stem-like cells. *Breast Cancer Res. Treat.* **2008**, *111*, 419–427. [CrossRef]
34. Tan, C.; Hu, W.; He, Y.; Zhang, Y.; Zhang, G.; Xu, Y.; Tang, J. Cytokine-mediated therapeutic resistance in breast cancer. *Cytokine* **2018**, *108*, 151–159. [CrossRef]
35. Zhao, M.; Liu, Y.; Liu, R.; Qi, J.; Hou, Y.; Chang, J.; Ren, L. Upregulation of IL-11, an IL-6 Family Cytokine, Promotes Tumor Progression and Correlates with Poor Prognosis in Non-Small Cell Lung Cancer. *Cell. Physiol. Biochem.* **2018**, *45*, 2213–2224. [CrossRef]
36. Johnson, D.E.; O'Keefe, R.A.; Grandis, J.R. Targeting the IL-6/JAK/STAT3 signalling axis in cancer. *Nat. Rev. Clin. Oncol.* **2018**, *15*, 234–248. [CrossRef]
37. Dominguez, C.; McCampbell, K.K.; David, J.M.; Palena, C. Neutralization of IL-8 decreases tumor PMN-MDSCs and reduces mesenchymalization of claudin-low triple-negative breast cancer. *JCI Insight* **2017**, *2*, e94296. [CrossRef]
38. Thomson, S.; Rice, C.A.; Zhang, T.; Edrada-Ebel, R.; Henriquez, F.L.; Roberts, C.W. Characterisation of sterol biosynthesis and validation of 14alpha-demethylase as a drug target in Acanthamoeba. *Sci. Rep.* **2017**, *7*, 8247. [CrossRef]

8

Oncofetal Chondroitin Sulfate: A Putative Therapeutic Target in Adult and Pediatric Solid Tumors

Nastaran Khazamipour [1,2], Nader Al-Nakouzi [1,2], Htoo Zarni Oo [1,2], Maj Ørum-Madsen [1,2], Anne Steino [2,3], Poul H Sorensen [3,4] and Mads Daugaard [1,2,*]

1 Department of Urologic Sciences, University of British Columbia, Vancouver, BC V5Z 1M9, Canada; nkhazamipour@prostatecentre.com (N.K.); nalnakouzi@prostatecentre.com (N.A.-N.); hoo@prostatecentre.com (H.Z.O.); moerum@prostatecentre.com (M.Ø.-M.)
2 Vancouver Prostate Centre, Vancouver, BC V6H 3Z6, Canada; asteino@bccrc.ca
3 Department of Pathology and Laboratory Medicine, University of British Columbia, Vancouver, BC V5Z 1M9, Canada; psor@mail.ubc.ca
4 Department of Molecular Oncology, British Columbia Cancer Research Centre, Vancouver, BC V5Z1L3, Canada
* Correspondence: mads.daugaard@ubc.ca

Abstract: Solid tumors remain a major challenge for targeted therapeutic intervention strategies such as antibody-drug conjugates and immunotherapy. At a minimum, clear and actionable solid tumor targets have to comply with the key biological requirement of being differentially over-expressed in solid tumors and metastasis, in contrast to healthy organs. Oncofetal chondroitin sulfate is a cancer-specific secondary glycosaminoglycan modification to proteoglycans expressed in a variety of solid tumors and metastasis. Normally, this modification is found to be exclusively expressed in the placenta, where it is thought to facilitate normal placental implantation during pregnancy. Informed by this biology, oncofetal chondroitin sulfate is currently under investigation as a broad and specific target in solid tumors. Here, we discuss oncofetal chondroitin sulfate as a potential therapeutic target in childhood solid tumors in the context of current knowhow obtained over the past five years in adult cancers.

Keywords: oncofetal chondroitin sulfate; chondroitin sulfate; cancer; solid tumors; target; pediatric cancer; VAR2

---

1. Oncofetal Similarities between the Fetal and Tumor Tissue Compartments

The placenta, an organ that develops during pregnancy, behaves in many ways like a tumor. In just 40 weeks, the placenta has to grow to a mass of ~500 grams, invade neighboring tissue, establish an elaborate vasculature, and escape the immune system, all key features of solid tumor development [1]. Moreover, similarities between placenta and cancer at the molecular level have been frequently observed. Several proto-oncogenes involved in malignant transformation and cancer progression, including c-*erbB1* family (*HER1*, *ERBB1* or *EGFR*), c-*myc*, *Fos* and c-*ras*, are preferentially expressed by trophoblast cells during the first week of pregnancy when the proliferative, migratory and invasive properties of these cells are at their peak [2,3]. For instance, c-*erbB1* is expressed exclusively by the cytotrophoblast in four- to five-week placentas and pre-dominantly in the syncytiotrophoblast compartment after six weeks of gestation [4–6]. It is also involved in the pathogenesis of numerous malignancies, including breast cancer [7] and some types of childhood cancer [8]. The c-*myc* (MYC) proto-oncogene displays strong expression in early placenta [9] and is also frequently increased in human cancers [10,11]. Hyperactivation of Ras signaling by mutations or overexpression of the *Ras* oncogenes is a powerful driver of solid tumor formation [12,13], and the *c-ras* proto-oncogene, a key player in signaling pathways that regulate cellular proliferation [14], is expressed in early villous trophoblasts [15,16]. Similarly, overexpression of the *Fos* proto-oncogene stimulates trophoblast invasion during placental implementation [17], while contributing to tumor metastasis in several types of cancer [18–20].

In addition to the expression of proto-oncogenes, a number of oncofetal proteins are also shared between placenta, tumors and fetal tissue, including pregnancy-associated plasma protein A (PAPP-A), PEG10, alpha-fetoprotein (AFP), carcinoembryonic antigen (CEA), trophoblast glycoprotein precursor (TPBG) and immature laminin receptor protein (iLRP). Based on their oncofetal properties, some of these proteins have since been pursued as potential therapeutic targets in solid tumors. For example, PAPP-A, which is produced by placental syncytiotrophoblasts and is essential for normal fetal development [21], has been shown to facilitate tumor growth and invasion in various malignancies [22]. Notably, PAPP-A has been investigated as a potent immunotherapeutic target in Ewing sarcoma [23]. Likewise, PEG10, an RNA splice factor that is crucial for placental and embryonic development [24], is reported to play a role in the progression of several types of human cancers, including leukemia, breast cancer, prostate cancer and hepatocellular carcinoma [25–27], and has been proposed as a therapeutic target for prostate cancer [26–28].

AFP is produced by the embryo during fetal development and is found in both fetal serum and amniotic fluid and is currently the most widely used prognostic marker in hepatocellular carcinoma [29,30]. Additionally, CEA produced during embryonal and fetal development is one of the most widely used tumor markers worldwide, especially in colorectal malignancies where it is used to detect and inform on the presence of liver metastasis [31]. In addition, TPBG is used as a prognostic tool in a broad spectrum of malignancies, including colorectal, ovarian and gastric cancers [32–34]. It is also the target of the cancer vaccine TroVax, currently in clinical trials for the treatment several solid tumor types [35–38]. iLRP, which is highly expressed in early fetal development, is re-expressed in many tumor types and has been associated with tumor progression and metastasis [39,40]. Moreover, iLRP has been investigated as a therapeutic target for patients with leukemic diseases and against metastatic spread of solid tumors [41]. There are thus numerous examples of oncofetal proteins that can be utilized as tumor targets.

To qualify as a tumor target, a protein must be differentially expressed between malignant and normal tissues. Inadequate differential expression of potential target proteins is a major concern for all targeted therapy approaches and there is therefore a high demand for discovery of new molecular targets, differentially expressed in malignant versus normal tissue. Post-translational modifications (PTMs) of proteins, including phosphorylation, glycosylation, ubiquitination, nitrosylation, methylation, acetylation, lipidation and proteolysis, increase the diversity of the proteome and influence almost all aspects of cell biology and pathogenesis [42]. Protein glycosylation has major effects on protein folding, conformation, distribution, stability and activity [43–47]. Given its critical role in expanding protein functionality and diversity, glycosylation is an attractive candidate source of molecular targets in cancer. Indeed, targeting the glycosylation component of a protein rather than the protein itself has clear advantages. Firstly, targeting of tumor-specific protein glycoforms could be a solution for increasing anti-tumor specificity while limiting off-target effects. Secondly, a specific glycosylation moiety or pattern can be present on several different proteins simultaneously across cell populations, including tumor stem cells, which may overcome challenges related to tumor heterogeneity and dormancy. Lastly, proteins that are not normally glycosylated may be subject to disease-specific glycosylations, thereby increasing the available tumor target reservoir [48–50].

2. Chondroitin Sulfate

Among the glycosylation components that play a critical role in protein functionality are glycosaminoglycans (GAGs). GAGs are large, linear, negatively-charged polysaccharides consisting of repeating disaccharide units that can be sulfated at different positions and to different extents [51,52]. Five GAG chains have been identified to date: Heparan sulfate (HS), chondroitin sulfate (CS), dermatan sulfate

(DS), and keratan sulfate, as well as the non-sulfated hyaluronic acid [51,52]. GAGs are expressed on virtually all mammalian cells and are usually covalently attached to proteins, forming proteoglycans (PG).

CS is the second most heterogenous GAG group after HS and functionally presented as CS proteoglycans (CSPGs) in the pericellular matrix, as well as the intracellular milieu and the extracellular matrix (ECM) [53–56]. CS interacts with multiple ligands, both soluble and insoluble, and modulates important roles in many physiological and pathophysiological processes [57,58]. CS consists of repeating N-acetylgalactosamine (GalNAc)-glucuronic acid (GlcA) disaccharide units. A complex biosynthetic machinery in the Golgi apparatus is responsible for the production and structure of CS chains [59]. Five enzymes catalyze a tetrasaccharide-linker region attached to a serine residue of the core protein and six additional CS enzymes produce the polymeric backbone. During elongation of the CS chain, the sulfation of hydroxyl groups in different positions can occur. CS may contain sulfate groups in both the carbon 4 (C4) and C6 positions of the GalNAc unit (CSE), but may also be predominantly C4-sulfated (CSA) or C6-sulfated (CSC). Four CS carbohydrate sulfotransferases (CHSTs: CHST11, CHST12, CHST13 and CHST14) can catalyze the 4-O-sulfation of GalNAc in CS [60]. The CHSTs involved in 6-O-sulfation of GalNAc include (CHST3, CHST7, CHST15). The GlcA unit can also be sulfated at the C2 position, giving rise to DS also known as CSB (4-sulfated GalNAc and 2-sulfated GlcA) and CSD (6-sulfated GalNAc and 2-sulfated GlcA) [61]. The role of CS modifications in cancer progression has been under investigation for decades. In solid tumors, CS participate in cell–cell and cell–ECM interactions that promote tumor cell adhesion and migration, thereby facilitating aggressive and metastatic behavior of malignant cells [62–65]. Increased production of CS is found in transformed fibroblasts and mammary carcinoma cells, where these polysaccharides contribute to cell proliferation, adhesion and migration [64,66,67]. Similarly during embryonic development, CS in the context of CSPGs has important morphogenetic functions, especially in relation to epithelial morphogenesis, cell migration and cell division rates [68–71]. Moreover, CS is indispensable for pluripotency and differentiation of embryonic stem cells [72]. The ECM of human placentas contain high levels of CSPGs [73]. Placental CSPGs are mainly located on trophoblast cells in the ECM surrounding the expanding syncytium [63], where they are involved in a number of physiological processes. For example, they are part of a glycocalyx double-barrier that prevents the migration of immune cells through the placenta, from the mother to the offspring [72,74].

3. Oncofetal Chondroitin Sulfate in Placenta

In pregnancy-associated malaria pathogenesis, CSPGs in the placenta mediate the sequestration of infected red blood cells (IRBCs) to the intervillous spaces of the placenta [63]. Upon infection and during the replication phase inside IRBCs, the malaria parasite *Plasmodium falciparum* expresses a specific lectin, VAR2CSA, on the surface of the IRBCs. VAR2CSA subsequently binds to CS chains expressed in the placental syncytium, thereby enabling *P. falciparum* IRBCs to exit blood circulation and avoid filtration and destruction in the spleen of the infected host [75–77]. The specific form of CS recognized by VAR2CSA is a type of CSA [78,79] presented as a PTM on PGs such as syndecan-1 [63]. Evident by the fact that VAR2CSA-positive *P. falciparum* IRBCs sequester to the placenta as the only organ in the human host, placental CSA is thought to be distinct from CSA found in other tissues. Perhaps due to the phenotypical similarities between the placenta and tumors, placental-type CSA is also found in the vast majority of solid tumors as a secondary oncofetal CS (ofCS) PTM to PGs [80]. While the exact structure and composition of ofCS is as yet poorly understood, it is clear that the ofCS GAG chain is highly sulfated on C4 of the vast majority of GalNAc residues [80], and this specific sulfation pattern is unique to CSPGs in placenta and solid tumor tissue [80]. Since ofCS is not found in other normal tissues but the placenta, this PTM constitutes an attractive tumor target.

4. Expression of Oncofetal Chondroitin Sulfate Proteoglycans in Adult Solid Tumors

Over the past five years, ofCS modifications of PGs have been described in multiple solid tumor indications [18,80–82]. Through binding and regulation of a large number of ligands, ofCS chains collaborate with other PG components to modulate cell behaviors such as proliferation, differentiation, migration and adhesion [63,80]. Although malignant tumors have individual CSPG profiles, they generally display strong ofCS expression [63]. Indeed, ~90% of breast tumors, 80% of melanomas [80], and 92% of bladder cancers [82], express ofCS-modified CSPGs on the cell surface and/or in the tumor stroma. Moreover, ofCS alterations are often linked to disease progression and outcome in cancer patients. For example, expression of ofCS in melanoma tumors is significantly increased in advanced tumors, Clark level 2–5 compared to level 1, and in metastatic/recurrent disease compared to newly diagnosed disease [80]. In non-small cell lung cancer, high expression of ofCS correlates with poor relapse-free survival [80]. In addition, high ofCS expression is correlated with advanced tumor stage, cisplatin resistance and poor overall survival of muscle-invasive bladder cancer (MIBC) patients [82]. In breast cancer, CHST11 is over-expressed in tumors as compared to normal tissues [62]. Also, high expression of the CHST11 predicts poor disease-free survival of lung, breast and colorectal cancer patients [80]. Contrarily, other studies have reported that expression of C4-S sulfotransferases including CHST11 seems to be downregulated in colorectal cancers [83]. This discrepancy between different cancers highlights a lack of knowledge about the regulation and maturation of CS chains, which is further complicated by tissue-specific expression patterns and redundancy among CS enzymes. Nevertheless, ofCS expression is currently being evaluated as a potential therapeutic target for several adult tumor types, including bladder cancer [82], prostate cancer, breast cancer and non-Hodgkin's lymphoma [80].

5. Expression of Oncofetal Chondroitin Sulfate Proteoglycans in Pediatric Solid Tumors

While the expression of ofCS and its correlation with disease progression and outcome has been demonstrated in a variety of adult tumors, the potential for utilizing ofCS expression as a therapeutic target in childhood tumors has been less explored. Pediatric solid tumors are non-hematologic malignancies that occur during childhood. This heterogeneous group of tumors represents approximately 40%–50% of all pediatric cancers [84]. The tumor distribution of malignant pediatric solid tumors in adolescents is different compared with that of younger children, in whom embryonal or developmental cancers, such as retinoblastoma, neuroblastoma, or hepatoblastoma, are more prevalent. The most common malignant solid tumors in adolescents are extracranial germ cell tumors, bone and soft tissue sarcomas, melanoma, and thyroid cancer [85]. Generally, the outcome for pediatric solid tumors depends on location of the specific disease and risk group such as histological finding, tumor stage and metastatic status.

Similar to adult tumors, childhood solid tumors express various CSPGs with diverse functions related to disease progression (Table 1). In osteosarcoma, versican upregulation promotes cell motility and correlates with disease progression [39]. In neuroblastoma (NB), the CSPG NCAN is highly expressed in the tumor ECM where it facilitates growth of NB cells and promotes disease progression [82]. Exogenous NCAN expression transforms adherent NB cells into spheroids with high malignancy potential both in vitro (anchorage-independent growth and chemoresistance) and in vivo (xenograft tumor growth) [82]. CSPG4 is a cell surface PG commonly modified with ofCS that has been exploited as a tumor target in several tumor indications [86–89]. High levels of CSPG4 are found on a variety of adult and pediatric solid tumors including melanoma [90,91], osteosarcoma [87], rhabdomyosarcoma [88] and some brain tumors [86,92]. The CSPG4 expression levels differ depending on tumor type but is often present in both high-grade and lower-grade pediatric brain tumors [93]. PTPRZ1 plays a key role in cell migration, and is a potential tumor target in glioblastoma multiforme (GBM) [94]. In Ewing sarcoma, overexpression of APLP2 results in lower sensitivity to radiotherapy-induced apoptosis and immunologic cell death [95].

Proteoglycans can harbor different and multiple GAGs at the same time. For instance, syndecans and glypicans are PGs containing both CS and HS chains [96]. Altered expression of these PGs has been reported in multiple cancers including pediatric tumors [97]. Glypican 3, for example, plays an important role in cellular growth and differentiation. It is absent or only minimally expressed in most adult tissues but highly expressed in a variety of non-central nervous system (CNS) pediatric tumors, including hepatoblastoma, Wilms tumor, rhabdomyosarcoma, and in atypical teratoid rhabdoid tumors [98,99]. Glypican 5 is expressed in rhabdomyosarcoma where it facilitates growth factor signaling, in particular FGF signaling [100]. High syndecan-1 levels are found in glioma, where it correlates with advanced clinicopathological features and poor patient survival [101]. Sarcomas commonly express ofCS chains in 50%–100% of cases, depending on subtypes. Overall, ~80% of bone sarcomas, and ~85% of soft-tissue sarcomas are positive for ofCS [80]. Pediatric sarcoma cell lines generally express high levels of ofCS, and ofCS is required for migration and invasion capacity of osteosarcoma and rhabdomyosarcoma cells [80,102]. Indeed, ofCS has also been found on pediatric glioma cells and circulating tumor cells (CTCs) from GBM patients [89], hinting that ofCS might be exploited for liquid diagnostic applications in pediatric brain cancers. Also, ofCS allows for EpCAM-independent detection of CTCs [81], which might provide access to circulating sarcoma cells. Combined, the broad expression of CSPGs and ofCS across multiple pediatric tumor indications, promotes ofCS as putative and attractive therapeutic target in pediatric solid tumors.

Table 1. Chondroitin sulfate proteoglycan (CSPG) expression in childhood solid tumors.

CS-Modified PG	Cancer Type	Function
NCAN	Neuroblastoma	Promotes cell division, undifferentiated state and malignant phenotypes [82] Provides a growth advantage to cancer cells [82]
Versican	Osteosarcoma [103] Glioblastoma multiforme (GBM) [89]	Involves in TGFß - induced cell migration and invasion [103] Relevant marker of osteosarcoma progression [103] Potential target in cancer treatment [103] Function is unknown in GBM [89]
Decorin	Osteosarcoma [104]	Necessary for MG63 cell migration [104] Counteracts the growth-limiting effects of TGF-β2 [104]
CSPG4	Osteosarcoma [87] Rhabdomyosarcomas (RMS) [88] Medulloblastoma [105] Neuroblastoma [105] Childhood diffuse intrinsic pontine glioma [86] GBM [86,89] Dysembryoplastic neuroepithelial tumors (DNETs) [86,93]	Correlates with shorter survival in osteosarcoma [87] Therapeutic option for the combination treatment of RMS [88] Potential target for immunotherapy [87,89,105] Impairs terminal differentiation [86] Increases the invasive and migratory capabilities of glioma cells by facilitating interactions with extracellular matrix proteins [86] Facilitates angiogenesis by sequestering angiostatin [86] Increases tumor growth [86] Potential therapeutic target for treating childhood CNS cancers [86,89]
CD44	GBM [89,106]	High CD44 expression identifies GBM with particular poor survival chance Promotes aggressive GBM growth [106]
PTPRZ1	GBM [89,94]	Potential anti-cancer targets in GBM [89,94] Plays critical role in GBM cell migration [94]
APLP2	GBM [89] Ewing sarcoma [95]	Function is unknown in GBM [89] Anti-apoptotic function within Ewing sarcoma cells [95]
Syndecan-1	Glioma [89,101]	Correlates with the advanced clinicopathological features and lower survival rate [101]
Glypican 3	Hepatoblastoma Wilms tumor Rhabdomyosarcoma Atypical teratoid rhabdoid tumors	Potential candidate for targeted therapies [98]
Glypican 5	Rhabdomyosarcoma	Facilitates growth factor signaling Increases cell proliferation Potential target for therapeutic approaches [100]
Testican-1	GBM [89]	Unknown
Neuropilin-1	Osteosarcoma [107] Neuroblastoma [108] GBM [89]	Regulates metastasis potency [107] Correlates with poor response to chemotherapy [107] Correlates with poor prognosis for osteosarcoma patients [107] Regulates angiogenesis [107,108] Increases tumor growth [108] Function is unknown in GBM [89]

6. Oncofetal Chondroitin Sulfate as a Therapeutic Target in Solid Tumors

As outlined above, ofCS has emerged as an attractive tumor target for both therapeutic and diagnostic applications [18,80–82]. VAR2CSA specifically recognizes and binds ofCS, and recombinant VAR2CSA (rVAR2) proteins have been utilized to probe and access the ofCS chain expressed in solid tumors [80,82]. rVAR2 has also been exploited as a delivery system to shuttle cytotoxic drugs directly into ofCS-expressing tumor cells. For example, rVAR2-DT, a recombinant protein drug consisting of the cytotoxic domain of diphtheria toxin (DT388) fused to rVAR2, is able to eliminate both epithelial and mesenchymal tumor cells without any deleterious effect to normal primary human endothelial cells (HUVEC) in vitro [80]. Moreover, rVAR2-DT can inhibit prostate tumor growth in xenograft mouse models [80]. However, because DT-fusion drugs historically have shown adverse toxicity in human clinical trials [80], other strategies for delivery of drugs to ofCS-positive tumors have been pursued, including a rVAR2 drug-conjugate, VDC886. VDC886 is comprised of a 72 kDa rVAR2 polypeptide conjugated with the hemiasterlin toxin analog KT886, derived from the marine sponge *Hemiasterella minor*. VDC886 contains an average payload of three KT886 toxins per rVAR2 protein and displays strong toxicity towards diverse tumor cell lines of both adult and pediatric origin [80]. In vivo, VDC886 significantly inhibits tumor growth and metastasis in non-Hodgkin's lymphoma, prostate cancer, and breast cancer xenograft models with no sign of adverse effects [80]. In a different study, VDC886 successfully targeted ofCS on cisplatin-resistant MIBC cells and suppressed tumor growth of MIBC in vivo [82]. Immunohistochemical analysis of two independent cohorts of matched pre- and post-neoadjuvant chemotherapy-treated MIBC patients, revealed that cisplatin-resistant residual tumors had elevated levels of ofCS expression, supporting ofCS as a marker for disease progression [82].

In summary, the broad expression of CSPGs across solid tumors, and of ofCS in particular, promotes ofCS as an attractive target for therapeutic intervention. Historically, targeted biologics-based therapies have been less successful in pediatric solid tumors as compared to adult cancers, largely due to low mutational burden and limited number of neoantigens [109]. Hence, targeting cancer-specific PTMs, such as ofCS, constitutes a novel opportunity to curb childhood solid tumors. Indeed, the ability of VDCs to target ofCS-positive solid tumors supports a rational for exploring additional ofCS-targeting strategies, such as chimeric antigen receptor (CAR) T cells and bi-specific immune-engagers (BiTEs).

Author Contributions: N.K., N.A.-N. and H.Z.O. performed the literature search and wrote the first draft of the manuscript. M.Ø.-M., A.S., P.H.S. and M.D. edited the manuscript and approved the content. All authors have read and agreed to the published version of the manuscript.

References

1. Holtan, S.G.; Creedon, D.J.; Haluska, P.; Markovic, S.N. Cancer and pregnancy: Parallels in growth, invasion, and immune modulation and implications for cancer therapeutic agents. *Mayo Clin. Proc.* **2009**, *84*, 985–1000. [CrossRef]
2. Quenby, S.; Brazeau, C.; Drakeley, A.; I Lewis-Jones, D.; Vince, G. Oncogene and tumour suppressor gene products during trophoblast differentiation in the first trimester. *Mol. Hum. Reprod.* **1998**, *4*, 477–481. [CrossRef] [PubMed]
3. Ferretti, C.; Bruni, L.; Dangles-Marie, V.; Pecking, A.; Bellet, D. Molecular circuits shared by placental and cancer cells, and their implications in the proliferative, invasive and migratory capacities of trophoblasts. *Hum. Reprod. Updat.* **2006**, *13*, 121–141. [CrossRef] [PubMed]

4. Maruo, T.; Mochizuki, M. Immunohistochemical localization of epidermal growth factor receptor and myc oncogene product in human placenta: Implication for trophoblast proliferation and differentiation. *Am. J. Obstet. Gynecol.* **1987**, *156*, 721–727. [CrossRef]
5. Maruo, T.; Matsuo, H.; Otani, T.; Mochizuki, M. Role of epidermal growth factor (EGF) and its receptor in the development of the human placenta. *Reprod. Fertil. Dev.* **1995**, *7*, 1465–1470. [CrossRef] [PubMed]
6. Sugawara, T.; Maruo, T.; Otani, T.; Mochizuki, M. Increase in the Expression of C-Erb-a and C-Erb-B Messenger-Rnas in the Human Placenta in Early Gestation—Their Roles in Trophoblast Proliferation and Differentiation. *Endoc. J.* **1994**, *41*, S127–S133. [CrossRef]
7. Chen, S.; Qiu, Y.; Guo, P.; Pu, T.; Feng, Y.; Bu, H. FGFR1 and HER1 or HER2 co-amplification in breast cancer indicate poor prognosis. *Oncol. Lett.* **2018**, *15*, 8206–8214. [CrossRef]
8. Bodey, B.; E Kaiser, H.; E Siegel, S. Epidermal growth factor receptor (EGFR) expression in childhood brain tumors. *In Vivo* **2005**, *19*, 931–941.
9. Pfeifer-Ohlsson, S.; Goustin, A.S.; Rydnert, J.; Wahlström, T.; Bjersing, L.; Stéhelin, D.; Ohlsson, R. Spatial and temporal pattern of cellular myc oncogene expression in developing human placenta: Implications for embryonic cell proliferation. *Cell* **1984**, *38*, 585–596. [CrossRef]
10. Dang, C.V.; O'Donnell, K.A.; Juopperi, T. The great MYC escape in tumorigenesis. *Cancer Cell* **2005**, *8*, 177–178. [CrossRef]
11. Schaub, F.X.; Trivedi, M.; Richardson, A.B.; Shaw, R.; Zhao, W.; Zhang, X.; Ventura, A.; Ayer, D.; Hurlin, P.J.; Eisenman, R.N.; et al. Pan-cancer Alterations of the MYC Oncogene and Its Proximal Network across the Cancer Genome Atlas. *Cell Syst.* **2018**, *6*, 282–300. [CrossRef] [PubMed]
12. Akao, Y.; Kumazaki, M.; Shinohara, H.; Sugito, N.; Kuranaga, Y.; Tsujino, T.; Yoshikawa, Y.; Kitade, Y. Impairment of K-Ras signaling networks and increased efficacy of epidermal growth factor receptor inhibitors by a novel synthetic miR-143. *Cancer Sci.* **2018**, *109*, 1455–1467. [CrossRef] [PubMed]
13. Díaz, R.; Lopez-Barcons, L.; Ahn, D.; Yoon, A.; Matthews, J.; Mangues, R.; Pellicer, A.; Garcia-España, A.; Perez-Soler, R. Complex effects of Ras proto-oncogenes in tumorigenesis. *Carcinogenesis* **2003**, *25*, 535–539. [CrossRef] [PubMed]
14. Yu, Q.; Ciemerych, M.A.; Sicinski, P. Ras and Myc can drive oncogenic cell proliferation through individual D-cyclins. *Oncogene* **2005**, *24*, 7114–7119. [CrossRef]
15. Kohorn, E.; Sarkar, S.; Kacinski, B.; Merino, M.; Carter, D.; Blakemore, K.; Summers, W. Demonstration of myc and ras oncogene expression by in situ hybridization in hydatidiform mole and in the choriocarcinoma cell line BeWo. *Gynecol. Oncol.* **1986**, *23*, 245. [CrossRef]
16. Lu, C.-W.; Yabuuchi, A.; Chen, L.; Viswanathan, S.; Kim, K.; Daley, G.Q. Ras-MAPK signaling promotes trophectoderm formation from embryonic stem cells and mouse embryos. *Nat. Genet.* **2008**, *40*, 921–926. [CrossRef]
17. Bischof, P. Endocrine, paracrine and autocrine regulation of trophoblastic metalloproteinases. *Early Pregnancy* **2001**, *5*, 30–31.
18. Ding, Y.; Hao, K.; Li, Z.; Ma, R.; Zhou, Y.; Zhou, Z.; Wei, M.; Liao, Y.; Dai, Y.; Yang, Y.; et al. c-Fos separation from Lamin A/C by GDF15 promotes colon cancer invasion and metastasis in inflammatory microenvironment. *J. Cell. Physiol.* **2019**, *235*, 4407–4421. [CrossRef]
19. Qu, X.; Yan, X.; Kong, C.; Zhu, Y.; Li, H.; Pan, D.; Zhang, X.; Liu, Y.; Yin, F.; Qin, H. c-Myb promotes growth and metastasis of colorectal cancer through c-fos-induced epithelial-mesenchymal transition. *Cancer Sci.* **2019**, *110*, 3183–3196. [CrossRef]
20. Weekes, D.; Kashima, T.G.; Zandueta, C.; Perurena, N.; Thomas, D.P.; Sunters, A.; Vuillier, C.; Bozec, A.; El-Emir, E.; Miletich, I.; et al. Regulation of osteosarcoma cell lung metastasis by the c-Fos/AP-1 target FGFR1. *Oncogene* **2016**, *35*, 2948. [CrossRef]
21. Kalousova, M.; Muravská, A.; Zima, T. Pregnancy-associated plasma protein A (PAPP-A) and preeclampsia. *Adv. Clin. Chem.* **2014**, *63*, 169–209. [PubMed]
22. Guo, Y.; Bao, Y.; Guo, D.; Yang, W. Pregnancy-associated plasma protein a in cancer: Expression, oncogenic functions and regulation. *Am. J. Cancer Res.* **2018**, *8*, 955–963. [PubMed]
23. Heitzeneder, S.; Sotillo, E.; Shern, J.F.; Sindiri, S.; Xu, P.; Jones, R.C.; Pollak, M.; Noer, P.R.; Lorette, J.; Fazli, L.; et al. Pregnancy-Associated Plasma Protein-A (PAPP-A) in Ewing Sarcoma: Role in Tumor Growth and Immune Evasion. *J. Natl. Cancer Inst.* **2019**, *111*, 970–982. [CrossRef] [PubMed]

24. Chen, H.; Sun, M.; Zhao, G.; Liu, J.; Gao, W.; Si, S.; Meng, T. Elevated expression of PEG10 in human placentas from preeclamptic pregnancies. *Acta Histochem.* **2012**, *114*, 589–593. [CrossRef]
25. Kainz, B.; Shehata, M.; Bilban, M.; Kienle, D.; Heintel, D.; Krömer-Holzinger, E.; Le, T.; Kröber, A.; Heller, G.; Schwarzinger, I.; et al. Overexpression of the paternally expressed gene10 (PEG10) from the imprinted locus on chromosome 7q21 in high-risk B-cell chronic lymphocytic leukemia. *Int. J. Cancer* **2007**, *121*, 1984–1993. [CrossRef]
26. Ip, W.-K.; Lai, P.B.; Wong, N.L.-Y.; Sy, M.H.; Beheshti, B.; Squire, J.; Wong, N. Identification of PEG10 as a progression related biomarker for hepatocellular carcinoma. *Cancer Lett.* **2007**, *250*, 284–291. [CrossRef]
27. Akamatsu, S.; Wyatt, A.W.; Lin, N.; Lysakowski, S.; Zhang, F.; Kim, S.; Tse, C.; Wang, K.; Mo, F.; Haegert, A.; et al. The Placental Gene PEG10 Promotes Progression of Neuroendocrine Prostate Cancer. *Cell Rep.* **2015**, *12*, 922–936. [CrossRef]
28. Kim, S.; Thaper, D.; Bidnur, S.; Toren, P.; Akamatsu, S.; Bishop, J.L.; Colins, C.; Vahid, S.; Zoubeidi, A. PEG10 is associated with treatment-induced neuroendocrine prostate cancer. *J. Mol. Endocrinol.* **2019**, *63*, 39–49. [CrossRef]
29. Bai, D.-S.; Zhang, C.; Chen, P.; Jin, S.-J.; Jiang, G.-Q. The prognostic correlation of AFP level at diagnosis with pathological grade, progression, and survival of patients with hepatocellular carcinoma. *Sci. Rep.* **2017**, *7*, 12870. [CrossRef]
30. Galle, P.R.; Foerster, F.; Kudo, M.; Chan, S.L.; Llovet, J.M.; Qin, S.; Schelman, W.R.; Chintharlapalli, S.; Abada, P.B.; Sherman, M.; et al. Biology and significance of alpha-fetoprotein in hepatocellular carcinoma. *Liver Int.* **2019**, *39*, 2214–2229. [CrossRef]
31. Peng, S.; Huang, P.; Yu, H.; Wen, Y.; Luo, Y.; Wang, X.; Zhou, J.; Qin, S.; Li, T.; Chen, Y.; et al. Prognostic value of carcinoembryonic antigen level in patients with colorectal cancer liver metastasis treated with percutaneous microwave ablation under ultrasound guidance. *Medicine* **2018**, *97*, e0044. [CrossRef] [PubMed]
32. Starzyńska, T.; Marsh, P.; Schofield, P.; Roberts, S.; Myers, K.; Stern, P. Prognostic significance of 5T4 oncofetal antigen expression in colorectal carcinoma. *Br. J. Cancer* **1994**, *69*, 899–902. [CrossRef] [PubMed]
33. Naganuma, H.; Kono, K.; Mori, Y.; Takayoshi, S.; Stern, P.L.; Tasaka, K.; Matsumoto, Y. Oncofetal antigen 5T4 expression as a prognostic factor in patients with gastric cancer. *Anticancer Res.* **2002**, *22*, 1033–1038. [PubMed]
34. Wrigley, E.; McGown, A.T.; Rennison, J.; Swindell, R.; Crowther, D.; Starzyńska, T.; Stern, P.L. 5T4 oncofetal antigen expression in ovarian carcinoma. *Int. J. Gynecol. Cancer* **1995**, *5*, 269–274. [CrossRef] [PubMed]
35. Harrop, R.; Connolly, N.; Redchenko, I.; Valle, J.W.; Saunders, M.; Ryan, M.G.; Myers, K.A.; Drury, N.; Kingsman, S.M.; Hawkins, R.E.; et al. Vaccination of Colorectal Cancer Patients with Modified Vaccinia Ankara Delivering the Tumor Antigen 5T4 (TroVax) Induces Immune Responses which Correlate with Disease Control: A Phase I/II Trial. *Clin. Cancer Res.* **2006**, *12*, 3416–3424. [CrossRef] [PubMed]
36. Elkord, E.; Dangoor, A.; Drury, N.L.; Harrop, R.; Burt, D.J.; Drijfhout, J.W.; Hamer, C.; Andrews, D.; Naylor, S.; Sherlock, D.; et al. An MVA-based Vaccine Targeting the Oncofetal Antigen 5T4 in Patients Undergoing Surgical Resection of Colorectal Cancer Liver Metastases. *J. Immunother.* **2008**, *31*, 820–829. [CrossRef]
37. Amato, R.J.; Drury, N.; Naylor, S.; Jac, J.; Saxena, S.; Cao, A.; et al. Vaccination of prostate cancer patients with modified vaccinia ankara delivering the tumor antigen 5T4 (TroVax): A phase 2 trial. *J. Immunother.* **2008**, *31*, 577–585. [CrossRef]
38. Amato, R.J.; Hawkins, R.E.; Kaufman, H.L.; Thompson, J.A.; Tomczak, P.; Szczylik, C.; McDonald, M.; Eastty, S.; Shingler, W.H.; De Belin, J.; et al. Vaccination of Metastatic Renal Cancer Patients with MVA-5T4: A Randomized, Double-Blind, Placebo-Controlled Phase III Study. *Clin. Cancer Res.* **2010**, *16*, 5539–5547. [CrossRef]
39. Barsoum, A.L.; Schwarzenberger, P.O. Oncofetal antigen/immature laminin receptor protein in pregnancy and cancer. *Cell. Mol. Boil. Lett.* **2014**, *19*, 393–406. [CrossRef]
40. Song, T.; Choi, C.H.; Cho, Y.J.; Sung, C.O.; Song, S.Y.; Kim, T.-J.; Bae, D.-S.; Lee, J.-W.; Kim, B.-G. Expression of 67-kDa laminin receptor was associated with tumor progression and poor prognosis in epithelial ovarian cancer. *Gynecol. Oncol.* **2012**, *125*, 427–432. [CrossRef]
41. McClintock, S.D.; Warner, R.L.; Ali, S.; Chekuri, A.; Dame, M.K.; Attili, D.; Knibbs, R.K.; Aslam, M.N.; Sinkule, J.; Morgan, A.C.; et al. Monoclonal antibodies specific for oncofetal antigen–immature laminin receptor protein: Effects on tumor growth and spread in two murine models. *Cancer Boil. Ther.* **2015**, *16*, 724–732. [CrossRef] [PubMed]

42. Duan, G.; Walther, D. The Roles of Post-translational Modifications in the Context of Protein Interaction Networks. *PLoS Comput. Boil.* **2015**, *11*, e1004049. [CrossRef] [PubMed]
43. Pol-Fachin, L.; Verli, H.; Lins, R.D. Extension and validation of the GROMOS 53A6glycparameter set for glycoproteins. *J. Comput. Chem.* **2014**, *35*, 2087–2095. [CrossRef] [PubMed]
44. Mitra, N.; Sharon, N.; Surolia, A. Role of N-Linked Glycan in the Unfolding Pathway ofErythrina corallodendron Lectin. *Biochemistry* **2003**, *42*, 12208–12216. [CrossRef]
45. Brandner, B.; Kurkela, R.; Vihko, P.; Kungl, A.J. Investigating the effect of VEGF glycosylation on glycosaminoglycan binding and protein unfolding. *Biochem. Biophys. Res. Commun.* **2006**, *340*, 836–839. [CrossRef]
46. Solá, R.J.; Griebenow, K. Effects of glycosylation on the stability of protein pharmaceuticals. *J. Pharm. Sci.* **2009**, *98*, 1223–1245. [CrossRef]
47. Dumez, M.-E.; Teller, N.; Mercier, F.; Tanaka, T.; Vandenberghe, I.; Vandenbranden, M.; Devreese, B.; Luxen, A.; Frère, J.-M.; Matagne, A.; et al. Activation mechanism of recombinant Der p 3 allergen zymogen: Contribution of cysteine protease Der p 1 and effect of propeptide glycosylation. *J. Boil. Chem.* **2008**, *283*, 30606–30617. [CrossRef]
48. Rossig, C.; Kailayangiri, S.; Jamitzky, S.; Altvater, B. Carbohydrate Targets for CAR T Cells in Solid Childhood Cancers. *Front. Oncol.* **2018**, *8*. [CrossRef]
49. Mereiter, S.; Balmaña, M.; Campos, D.; Gomes, J.; Reis, C.A. Glycosylation in the Era of Cancer-Targeted Therapy: Where Are We Heading? *Cancer Cell* **2019**, *36*, 6–16. [CrossRef]
50. Steentoft, C.; Migliorini, D.; King, T.R.; Mandel, U.; June, C.H.; Posey, A.D. Glycan-directed CAR-T cells. *Glycobiology* **2018**, *28*, 656–669. [CrossRef]
51. Esko, J.D.; Kimata, K.; Lindahl, U. *Proteoglycans and Sulfated Glycosaminoglycans*; Varki, A., Cummings, R.D., Esko, J.D., Freeze, H.H., Stanley, P., Eds.; Essentials of Glycobiology: Cold Spring Harbor, NY, USA, 2009.
52. Pomin, V.H.; Mulloy, B. Glycosaminoglycans and Proteoglycans. *Pharmaceuticals* **2018**, *27*, 11.
53. Wang, Q.G.; El Haj, A.J.; Kuiper, N.J. Glycosaminoglycans in the pericellular matrix of chondrons and chondrocytes. *J. Anat.* **2008**, *213*, 266–273. [CrossRef] [PubMed]
54. Hedman, K.; Johansson, S.; Vartio, T.; Kjellén, L.; Vaheri, A.; Höök, M. Structure of the pericellular matrix: Association of heparan and chondroitin sulfates with fibronectin-procollagen fibers. *Cell* **1982**, *28*, 663–671. [CrossRef]
55. Munakata, H.; Takagaki, K.; Majima, M.; Endo, M. Interaction between collagens and glycosaminoglycans investigated using a surface plasmon resonance biosensor. *Glycobiology* **1999**, *9*, 1023–1027. [CrossRef] [PubMed]
56. Wu, Y.J.; La Pierre, D.P.; Wu, J.; Yee, A.J.; Yang, B.B. The interaction of versican with its binding partners. *Cell Res.* **2005**, *15*, 483–494. [CrossRef] [PubMed]
57. Zhou, Z.-H.; Karnaukhova, E.; Rajabi, M.; Reeder, K.; Chen, T.; Dhawan, S.; Kozlowski, S. Oversulfated Chondroitin Sulfate Binds to Chemokines and Inhibits Stromal Cell-Derived Factor-1 Mediated Signaling in Activated T Cells. *PLoS ONE* **2014**, *9*, e94402. [CrossRef] [PubMed]
58. García-Suárez, O.; Garcia, B.; Fernandez-Vega, I.; Astudillo, A.; Quiros-Fernandez, L.M. Neuroendocrine Tumors Show Altered Expression of Chondroitin Sulfate, Glypican 1, Glypican 5, and Syndecan 2 Depending on Their Differentiation Grade. *Front. Oncol.* **2014**, *4*, 15. [CrossRef]
59. Prabhakar, V.; Sasisekharan, R. The Biosynthesis and Catabolism of Galactosaminoglycans. *Adv. Pharmacol.* **2006**, *53*, 69–115.
60. Mikami, T.; Kitagawa, H. Biosynthesis and function of chondroitin sulfate. *Biochim. Biophys. Acta Gen. Subj.* **2013**, *1830*, 4719–4733. [CrossRef]
61. Da Costa, D.S.; Reis, R.L.; Pashkuleva, I. Sulfation of Glycosaminoglycans and Its Implications in Human Health and Disorders. *Annu. Rev. Biomed. Eng.* **2017**, *19*, 1–26. [CrossRef]
62. Cooney, C.; Jousheghany, F.; Yao-Borengasser, A.; Phanavanh, B.; Gomes, T.; Kieber-Emmons, A.M.; Siegel, E.R.; Suva, L.J.; Ferrone, S.; Kieber-Emmons, T.; et al. Chondroitin sulfates play a major role in breast cancer metastasis: A role for CSPG4 and CHST11gene expression in forming surface P-selectin ligands in aggressive breast cancer cells. *Breast Cancer Res.* **2011**, *13*, R58. [CrossRef] [PubMed]

63. Pereira, M.M.B.A.; Clausen, T.M.; Pehrson, C.; Mao, Y.; Resende, M.; Daugaard, M.; Kristensen, A.R.; Spliid, C.; Mathiesen, L.; Knudsen, L.E.; et al. Placental Sequestration of Plasmodium falciparum Malaria Parasites Is Mediated by the Interaction Between VAR2CSA and Chondroitin Sulfate A on Syndecan-1. *PLoS Pathog.* **2016**, *12*, e1005831.
64. Nadanaka, S.; Kinouchi, H.; Kitagawa, H. Chondroitin sulfate-mediated N-cadherin/beta-catenin signaling is associated with basal-like breast cancer cell invasion. *J. Biol. Chem.* **2018**, *293*, 444–465. [CrossRef] [PubMed]
65. Pudełko, A.; Wisowski, G.; Olczyk, K.; Koźma, E.M. The dual role of the glycosaminoglycan chondroitin-6-sulfate in the development, progression and metastasis of cancer. *FEBS J.* **2019**, *286*, 1815–1837. [CrossRef]
66. Fthenou, E.; Zong, F.; Zafiropoulos, A.; Dobra, K.; Hjerpe, A.; Tzanakakis, G.N. Chondroitin sulfate A regulates fibrosarcoma cell adhesion, motility and migration through JNK and tyrosine kinase signaling pathways. *In Vivo* **2009**, 23.
67. Chiarugi, V.P.; Dietrich, C.P. Sulfated mucopolysaccharides from normal and virus transformed rodent fibroblasts. *J. Cell. Physiol.* **1979**, *99*, 201–206. [CrossRef]
68. Kramer, K.L. Specific sides to multifaceted glycosaminoglycans are observed in embryonic development. *Semin. Cell Dev. Boil.* **2010**, *21*, 631–637. [CrossRef]
69. Shannon, J.M.; McCormick-Shannon, K.; Burhans, M.S.; Shangguan, X.; Srivastava, K.; Hyatt, B.A. Chondroitin sulfate proteoglycans are required for lung growth and morphogenesis in vitro. *Am. J. Physiol. Cell. Mol. Physiol.* **2003**, *285*, L1323–L1336. [CrossRef]
70. Long, K.R.; Huttner, W.B. How the extracellular matrix shapes neural development. *Open Boil.* **2019**, *9*, 180216. [CrossRef]
71. Djerbal, L.; Lortat-Jacob, H.; Kwok, J. Chondroitin sulfates and their binding molecules in the central nervous system. *Glycoconj. J.* **2017**, *34*, 363–376. [CrossRef]
72. Izumikawa, T.; Sato, B.; Kitagawa, H. Chondroitin Sulfate Is Indispensable for Pluripotency and Differentiation of Mouse Embryonic Stem Cells. *Sci. Rep.* **2014**, *4*, 3701. [CrossRef] [PubMed]
73. Lee, T.-Y.; Jamieson, A.M.; A Schafer, I. Changes in the Composition and Structure of Glycosaminoglycans in the Human Placenta during Development. *Pediatr. Res.* **1973**, *7*, 965–977. [CrossRef] [PubMed]
74. Blois, S.; Dveksler, G.; Vasta, G.R.; Freitag, N.; Blanchard, V.; Barrientos, G. Pregnancy Galectinology: Insights Into a Complex Network of Glycan Binding Proteins. *Front. Immunol.* **2019**, *10*, 1166. [CrossRef] [PubMed]
75. Salanti, A.; Dahlbaäck, M.; Turner, L.; Nielsen, M.A.; Barfod, L.; Magistrado, P.; Jensen, A.R.; Lavstsen, T.; Ofori, M.F.; Marsh, K.; et al. Evidence for the Involvement of VAR2CSA in Pregnancy-associated Malaria. *J. Exp. Med.* **2004**, *200*, 1197–1203. [CrossRef]
76. Clausen, T.; Christoffersen, S.; Dahlbäck, M.; Langkilde, A.E.; Jensen, K.E.; Resende, M.; Agerbæk, M.Ø.; Andersen, D.; Berisha, B.; Ditlev, S.B.; et al. Structural and Functional Insight into How the Plasmodium falciparum VAR2CSA Protein Mediates Binding to Chondroitin Sulfate A in Placental Malaria*. *J. Boil. Chem.* **2012**, *287*, 23332–23345. [CrossRef]
77. Fried, M.; Duffy, P.E. Adherence of Plasmodium falciparum to Chondroitin Sulfate A in the Human Placenta. *Science* **1996**, *272*, 1502–1504. [CrossRef]
78. Resende, M.; Nielsen, M.A.; Dahlbäck, M.; Ditlev, S.B.; Andersen, P.; Sander, A.F.; Ndam, N.T.; Theander, T.G.; Salanti, A. Identification of glycosaminoglycan binding regions in the Plasmodium falciparum encoded placental sequestration ligand, VAR2CSA. *Malar. J.* **2008**, *7*, 104. [CrossRef]
79. Gangnard, S.; Chêne, A.; Dechavanne, S.; Srivastava, A.; Avril, M.; Smith, J.D.; Gamain, B. VAR2CSA binding phenotype has ancient origin and arose before Plasmodium falciparum crossed to humans: Implications in placental malaria vaccine design. *Sci. Rep.* **2019**, *9*, 1–10. [CrossRef]
80. Salanti, A.; Clausen, T.M.; Agerbæk, M.Ø.; Al Nakouzi, N.; Dahlbäck, M.; Oo, H.Z.; Lee, S.; Gustavsson, T.; Rich, J.R.; Hedberg, B.J.; et al. Targeting Human Cancer by a Glycosaminoglycan Binding Malaria Protein. *Cancer Cell* **2015**, *28*, 500–514. [CrossRef]
81. Agerbæk, M.Ø.; Bang-Christensen, S.R.; Yang, M.-H.; Clausen, T.M.; Pereira, M.M.B.A.; Sharma, S.; Ditlev, S.B.; Nielsen, M.A.; Choudhary, S.; Gustavsson, T.; et al. The VAR2CSA malaria protein efficiently retrieves circulating tumor cells in an EpCAM-independent manner. *Nat. Commun.* **2018**, *9*, 3279.
82. Seiler, R.; Oo, H.Z.; Tortora, D.; Clausen, T.; Wang, C.K.; Kumar, G.; Pereira, M.M.B.A.; Ørum-Madsen, M.S.; Agerbæk, M.Ø.; Gustavsson, T.; et al. An Oncofetal Glycosaminoglycan Modification Provides Therapeutic Access to Cisplatin-resistant Bladder Cancer. *Eur. Urol.* **2017**, *72*, 142–150. [CrossRef] [PubMed]

83. Fernandez-Vega, I.; García-Suarez, O.; García, B.; Crespo, A.; Astudillo, A.; Quiros-Fernandez, L.M. Heparan sulfate proteoglycans undergo differential expression alterations in right sided colorectal cancer, depending on their metastatic character. *BMC Cancer* **2015**, *15*, 742. [CrossRef] [PubMed]
84. Allen-Rhoades, W.; Whittle, S.B.; Rainusso, N. Pediatric Solid Tumors of Infancy: An Overview. *Pediatr. Rev.* **2018**, *39*, 57–67. [CrossRef] [PubMed]
85. Allen-Rhoades, W.; Whittle, S.B.; Rainusso, N. Pediatric Solid Tumors in Children and Adolescents: An Overview. *Pediatr. Rev.* **2018**, *39*, 444–453. [CrossRef] [PubMed]
86. Yadavilli, S.; Hwang, E.I.; Packer, R.J.; Nazarian, J. The Role of NG2 Proteoglycan in Glioma. *Transl. Oncol.* **2016**, *9*, 57–63. [CrossRef]
87. Riccardo, F.; Tarone, L.; Iussich, S.; Giacobino, D.; Arigoni, M.; Sammartano, F.; Morello, E.; Martano, M.; Gattino, F.; De Maria, R.; et al. Identification of CSPG4 as a promising target for translational combinatorial approaches in osteosarcoma. *Ther. Adv. Med Oncol.* **2019**, *11*. [CrossRef]
88. Brehm, H.; Niesen, J.; Mladenov, R.; Stein, C.; Pardo, A.; Fey, G.; Helfrich, W.; Fischer, R.; Gattenlöhner, S.; Barth, S. A CSPG4-specific immunotoxin kills rhabdomyosarcoma cells and binds to primary tumor tissues. *Cancer Lett.* **2014**, *352*, 228–235. [CrossRef]
89. Bang-Christensen, S.R.; Pedersen, R.S.; Pereira, M.M.B.A.; Clausen, T.; Løppke, C.; Sand, N.T.; Ahrens, T.D.; Jørgensen, A.M.; Lim, Y.C.; Goksøyr, L.; et al. Capture and Detection of Circulating Glioma Cells Using the Recombinant VAR2CSA Malaria Protein. *Cells* **2019**, *8*, 998. [CrossRef]
90. Price, M.A.; Wanshura, L.E.C.; Yang, J.; Carlson, J.; Xiang, B.; Li, G.; Ferrone, S.; Dudek, A.Z.; Turley, E.A.; McCarthy, J.B. CSPG4, a potential therapeutic target, facilitates malignant progression of melanoma. *Pigment. Cell Melanoma Res.* **2011**, *24*, 1148–1157. [CrossRef]
91. Rolih, V.; Barutello, G.; Iussich, S.; De Maria, R.; Quaglino, E.; Buracco, P.; Cavallo, F.; Riccardo, F. CSPG4: A prototype oncoantigen for translational immunotherapy studies. *J. Transl. Med.* **2017**, *15*, 151. [CrossRef]
92. Sood, D.; Tang-Schomer, M.; Pouli, D.; Mizzoni, C.; Raia, N.; Tai, A.; Arkun, K.; Wu, J.; Black, L.D.; Scheffler, B.; et al. 3D extracellular matrix microenvironment in bioengineered tissue models of primary pediatric and adult brain tumors. *Nat. Commun.* **2019**, *10*, 1–14. [CrossRef] [PubMed]
93. Higgins, S.C.; Bolteus, A.J.; Donovan, L.K.; Hasegawa, H.; Doey, L.; Al-Sarraj, S.; King, A.; Ashkan, K.; Roncaroli, F.; Fillmore, H.L.; et al. Expression of the chondroitin sulphate proteoglycan, NG2, in paediatric brain tumors. *Anticancer Res.* **2014**, 34.
94. Müller, S.; Kunkel, P.; Lamszus, K.; Ulbricht, U.; Lorente, G.A.; Nelson, A.M.; von Schack, D.; Chin, D.J.; Lohr, S.C.; Westphal, M.; et al. A role for receptor tyrosine phosphatase zeta in glioma cell migration. *Oncogene* **2003**, *22*, 6661–6668. [CrossRef] [PubMed]
95. Peters, H.L.; Yan, Y.; Nordgren, T.; Cutucache, C.; Joshi, S.S.; Solheim, J.C. Amyloid precursor-like protein 2 suppresses irradiation-induced apoptosis in Ewing sarcoma cells and is elevated in immune-evasive Ewing sarcoma cells. *Cancer Boil. Ther.* **2013**, *14*, 752–760. [CrossRef]
96. Nikitovic, D.; Berdiaki, A.; Spyridaki, I.; Krasanakis, T.; Aristidis, T.; Tzanakakis, G.N. Proteoglycans—Biomarkers and Targets in Cancer Therapy. *Front. Endocrinol.* **2018**, *9*. [CrossRef]
97. Iozzo, R.V.; Sanderson, R.D. Proteoglycans in cancer biology, tumour microenvironment and angiogenesis. *J. Cell. Mol. Med.* **2011**, *15*, 1013–1031. [CrossRef]
98. Ortiz, M.; Roberts, S.S.; Bender, J.G.; Shukla, N.; Wexler, L.H. Immunotherapeutic Targeting of GPC3 in Pediatric Solid Embryonal Tumors. *Front. Oncol.* **2019**, *9*, 108. [CrossRef]
99. Chan, E.S.; Pawel, B.R.; A Corao, D.; Venneti, S.; Russo, P.; Santi, M.; Sullivan, L. Immunohistochemical Expression of Glypican-3 in Pediatric Tumors: An Analysis of 414 Cases. *Pediatr. Dev. Pathol.* **2013**, *16*, 272–277. [CrossRef]
100. Williamson, D.; Selfe, J.; Gordon, T.; Lu, Y.-J.; Pritchard-Jones, K.; Murai, K.; Jones, P.H.; Workman, P.; Shipley, J.M. Role for Amplification and Expression ofGlypican-5in Rhabdomyosarcoma. *Cancer Res.* **2007**, *67*, 57–65. [CrossRef]
101. Xu, Y.; Yuan, J.; Zhang, Z.; Lin, L.; Xu, S. Syndecan-1 expression in human glioma is correlated with advanced tumor progression and poor prognosis. *Mol. Boil. Rep.* **2012**, *39*, 8979–8985. [CrossRef]
102. Clausen, T.M.; Pereira, M.M.B.A.; Al Nakouzi, N.; Oo, H.Z.; Agerbæk, M.Ø.; Lee, S.; Ørum-Madsen, M.S.; Kristensen, A.R.; El-Naggar, A.; Grandgenett, P.M.; et al. Oncofetal Chondroitin Sulfate Glycosaminoglycans Are Key Players in Integrin Signaling and Tumor Cell Motility. *Mol. Cancer Res.* **2016**, *14*, 1288–1299. [CrossRef] [PubMed]

103. Li, F.; Li, S.; Cheng, T. TGF-beta1 promotes osteosarcoma cell migration and invasion through the miR-143-versican pathway. *Cell. Phys. Biochem.* **2014**, *34*, 2169–2179. [CrossRef] [PubMed]
104. Zafiropoulos, A.; Nikitovic, D.; Katonis, P.; Aristidis, T.; Karamanos, N.K.; Tzanakakis, G.N. Decorin-Induced Growth Inhibition Is Overcome through Protracted Expression and Activation of Epidermal Growth Factor Receptors in Osteosarcoma Cells. *Mol. Cancer Res.* **2008**, *6*, 785–794. [CrossRef] [PubMed]
105. Rota, C.M.; Tschernia, N.; Feldman, S.; Mackall, C.; Lee, D.W. Abstract 3151: T cells engineered to express a chimeric antigen receptor targeting chondroitin sulfate proteoglycan 4 (CSPG4) specifically kill medulloblastoma and produce inflammatory cytokines. *Immunology* **2015**, *75*, 3151.
106. Pietras, E.J.; Katz, A.M.; Ekström, E.J.; Wee, B.; Halliday, J.J.; Pitter, K.L.; Werbeck, J.L.; Amankulor, N.M.; Huse, J.T.; Holland, E.C. Osteopontin-CD44 signaling in the glioma perivascular niche enhances cancer stem cell phenotypes and promotes aggressive tumor growth. *Cell Stem Cell* **2014**, *14*, 357–369. [CrossRef] [PubMed]
107. Zhu, H.; Cai, H.; Tang, M.; Tang, J. Neuropilin-1 is overexpressed in osteosarcoma and contributes to tumor progression and poor prognosis. *Clin. Transl. Oncol.* **2013**, *16*, 732–738. [CrossRef] [PubMed]
108. Marcus, K.; Johnson, M.; Adam, R.; O'Reilly, M.S.; Donovan, M.; Atala, A.; Freeman, M.R.; Soker, S. Tumor cell-associated neuropilin-1 and vascular endothelial growth factor expression as determinants of tumor growth in neuroblastoma. *Neuropathology* **2005**, *25*, 178–187. [CrossRef]
109. Downing, J.R.; Wilson, R.K.; Zhang, J.; Mardis, E.R.; Pui, C.-H.; Ding, L.; Ley, T.J.; Evans, W.E. The Pediatric Cancer Genome Project. *Nat. Genet.* **2012**, *44*, 619–622. [CrossRef]

9

The Pyrazolo[3,4-d]pyrimidine Derivative, SCO-201, Reverses Multidrug Resistance Mediated by ABCG2/BCRP

Sophie E. B. Ambjørner [1], Michael Wiese [2], Sebastian Christoph Köhler [2], Joen Svindt [3], Xamuel Loft Lund [1], Michael Gajhede [1], Lasse Saaby [4], Birger Brodin [4], Steffen Rump [5], Henning Weigt [6], Nils Brünner [1,7] and Jan Stenvang [1,7,*]

1 Department of Drug Design and Pharmacology, University of Copenhagen, 1353 Copenhagen, Denmark; sophie.ambjoerner@gmail.com (S.E.B.A.); lxs184@alumni.ku.dk (X.L.L.); mig@sund.ku.dk (M.G.); nb@scandiononcology.com (N.B.)
2 Pharmaceutical Institute, University of Bonn, 53012 Bonn, Germany; mwiese@uni-bonn.de (M.W.); skoehler@uni-bonn.de (S.C.K.)
3 Department of Biology, University of Copenhagen, 1353 Copenhagen, Denmark; joen.svindt@gmail.com
4 Department of Pharmacy, University of Copenhagen, 1353 Copenhagen, Denmark; lasse.saaby@sund.ku.dk (L.S.); birger.brodin@sund.ku.dk (B.B.)
5 SRConsulting, 31319 Sehnde, Germany; rump@s-r-consulting.com
6 Division of Chemical Safety and Toxicity, Fraunhofer Institute of Toxicology and Experimental Medicine, 30625 Hannover, Germany; henning.weigt@item.fraunhofer.de
7 Scandion Oncology A/S, Symbion, 1353 Copenhagen, Denmark
* Correspondence: js@scandiononcology.com

Abstract: ATP-binding cassette (ABC) transporters, such as breast cancer resistance protein (BCRP), are key players in resistance to multiple anti-cancer drugs, leading to cancer treatment failure and cancer-related death. Currently, there are no clinically approved drugs for reversal of cancer drug resistance caused by ABC transporters. This study investigated if a novel drug candidate, SCO-201, could inhibit BCRP and reverse BCRP-mediated drug resistance. We applied in vitro cell viability assays in SN-38 (7-Ethyl-10-hydroxycamptothecin)-resistant colon cancer cells and in non-cancer cells with ectopic expression of BCRP. SCO-201 reversed resistance to SN-38 (active metabolite of irinotecan) in both model systems. Dye efflux assays, bidirectional transport assays, and ATPase assays demonstrated that SCO-201 inhibits BCRP. In silico interaction analyses supported the ATPase assay data and suggest that SCO-201 competes with SN-38 for the BCRP drug-binding site. To analyze for inhibition of other transporters or cytochrome P450 (CYP) enzymes, we performed enzyme and transporter assays by in vitro drug metabolism and pharmacokinetics studies, which demonstrated that SCO-201 selectively inhibited BCRP and neither inhibited nor induced CYPs. We conclude that SCO-201 is a specific, potent, and potentially non-toxic drug candidate for the reversal of BCRP-mediated resistance in cancer cells.

Keywords: multidrug resistance in cancer; drug efflux pumps; ATP-binding cassette transporter; breast cancer resistance protein (BCRP); ABCG2; pyrazolo-pyrimidine derivative; SCO-201

---

1. Introduction

Chemotherapy resistance is considered the single most important obstacle to greater success with chemotherapy for cancer patients [1–3]. Although many cancer patients initially benefit from chemotherapy treatment, a large proportion of treatments fail due to acquisition of resistance to multiple anti-cancer drugs. This phenomenon is known as multidrug resistance (MDR) and refers to the concurrent development of cross-resistance to many chemically diverse anti-cancer agents [4]. MDR results in poor prognosis and decreased survival rate of cancer patients, and strategies to circumvent MDR are therefore highly needed [3,5]. The mechanisms underlying MDR are complex and include many different tumor survival mechanisms [6]. Overexpression of drug expelling ATP-binding cassette (ABC) transporters seems to be an important mechanism of MDR in cancer cells [7]. Today, the most extensively studied and characterized ABC transporters, found to be involved in cancer MDR, are (a) multidrug resistance protein 1/P-glycoprotein (MDR1/P-gp), encoded by the *ABCB1* gene; (b) multidrug resistance-associated protein 1 (MRP1), encoded by the *ABCC1* gene; and (c) breast cancer resistance protein (BCRP), encoded by the *ABCG2* gene [8]. ABC transporters are normally expressed in tissues such as the intestines, brain, liver, and placenta, where they prevent xenobiotic substrates from accumulating [7]. The ABC transporters are transmembrane proteins that utilize ATP hydrolysis to drive the active transport of substrates from the cytoplasmic site to the extracellular space [9]. The transporters consist of two transmembrane domains (TMDs), able to undergo a conformational change that triggers the removal of the substrate, and two cytoplasmic nucleotide-binding domains (NBDs) that bind and hydrolyze ATP [10]. Due to a broad drug specificity, ABC transporters can efflux many different anticancer agents, thus resulting in MDR [7,9]. BCRP (ABCG2) is a 72 kDa half-transporter that acts as a homomeric dimer, and so far, BCRP is known to mediate resistance to a variety of anti-cancer agents, among these the chemotherapeutic agents SN-38, topotecan, mitoxantrone, doxorubicin, and daunorubicin [11–16]. SN-38 (Figure 1) is the active metabolite of irinotecan (Camptosar) and is especially important in the treatment of gastrointestinal cancers such as colorectal cancer [17] and pancreatic cancer (European Society for Medical Oncology (ESMO) guidelines for pancreatic cancer). Several studies have indicated that high cancer cell levels of BCRP is the key player in SN-38 resistance, and BCRP thus hinders successful treatment of metastatic gastrointestinal cancer patients [11–16]. Mitoxantrone was the first chemotherapy to be identified as a substrate of BCRP, and BCRP was found to be involved in mitoxantrone-resistant breast cancer, thus giving BCRP its name [13].

During the last 40 years, researchers have tried to develop non-toxic, highly potent, and efficacious drugs that are able to reverse ABC-transporter-mediated MDR [7,9,17–19]. These MDR-reversing agents, also known as re-sensitizing agents or chemo-sensitizers, act by either inhibiting the expression of ABC transporters or by directly inhibiting the transport function, and thereby restore the sensitivity of the cancer cells to anti-cancer agents [9,10]. The compound fumitremorgin C was the first BCRP inhibitor to be identified, and although it was found to have a high inhibitory potency, neurotoxic side effects prevented the clinical use of this compound [20,21]. To prevent these side effects, researchers synthesized new different fumitremorgin C analogues, for instance, the potent BCRP inhibitor Ko143 [22,23]. Nonetheless, these analogues, including Ko143, were not stable in plasma, still caused the side effects, and could not be used in the clinic [23]. Other known ABC transporter inhibitors include verapamil, tariquidar, and valspodar (PSC833), which all inhibit MDR1/P-gp [9]. However, despite a long list of different potent inhibitors, none of these have been approved for clinical use. The lack of ABC transporter inhibitors in clinical use can be attributed to several issues: (1) the inhibitors specifically only inhibit one transporter, (2) the inhibitors exhibit a significant degree of toxicity, (3) clinical studies were poorly designed—inhibitors were not combined with the drug that the patients had proved to be resistant to—and the studies lacked randomization, and (4) lack of companion diagnostic tests to optimize patients' selection and treatment [1,7,9]. Thus, new strategies are greatly needed to improve the treatment success and survival rate of cancer patients with MDR.

To identify potential new compounds that interfere with common drug resistance mechanisms, such as the overexpression of BCRP, we previously established the DEN-50R screening platform. This platform consists of isogenic pairs of drug-sensitive and drug-resistant patient-derived cancer cell lines, for instance, colorectal, breast, prostate, and pancreatic cancer [24]. These resistant cell lines were established by exposing chemotherapy-sensitive cells to gradually increasing concentrations of chemotherapy over a period of 8–10 months [25]. We thoroughly characterized these drug-resistant cell lines to identify important drug resistance mechanisms [25–30]. In accordance with several other studies with in vitro model systems [31], we found that BCRP overexpression was a key player of resistance to SN-38 [25]. Using our DEN-50R screening platform, we found that pyrazolo-pyrimidine derivatives might serve as potential inhibitors of drug resistance in these cell lines. One of the hits from the drug screening was the pyrazolo-pyrimidine derivative SCO-201 (previously OBR-5-340) (Figure 1). These preliminary data indicated that SCO-201, which is previously known as a potent viral capsid inhibitor, might serve as a potential inhibitor of drug resistance [32,33]. Interestingly, in a study by Burkhart et al. (2009) [34], it was demonstrated that pyrazolo-pyrimidine derivatives comprise a prominent structural class of selective and potent ABC transporter inhibitors, with low toxicity and low risk of increased chemotherapy-mediated toxicity [19,34].

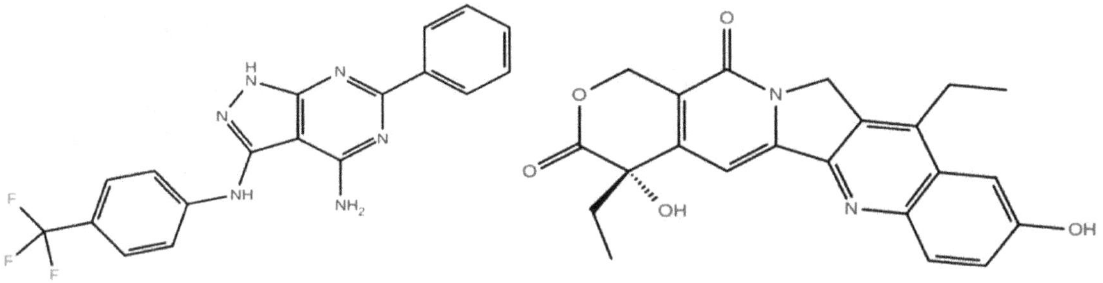

Figure 1. Chemical structures of the pyrazolo[3,4-d]pyrimidine derivative SCO-201 and the active metabolite of irinotecan, SN-38. Graphics produced using Maestro, Schrödinger 2019-3, limited liability company (LLC), New York, NY, 2019. SN-38 structure obtained from PubChem Database [35,36].

On the basis of these findings, the aim of this study was to clarify if SCO-201 re-sensitizes cancer cells to chemotherapy substrates of BCRP. An additional aim was to investigate any potential risks of pharmacokinetic interactions of SCO-201, which was investigated by testing the effect of SCO-201 on cytochrome P450 enzymes and efflux/uptake transporters. Our study is the first to show that SCO-201 competitively inhibits the transport activity of BCRP, triggers the accumulation of BCRP dye substrate, and re-sensitizes cancer cells to chemotherapy in two different in vitro models of BCRP-mediated resistance. Moreover, in vitro drug metabolism and pharmacokinetics (DMPK) data suggest that SCO-201 will not influence metabolism of other drugs by the cytochrome P450 (CYP) system. This indicates that SCO-201 is not likely to increase the risk of pharmacokinetic interactions with chemotherapy that are metabolized by the CYP system. The present data warrant further studies including regulatory toxicity and ADME (absorption, distribution, metabolism, and excretion) studies according to good laboratory practice (GLP) in order to initiate clinical development [35,36].

2. Materials and Methods

2.1. Reagents and Antibodies

DMSO, SN-38, Ko143, topotecan, mitoxantrone, Hoechst 33342, MTT reagent (3-(4,5-dimethylthiazol-2-yl)-2,5-diphenyltetrazolium bromide), primary antibody for β-actin (mAb A5441), PREDEASY SB-MDR1/P-gp Hi5, and SB-BCRP-M ATPase assays kits (Solvo Biotechnology) were all purchased from Sigma-Aldrich/Merck (Schnelldorf, Germany). PSC833 was purchased from Tocris/Bio-techne (Abingdon, UK). The primary antibody for BCRP (mAb BXP-21) was purchased from Abcam (Cambridge, UK).

Plasticware, such as T-75 culture flasks and Transwell permeable supports (1.12 cm^2, 0.4 μm pores), were purchased from Corning, Fisher Scientific (Slangerup, Denmark). Cell culture reagents such as Hank's balanced salt solution (HBSS) was purchased from Life Technologies (Taastrup, Denmark); fetal bovine serum (FBS) from Gibco, Fischer Scientific (Slangerup, Denmark); penicillin and streptomycin were acquired from Bio Whittaker Cambrex (Vallensbaek, Denmark); Dulbecco's modified Eagle's medium, bovine serum albumin (BSA), and Minimum Essential Media (MEM) nonessential amino acids were purchased from Sigma-Aldrich (Brøndby, Denmark); whereas 2-[4-(2-hydroxyethyl)piperazin-1-yl] ethanesulfonic acid (HEPES) was purchased from AppliChem GmbH (Darmstadt, Germany). [3H]-Estrone-3-sulfate (51.8 Ci/mmol), [14C]-mannitol (0.06 Ci/mmol), and Ultima Gold scintillation fluid was purchased from PerkinElmer (Boston, MA, USA).

All drugs were dissolved in DMSO, except mitoxantrone, which was dissolved in ethanol.

2.2. Cell Lines and Culture Conditions

All cell lines were maintained at 37 °C in a humidified 5% CO_2 atmosphere. The Madin-Darby Canine Kidney (MDCK)-II-BCRP cell line was a kind gift from Dr. A. Schinkel (The Netherlands Cancer Institute, Amsterdam, The Netherlands [29,30]) and cultured in Dulbecco's modified Eagle's medium (DMEM) supplemented with 10% fetal calf serum (FCS), 50 μg/mL streptomycin, 50 U/mL penicillin G, and 2 mM L-glutamine. The parental drug-sensitive ($HT29_{PAR}$), obtained from the National Cancer Institute (NCI)/Development Therapeutics Program, and SN-38-resistant ($HT29_{SN\text{-}38\text{-}RES}$) cell lines were cultured in Gibco Roswell Park Memorial Institute (RPMI) 1640–GlutaMAX medium supplemented with 10% FCS [25].

2.3. Western Blot Analysis

The proteins of HT29 cell lysates were separated with SDS-PAGE and transferred to nitrocellulose membranes. After blocking the membrane with 5% skimmed milk in 1× Tris-Buffered Saline, 0.1% Tween® 20 Detergent (TBS-T), the membrane were incubated with primary monoclonal antibodies: anti-BCRP (BXP-21; 1:1000) and β-actin (1:500,000) overnight at 4 °C, and thereafter with HRP-conjugated secondary antibody (1:4000) for 1 h. Bands were detected using Enhanced Chemiluminescence (ECL) peroxide solution and luminol/enhancer solution (Clarity Western ECL Substrate, Bio-Rad Laboratories (Copenhagen, Denmark)) for 5 min. Images were obtained with the UVP Biospectrum imaging system (VisionWorks software, version LS 7.0.1).

2.4. MDR Reversal Analysis with MTT Assay

Cells were seeded in Nunc 96-well plates (2000 or 8000 cells/well for the MDCK-II and HT29 cells, respectively). Following cell attachment (12–24 h), drugs were added to a total volume of 200 μL. Control conditions consisted of full growth medium. All treatments were performed in triplicate. Following 72 h of drug exposure, MTT reagent was added for either 1 h (MDCK-II) or 3 h (HT29). For cell lysis and solubilization of the formazan crystals, DMSO was added to the MDCK-II cells, whereas acidified (0.02 M HCl) sodium dodecyl sulphate was added to the HT29 cells. Optical densities were measured with a microplate spectrophotometer at either 544 nm and 710 nm (background) for the MDCK-II cells or 570 nm and 670 nm (background) for the HT29 cells. Background optical density values were subtracted, and the average optical densities were calculated. Cell viability was calculated as percentage of untreated control cells. The mean IC_{50} values were determined using GraphPad Prism (version 6.0, San Diego, CA, USA). The drug sensitivity analysis was carried out at least three independent times and representative data is shown.

2.5. Bidirectional Transport Assay

Bidirectional transport experiments with [3H]-estrone-3-sulfate were completed with monolayers of Caco-2 cells from the American Type Culture Collection (ATCC) cultured on Transwell permeable supports for 27 days in Dulbecco's modified Eagle's medium, supplemented with 10% FBS, 10 $\mu L \cdot mL^{-1}$ nonessential amino acids (×100), and 100 $U \cdot mL^{-1}$ to 100 $\mu g \cdot mL^{-1}$ penicillin-streptomycin solution. The transepithelial electrical resistance was measured across Caco-2 cell monolayers with an Endohm 12-cup electrode chamber (World Precision Instruments Inc., Sarasota, FL, USA) connected volt meter (EVOM, World Precision Instruments Inc., Sarasota, FL, USA) to ensure that cell monolayers were electrically tight before initiating transport experiments. Cell monolayers were allowed to equilibrate to room temperature before the resistance was measured. Prior to initiating the transport experiments, the cell monolayers were pre-incubated in transport buffer (HBSS supplemented with 10 mM HEPES, pH 7.4, and 0.05 % BSA) for 30 min. Transport experiments were started by replacing the blank transport buffer in the donor compartment with transport buffer containing [3H]-estrone-3-sulfate (1 μCi/mL) and [14C]-mannitol (0.8 μCi/mL) with or without 10 μM SCO-201. For transport experiments in the apical to basolateral direction, samples of 100 μL were taken from the basoteral compartment (volume 1 mL) at t = 15, 30, 45, 60, 90, and 120 min. From transport experiments in the basolateral to apical direction, samples of 50 μL were taken from the apical compartment (volume 0.5 mL) at the same time points. The withdrawn sample volume from the acceptor compartments were immediately replaced with an equal volume of blank transport buffer. The withdrawn samples were pipetted into scintillation vials and mixed with 2 mL of scintillation fluid. The radioactivity of the samples was determined by means of liquid scintillation (Packard Tri-Carb 2910 TR, PerkinElmer, Waltham, MA, USA). Transport of mannitol was measured to validate the barrier integrity of the Caco-2 cell monolayers. The overall average apparent permeability of mannitol across Caco-2 cell monolayers was $2.1 \pm 0.4 \times 10^{-7}$ cm·s^{-1} ($n = 3$, total $N = 9$), which is within the expected range for mannitol permeability across intact monolayers of Caco-2 cells.

Data treatment: The accumulated amount of compound (Qt, nmol) appearing in the donor compartment was plotted against time. The steady-state flux of compound was calculated as the slope of the linear part of this plot, thus correcting for lag-time effects. The apparent permeability was subsequently calculated with Equation (1):

$$P = \frac{J}{C\_0} = \frac{Q\_t}{(C_0 * A\_t)} \tag{1}$$

where J represents the steady state flux (nmol·cm^{-2}·min^{-1}), C_0 represents the initial concentration in the donor compartment, A_t denotes the area of the permeable support (1.12 cm^2), and Q_t is the accumulated amount of compound (nmol) in the receiver compartment at time t (min).

The ratio between apparent permeability in the basolateral to apical direction and the apparent permeability in the opposite direction (efflux ratio = $\frac{PB-A}{PA-B}$) was used as a measure of active efflux transport.

2.6. Cellular Dye Efflux Assay

2.6.1. HT29 Cells

HT29 cells were seeded either into a 96-well Nunclon plate (Thermo Fisher Scientific, Roskilde, Denmark) at a density of 6000 cells/well (for Celigo Imaging Cytometry) or into a Nunc 6-well plate at a density of 150,000 cells/well (for fluorescence microscopy). After 24 h incubation for cell attachment, the cells were incubated with either drug, DMSO or medium for 1 h, then stained with 5 μg/mL Hoechst 33,342 and incubated for 1 h at 37 °C. Then, the cells were washed with ice-cold PBS to remove excess Hoechst dye. Drugs were added again and the cells were incubated for 1h at 37 °C. The plates were analyzed with either fluorescence microscopy (6-well plates) or imaging cytometry (96-well plates). For the Celigo Imaging Cytometry (Lawrence, MA, USA), the application "Target 1 + 2 (merge)" was used, and the mean fluorescence intensities were measured and data presented as percentage of parental control.

2.6.2. MDCK-II-BCRP Cells

The inhibitory effect of SCO-201 on BCRP was determined in the Hoechst 33,342 accumulation assay as described earlier [37]. Briefly, cells were pre-incubated with SCO-201 for 30 min and then Hoechst 33,342 was added to a final concentration of 1 mM. Fluorescence was measured immediately in constant intervals (60 s) for a period of 120 min with an excitation of 355 nm and an emission wavelength of 460 nm at 37 °C using microplate readers (POLARstar and FLUOstar optima by BMG Labtech, Offenburg, Germany). Background fluorescence was subtracted and the average fluorescence between 100 and 109 min obtained in the steady state was calculated and plotted against the logarithm of the compound concentration. Dose–response curves were fitted by nonlinear regression using the four-parameter or three-parameter logistic equation, whichever was statistically preferred (GraphPad Prism, version 6.0, San Diego, CA, USA).

2.7. ATPase Assay

The effect of SCO-201 on the ATPase activity of human BCRP was measured using the PREDEASY ATPase assay system (Solvo Biotechnology, (Sigma-Aldrich/Merck, Schnelldorf, Germany). The assay is a modification of the method of Müller and Sarkardi et al. [38], and the procedure was carried out according to the instructions provided by the manufacturer. Briefly, recombinant BCRP membranes (provided by Solvo Biotechnology) were incubated in the presence or absence of vanadate and different concentrations of either SCO-201 or SN-38, and incubated at 37 °C for 10 min. To test the effect of SCO-201 on the sulfasalazine-stimulated ATPase activity of BCRP, the membranes were prepared with sulfasalazine, prior to the incubation with SCO-201. To test the ability of SCO-201 to hinder the stimulation of BCRP by SN-38, the membranes were prepared with either 0.5 or 1.5 μM SCO-201 and then incubated with different concentrations of SN-38. After incubation with test compounds, MgATP was added to each well and incubated at 37 °C for 10 min. The ATPase reaction was stopped by the addition of 1x Developer solution at room temperature (RT). Two minutes after, 100 μL Blocker solution was added and the plate was incubated for 30 min at 37 °C for 30 min. The optical densities were measured at 620 nm using a PowerWave X Microplate spectrophotometer (BioTek, Bad Friedrichshall, Germany).

2.8. Molecular Interaction Modelling

Docking of SCO-201 and SN-38 in human BCRP transporter were performed using Glide, Schrödinger Release, 2019-3, limited liability company (LLC) [39–41]. The 3D structure of BCRP was obtained from the Research Collaboratory for Structural Bioinformatics (RCSB) Protein Data Bank (PDB ID: 6ETI) [16] and prepared using Protein Preparation Wizard, Schrödinger 2019-3, LLC [42]. SCO-201 and SN-38 were prepared using Ligprep, Schrödinger 2019-3, LLC, and docked using flexible XP docking with sampling of both nitrogen inversions and ring conformations. Further characterization of the binding between BCRP and the ligands were performed using the Desmond Molecular Dynamics System, D.E. Shaw Research, Schrödinger, 2019-2, LLC [43]. A standard membrane was fitted to the transmembrane domain of the transporter, and the system was saturated with ions and water molecules. Simulation was run for 10ns and analyzed visually and using the Simulations Interactions Diagram, Desmond, Schrödinger, 2019-2, LLC [43]. 2D docking graphics were produced from Desmond, Schrödinger, 2019-2, LLC, and 3D molecular graphic images of docking were established using the PyMOL Molecular Graphics System, Version 2.0, Schrödinger, LLC.

2.9. In Vitro DMPK Analysis: Transporter Inhibition Analysis

Cells were seeded in a 96-well plate (20,000 cells/well) and used on days 2 or 3 post-seeding. SCO-201 was prepared in assay buffer (HBSS-HEPES, pH 7.4), added to the cell plate and pre-incubated at 37 °C for 15 min. SCO-201 was tested at either a single concentration (10 μM by default) or multiple concentrations (0.03, 0.1, 0.3, 1, 3, 10, 30, and 100 μM by default), with a final DMSO concentration of 1%. Subsequently, substrate was added to the plate followed by 20 min incubation at 37 °C. The plate was then washed with cold assay buffer followed by fluorescence reading on a plate reader. The tested transporters, cell lines, substrates, and reference inhibitors are shown in the Supplementary Materials (Tables S1 and S2).

2.10. In Vitro DMPK Analysis: CYP Inhibition

The following procedure was used to asses if SCO-201 inhibits the activity of common CYP enzymes in pooled human liver microsomes in 96-well plate format. SCO-201 was pre-incubated with substrate and human liver microsomes (mixed gender, pool of 50 donors, 0.1 mg/mL) in phosphate buffer (pH 7.4) for 5 min in a 37 °C shaking waterbath. SCO-201 was tested at either a single concentration (10 µM by default) with 0.1% DMSO or multiple concentrations (0.03, 0.1, 0.3, 1, 3, 10, 30, and 100 µM by default) with up to 1% DMSO for IC_{50} determination. The reaction was initiated by adding a Nicotinamide adenine dinucleotide phosphate (NADPH)-generating system. The reaction was allowed for 10 min and stopped by transferring the reaction mixture to acetonitrile/methanol. Samples were mixed and centrifuged. Supernatants were used for HPLC-MS/MS of the respective metabolite. Tested CYP enzymes, substrates, metabolites, and reference inhibitors are shown in the Supplementary Materials (Tables S2 and S3).

Data analysis: Peak areas corresponding to the metabolite were recorded. The percent of control activity was calculated by comparing the peak area in the presence of the test compound to the control samples containing the same solvent. Subsequently, the percent inhibition was calculated by subtracting the percent control activity from 100. The IC_{50} value (concentration causing a half-maximal inhibition of the control value) was determined by non-linear regression analysis of the concentration–response curve using the Hill equation.

2.11. *In Vitro DMPK Analysis: CYP Induction*

The following procedure was carried out to test whether SCO-201 induces CYP1A, CYP2B6, and CYP3A activities in human hepatocytes. The procedure was designed in accordance with the FDA Guidance for Industry on Drug Interaction Studies (2006). Male and female human hepatocytes were thawed and plated into collagen-coated 96-well plates in serum-containing medium (plating medium) at a density of 0.7×10^6 viable cells/mL. The hepatocytes were cultured in a humidified incubator at 37 °C and 5% CO_2. At 4 h post plating, human hepatocytes were washed once with fresh plating medium, followed by overnight incubation. At 24 h after plating, the plating medium was removed, and the hepatocytes were overlaid with extracellular matrix (ECM) (Sigma) or Matrigel (BD) in the serum-free medium (incubation medium), and then incubated for another 24 h. Incubation medium with 0.1% DMSO was used as the negative control. After the 2-day recovery period, the hepatocytes were treated with SCO-201 or a known inducer (Table S3) in the incubation medium on day 3 and day 4. The known inducer was tested as the positive control. On day 5, the medium was removed, and the cells were incubated with the respective CYP substrate in Krebs–Henseleit buffer (pH 7.4) containing 3 mM salicylamide for 30 min. The reaction was terminated by transferring the incubation mixture to an equal volume of acetonitrile/methanol mixture (1/1, *v*/*v*). Samples were mixed and centrifuged. Supernatants are used for HPLC-MS/MS analysis of the corresponding metabolite. Peak areas corresponding to the metabolite were recorded. The assay was rendered valid if enzyme activity with the positive control was at least twofold greater than negative control.

2.12. *Statistical Analyses*

Statistical analyses were performed using Microsoft Excel. Means and standard deviations were calculated for all quantitative data. For data represented in percentage (i.e., cell viability), the standard deviations, determined from triplicate experiments, were calculated and displayed on the graphs as standard deviation percentages: $Stdv\% = Stdv * \left(\frac{\%of control}{ODaverage}\right)$. Two-tailed, type 3 Student's *t*-tests were applied on datasets where relevant, in order to determine any significant statistical differences. Statistical analysis of the data in the bidirectional transport assay was performed by comparing group means with a Student's *t*-test (two-tailed) or ANOVA, followed by Bonferroni's multiple comparisons test. The significance level was set to 5%, and thus *p*-values less than 0.05 were considered significant.

3. Results

3.1. SCO-201 Reversed BCRP-mediated Drug Resistance in Chemotherapy Resistant Cells

To assess the potential BCRP-dependent re-sensitizing effects of SCO-201, we used the BCRP-transduced canine kidney subline, MDCK-II-BCRP, which in several studies has been shown to express high levels of BCRP [37,44]. The MDCK-II-BCRP cells are known to be less sensitive to chemotherapy substrates of BCRP, such as SN-38, topotecan, and mitoxantrone, compared to their parental counterpart, MDCK-II-WT [37,44]. We therefore tested the potential of SCO-201 to restore the drug sensitivity of the MDCK-II-BCRP cells to SN-38 and mitoxantrone by treating the cells with either chemotherapy alone or in combination with SCO-201, or the BCRP inhibitor Ko143 for comparison. As seen in Figure 2A-C, SCO-201 was able to completely restore the response to SN-38 and mitoxantrone in the MDCK-II-BCRP cells similar to the BCRP-inhibitor Ko143. The IC_{50} values are shown in Table 1. Treatment with SCO-201 and SN-38 or mitoxantrone resulted in decreased IC_{50} values for the MDCK-II-BCRP cells that were comparable to the IC_{50} values found for the MDCK-II-WT cells. Altogether, these results show that SCO-201 significantly re-sensitized MDCK-II-BCRP cells to both SN-38 and mitoxantrone. This is proof-of-concept that SCO-201 can affect BCRP-mediated resistance in a model system where the resistance is engineered by ectopic overexpression of BCRP.

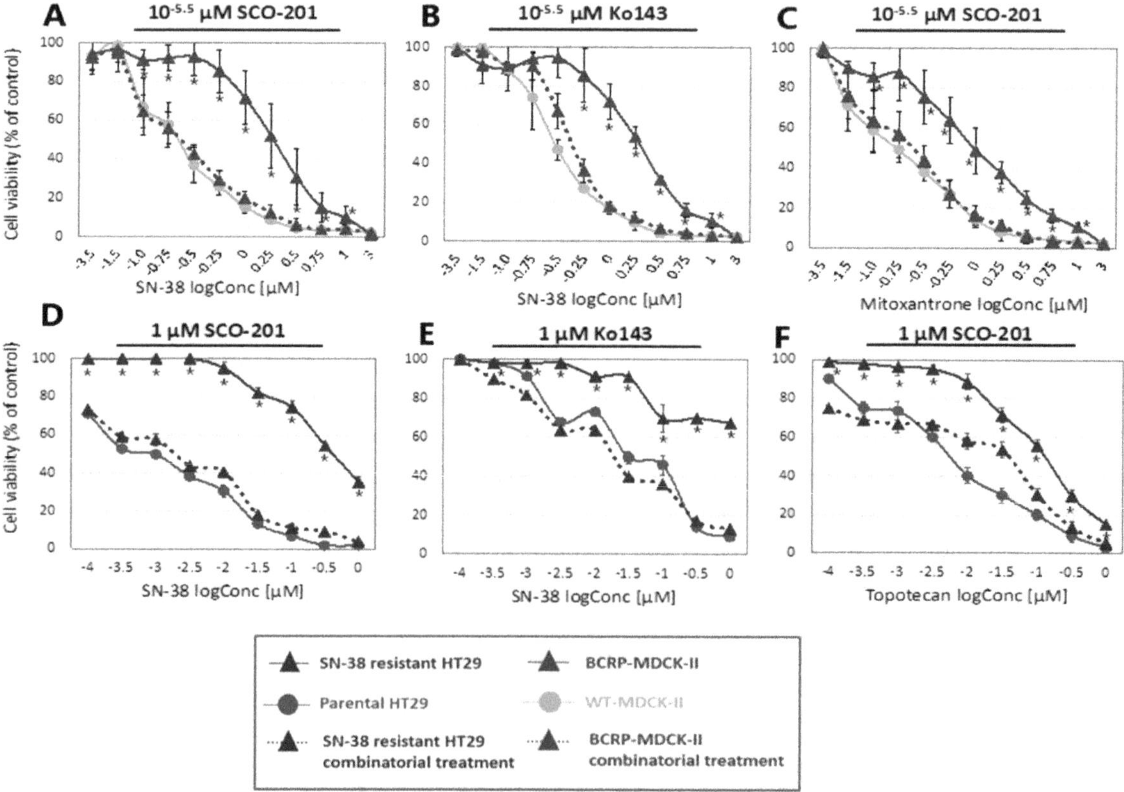

Figure 2. SCO-201 reversed drug resistance in multidrug resistance (MDR) cells. Cell viability of wild-type or breast cancer resistance protein (BCRP)-overexpressing MDCK-II cells and SN-38-sensitive or -resistant HT29 cells. Cell viability is indicated as percentage of untreated control, and error bars indicate percentage SD determined on the basis of $n = 3$–4. Note that some error bars might be invisible due to the size of the data labels. Control conditions consisted of full growth medium. (**A–C**) Wild-type and BCRP-overexpressing MDCK-II cells treated with either chemotherapy alone or in combination with $10^{-5.5}$ µM SCO-201 or Ko143. (**D–F**) Parental and SN-38-resistant HT29 cells treated with either chemotherapy alone or in combination with 1 µM SCO-201 or Ko143. Statistical difference ($p < 0.05$) between mono-treatment and combination treatment of the resistant cell lines is marked by * (Student's *t*-test (two-tailed, type 3)).

Table 1. IC_{50} values of anti-cancer drugs in the presence/absence of SCO-201 or Ko143.

	IC_{50} Value (μM) for Each Cell Line			
Drug/Drug Combination	**MDCK-II-WT**	**MDCK-II-BCRP**	**$HT29_{PAR}$**	**$HT29_{SN\text{-}38\text{-}RES}$**
SN-38	0.214 ± 0.023	1.956 ± 0.080	0.016 ± 0.010	0.463 ± 0.363
SN-38 + SCO-201		0.238 ± 0.029		0.007 ± 0.005
SN-38 + Ko143		0.437 ± 0.020		0.014 ± 0.021
Mitoxantrone	0.157 ± 0.023	1.060 ± 0.095		
Mitoxantrone + SCO-201		0.214 ± 0.030		
Topotecan			0.008 ± 0.003	0.121 ± 0.024
Topotecan + SCO-201				0.088 ± 0.030

Taken together, our results show that SCO-201 could successfully reverse resistance to the anti-cancer BCRP substrates, SN-38, topotecan, and mitoxantrone, similarly to the BCRP inhibitor Ko143 in BCRP over-expressing MDCK-II-BCRP and $HT29_{SN\text{-}38\text{-}RES}$ cells. This indicates that SCO-201 could be a modulator of BCRP activity. Supplementary studies showed that SCO-201 has a dose-dependent effect with SN-38 in both MDCK-II-BCRP and $HT29_{SN\text{-}38\text{-}RES}$ cells (Figures S3 and S4).

To further investigate the re-sensitizing effects of SCO-201 and to apply a more complex model system of resistance, we tested the effects of SCO-201 in our DEN-50R in vitro model system of acquired SN-38 resistance in colorectal cancer. To generate this system, the colorectal adenocarcinoma cell line, HT29, was subjected to gradually increasing SN-38 concentrations for a period of ≈10 months, resulting in an SN-38-resistant cell line ($HT29_{SN\text{-}38\text{-}RES}$). Genome-wide expression mRNA profiling revealed that BCRP was highly upregulated (25-fold) in the $HT29_{SN\text{-}38\text{-}RES}$ cells, compared to their parental counterpart ($HT29_{PAR}$) (GEO—Gene Expression Omnibus, NCBI, accession number GSE42387) [25]. We confirmed the BCRP overexpression with Western blot analysis (Figure S1). As seen in the blot, two bands could be observed for BCRP in the $HT29_{SN\text{-}38\text{-}RES}$ cells, most likely due to the glycosylation states of BCRP [45].

We tested the potential re-sensitizing effects of SCO-201 in the $HT29_{SN\text{-}38\text{-}RES}$ cells by treating the cells with either chemotherapy alone or in combination with SCO-201 or Ko143. As seen in Figure 2D–F, SCO-201 was able to significantly restore the response to both SN-38 and topotecan in the $HT29_{SN\text{-}38\text{-}RES}$ cells, similar to the response observed for combinatorial treatment with Ko143. The IC_{50} values are shown in Table 1. The IC_{50} values of SN-38 and topotecan decreased several folds for the $HT29_{SN\text{-}38\text{-}RES}$ cells, following treatment with SCO-201, and they almost completely reached the IC_{50} values for the $HT29_{PAR}$ cells (Table 1).

To investigate if these observations were due to general damaging effects on the cells that could lead to general increase in sensitivity to chemotherapy, we applied oxaliplatin, which is not a substrate for BCRP. When oxaliplatin was combined with either SCO-201 or Ko143 in the $HT29_{SN\text{-}38\text{-}RES}$ cells, no added effects were observed (Figure S2). This suggests that the re-sensitizing effects were not due to general cellular effects of either SCO-201 or Ko143.

3.2. SCO-201 Inhibited the BCRP-Mediated Flux Across Cell Membranes

To more directly investigate whether SCO-201 inhibits BCRP-mediated efflux transport, a series of bidirectional transport experiments with the prototypical BCRP substrate [^{3}H]-estrone-3-sulfate were completed across monolayers of Caco-2 cells (Figure 3). In the absence of SCO-201, the apparent permeability of [^{3}H]-estrone-3-sulfate in the efflux direction (basolateral to apical) was $2.7 \pm 0.2 \times 10^{-5}$ cm/second, whereas it was considerably lower in the opposite direction with an apparent permeability of $2.2 \pm 0.01 \times 10^{-6}$ cm/second. The resulting efflux ratio in the absence of SCO-201 was 12.2, which indicated a marked polarized transport in the efflux direction for [^{3}H]-estrone-3-sulfate across monolayers of Caco-2 cells. In the presence of 10 μM SCO-201, the apparent B-A (basolateral to apical) permeability was significantly reduced to $9.6 \pm 0.7 \times 10^{-6}$ cm/second ($p < 0.0001$), whereas the apparent permeability in the A-B (apical to basolateral) direction was significantly increased to $3.2 \pm 0.3 \times 10^{-6}$ cm/second ($p = 0.0061$). Correspondingly, the calculated efflux ratio was markedly reduced to 2.9, which together with the reduction in efflux transport of [^{3}H]-estrone-3-sulfate were clear indications that SCO-201 had an inhibitory effect on BCRP-mediated efflux transport of [^{3}H]-estrone-3-sulfate across Caco-2 cell monolayers (Figure 3).

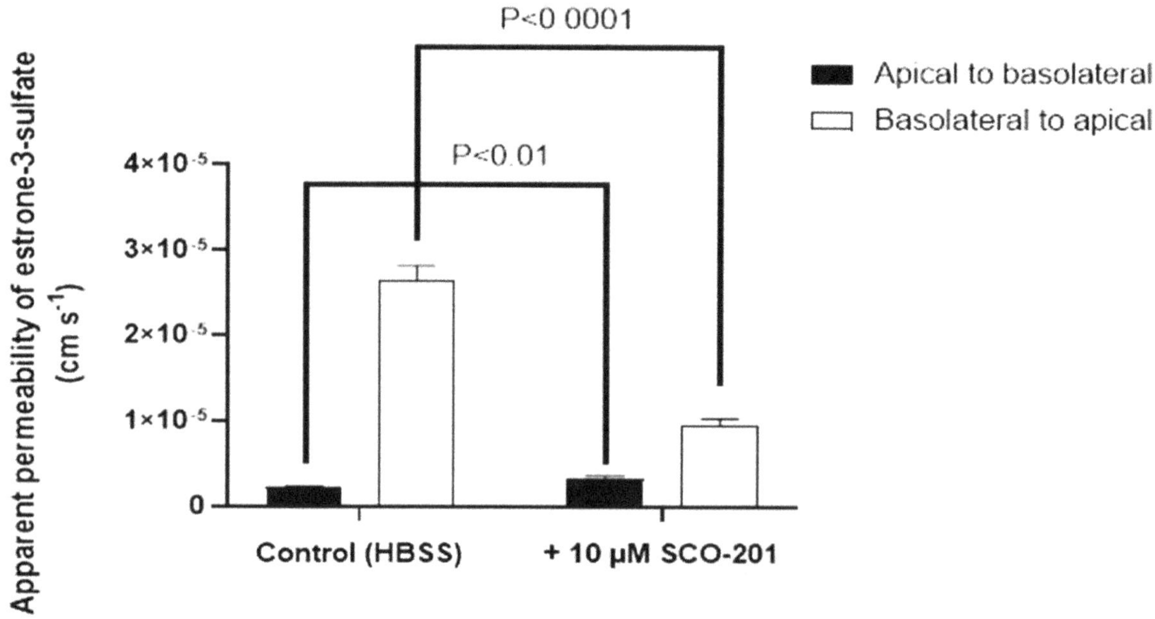

Figure 3. Bidirectional transport of estrone-3-sulfate across Caco-2 cell monolayers in the presence or absence of 10 μM SCO-201. Permeability (Papp) values were calculated from steady-state fluxes as described the in the Methods section (Section 2.5). Filled bars show PA-B (apical to basolateral) values, open bars show PB-A (basolateral to apical) values. Values are means ± SD of three individual passages, with three individual permeable supports for each transport direction per passage (n = 3–5, total N = 9). The p-values are indicated in the figure.

To further elucidate whether SCO-201 modulates BCRP and in this way triggers intracellular accumulation of chemotherapy, we conducted dye efflux studies on wild-type and SN-38-resistant HT29 cells, the latter of which overexpresses BCRP. The cells were stained with Hoechst in the presence or absence of SCO-201, Ko143, or the MDR1/P-gp inhibitor PSC833 as a negative control. Figure 4 presents results from fluorescence microscopy and imaging cytometry analysis. Accumulation of Hoechst could clearly be detected in the parental cells, whereas only low levels of Hoechst accumulation could be detected in the BCRP-overexpressing chemotherapy-resistant cells (Figure 4A,B). When the resistant cells were treated with either SCO-201 or Ko143, Hoechst accumulated to the level of the parental control cells, whereas treatment with PSC833 did not have any effects (Figure 4A,B). In a similar experiment, we quantified the dose-dependent effects of SCO-201 compared with Ko143 and evaluated the outcome with imaging cytometry. Figure 4C shows the dose-dependent effect of SCO-201 on intracellular accumulation of dye in Hoechst-stained cells compared to Ko143. As seen from the IC_{50} values, the potency of Ko143 (IC_{50} = 0.37 μM) and SCO-201 (IC_{50} = 0.45 μM) was almost identical. Altogether, these results indicate that SCO-201, like Ko143, modulates the efflux of dye via BCRP, resulting in an accumulation of Hoechst dye in the $HT29_{SN\text{-}38\text{-}RES}$ cells. The same tendency could be observed when we quantified the effect of SCO-201 on the accumulation of Hoechst or Pheophorbic A in the MDCK-II-BCRP cells (Figure S5 and S6). These Supplementary studies also indicated that SCO-201 is likely not an inhibitor of MDR1/P-gp.

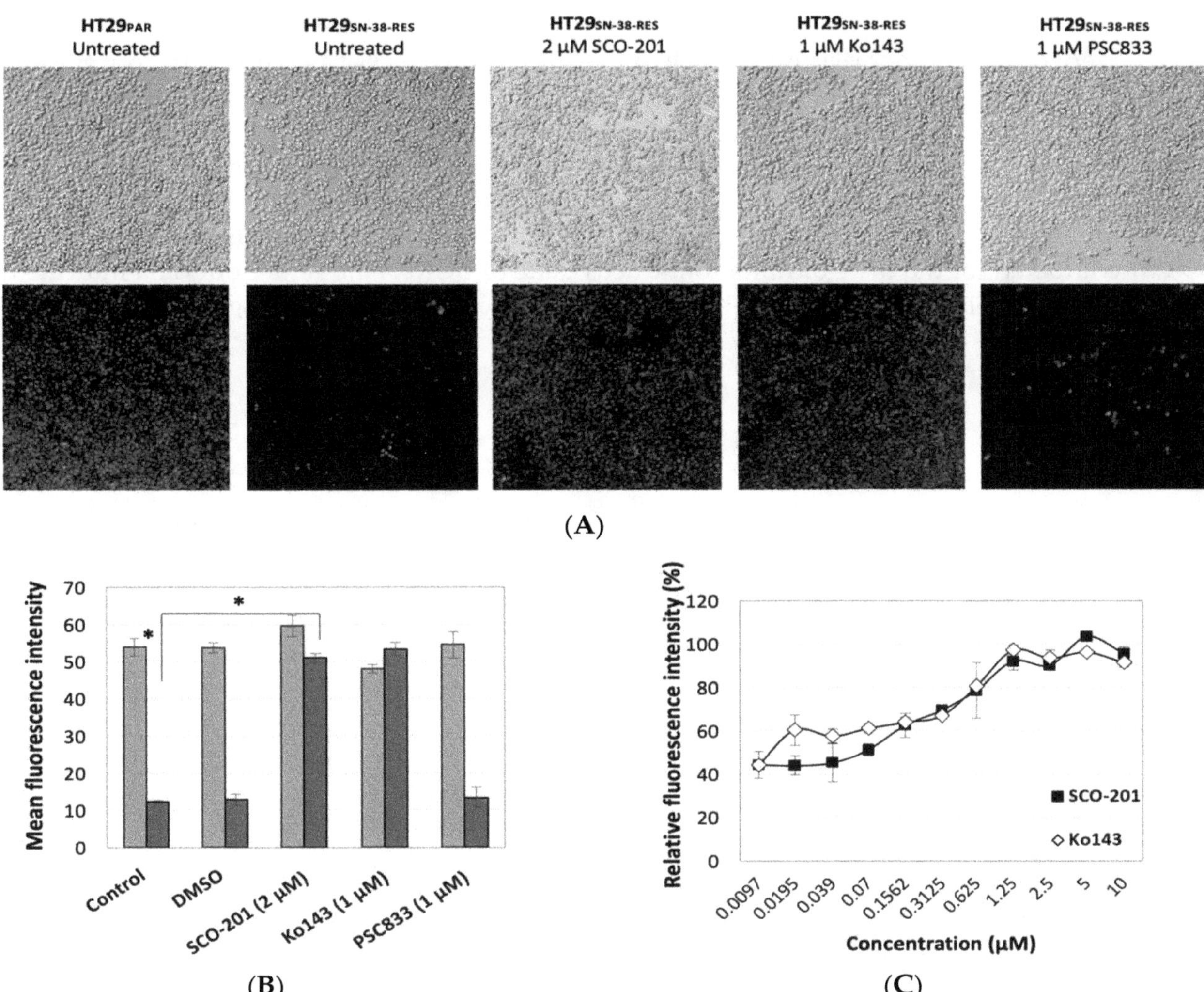

Figure 4. SCO-201 inhibited the efflux of Hoechst 33,342 from $HT29_{SN\text{-}38\text{-}RES}$ cells. (**A**) Fluorescence micrographs of Hoechst-stained parental HT29 cells ($HT29_{PAR}$) and $HT29_{SN\text{-}38\text{-}RES}$ cells that were incubated with either SCO-201, the BCRP-inhibitor Ko143, or the MDR1-inhibitor valspodar (PSC833). Full growth medium was used for the control condition. Untreated parental HT29 cells were included as a positive control, indicating the maximal accumulation of Hoechst dye, as these cells do not overexpress BCRP. (**B**) Mean fluorescence intensity of Hoechst-stained SN-38-sensitive (light grey) and SN-38 resistant (dark grey) HT29 cells treated with either DMSO, SCO-201, Ko143, or PSC833. Full growth medium was used for the control condition. The asterisks (*) indicate statistical significance ($p < 0.05$). (**C**) The dose-dependent effects of SCO-201 and Ko143 on the accumulation of Hoechst, indicated by the increase in relative fluorescence intensity of Hoechst-stained $HT29_{SN\text{-}38\text{-}RES}$ cells. Error bars in (**B**,**C**) indicate SD determined from triplicate experiments.

3.3. The Drug-Stimulated ATPase Activity of BCRP Was Competitively Inhibited by SCO-201

Following our results from the flux studies (Figures 3 and 4), we further evaluated whether SCO-201 indeed is a modulator of BCRP transport activity. To evaluate the modulatory effects of SCO-201, we conducted ATPase studies to test the effect of SCO-201 on the ATPase activity of BCRP in the presence or absence of another activating BCRP substrate. Figure 5A shows the relative ATPase activities of BCRP incubated with either SCO-201 alone, or in the presence of the strong BCRP activator, sulfasalazine. Sulfasalazine alone resulted in a maximal ATPase activity of 104.8 nmol Pi/mg protein/min compared to the basal activity of 50.68 nmol Pi/mg protein/min (data not shown). As seen on Figure 5A, SCO-201 was not in itself a stimulator of BCRP ATPase activity, and in the absence of sulfasalazine, the ATPase activity of BCRP decreased dose-dependently upon incubation with SCO-201.

When SCO-201 was added to sulfasalazine-stimulated BCRP, the ATPase activity of BCRP decreased in a dose-dependent manner (Figure 5A). Then, we tested the effect of two different concentrations of SCO-201 on SN-38-stimulated BCRP. Figure 5B,C shows the relative SN-38-stimulated ATPase activity of BCRP in the presence or absence of either 0.5 μM or 1.5 μM SCO-201. In the presence of SCO-201, the SN-38-stimulated ATPase activity of BCRP was shifted downwards, and the higher the SCO-201 concentration, the higher the SN-38 concentration was needed to reach the maximal activity of SN-38-stimulated BCRP. This revealed a typical competitive inhibition mechanism, showing that SCO-201 competed for the drug binding to the active site of BCRP. Altogether our data indicate that SCO-201 competitively inhibits the drug-stimulated ATPase activity of BCRP, suggesting that SCO-201 is a direct modulator of BCRP.

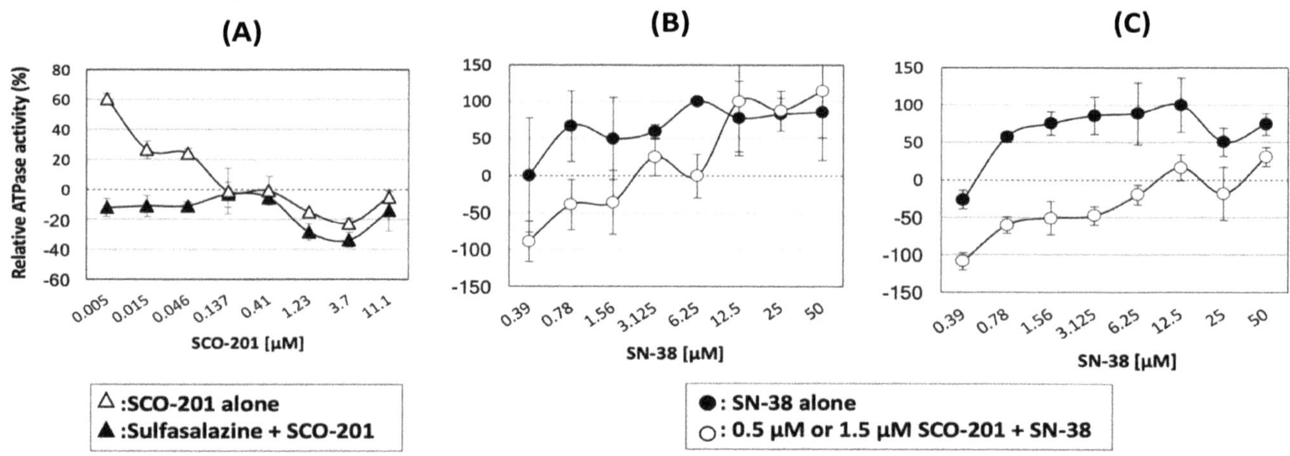

Figure 5. SCO-201 inhibited drug-stimulated ATPase activity of BCRP. (**A**) The effect of increasing concentrations of SCO-201 on basal and sulfasalazine-stimulated ATPase activity of BCRP. The data are indicated as relative ATPase activity, normalized with respect to basal (untreated) and maximal (sulfasalazine-stimulated) ATPase activity of BCRP. Sulfasalazine alone resulted in a maximal ATPase activity of 104.8 nmol Pi/mg protein/min compared to the baseline activity of 50.68 nmol Pi/mg protein/min. (**B**,**C**) The effect of 0.5 μM (B) and 1.5 μM (C) SCO-201 on SN-38-stimulated ATPase activity of BCRP. Error bars on all graphs represent SD determined from duplicates.

3.4. Molecular Binding Model Further Supported a Competitive Action of SCO-201

Thus far, our results have indicated that SCO-201 competitively inhibits the transport of BCRP substrates, such as SN-38, and that SCO-201 directly interacts with BCRP. To further support these results, we performed in silico molecular docking simulations to identify the binding sites of SCO-201 or SN-38 in BCRP. SN-38 and SCO-201 were successfully docked into the 3D structure of the BCRP and the resulting models showed that both SN-38 and SCO-201 were predicted to bind in the same binding cavity (Figure 6). Docking scores were -12.24 for SN-38 and -8.66 for SCO-201, indicating that both ligands could bind in the ligand binding site of the transporter.

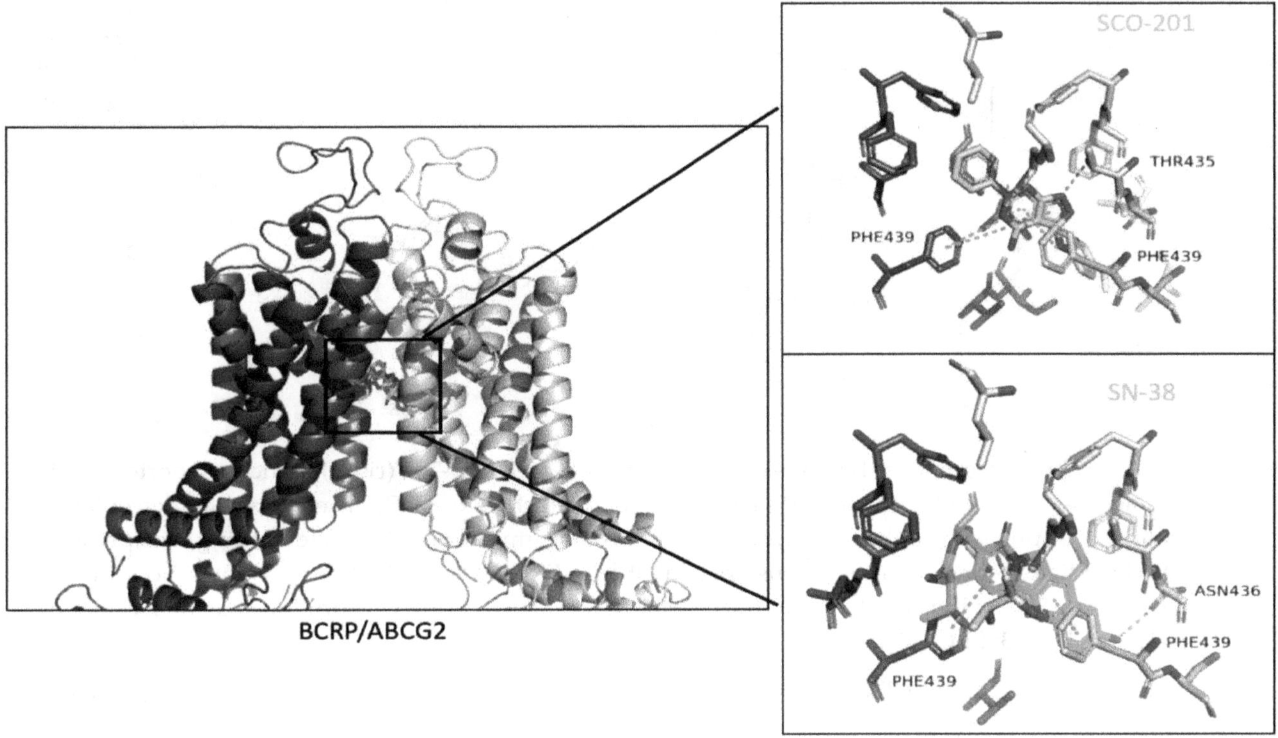

Figure 6. Docking of SN-38 and SCO-201 in the human BCRP transporter. The transporter is a homomeric dimer with chain A (dark grey) and chain B (light grey). SN-38 (green) and SCO-201 (orange) bind in the same binding cavity when docked using Glide, Schrödinger, 2019-3, LLC [39–41]. Both the substrate SN-38 and the proposed inhibitor SCO-201 interacted with Phenylalanine (PHE)-439 in both chains of the protein through hydrophobic Pi-stacking interactions. SCO-201 formed a hydrogen bond to Threonine (THR)-435, whereas SN-38 formed a hydrogen bond to Aspargine (ASN)-436. Pi-stacking interactions are colored green and hydrogen bonds are colored violet.

The molecular dynamic simulations demonstrated that both ligands remained in the binding sites throughout the sampled time period (Videos S1 and S2). The simulation interaction diagram (Figure 7) showed that SN-38 interacted through pi-stacking interactions with Phenylalanine (PHE)-439 of both protein chains, whereas SCO-201 predominantly interacted with the PHE-439 residue of the B chain and only to a lesser extent with the residue of the A protein chain (Figure 7; Figures S7 and S8). SN-38 further formed a hydrogen bond to Aspargine (ASN)-436 residue of the B chain of the transporter, whereas SCO-201 formed a hydrogen bond to both the Threonine (THR)-435 and ASN-436 residues of the B chain (Figure 7). As SCO-201 binds in the same binding cavity and interacts with some of the residues that the substrate SN-38 interacts with, it is likely that SCO-201 is a competitive inhibitor of the BCRP transporter by blocking substrate access.

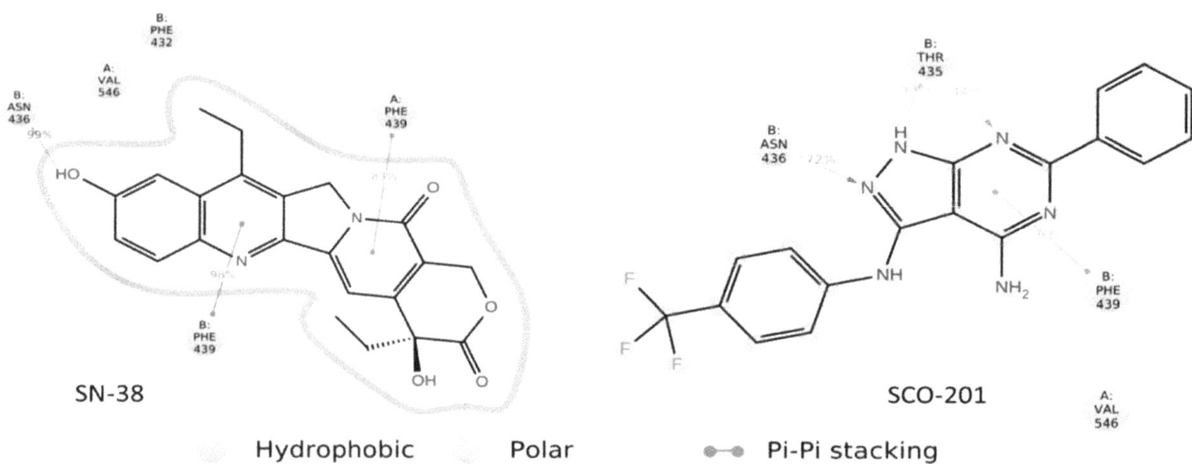

Figure 7. Binding interactions shown between SN-38 (left) and SCO-201 (right) to the transporter BCRP. Both molecules interacted with the PHE-439 residue of the B chain of BCRP. The interaction percentages indicate accounting for number of frames over the 10 ns simulation where the binding was present. Timetable of ligand–protein interactions are available in Figures S7 and S8. Interactions shown were present in over 30% of the simulation frames. Graphical representation was produced using Desmond, Schrödinger, 2019-3, LLC [43].

3.5. *In Vitro DMPK Data Suggest That SCO-201 Is Not Likely to Increase The Risk of Pharmacokinetic Interactions*

In clinical trials with ABC transporter inhibitors, pharmacokinetic interactions gave rise to increased serum levels of chemotherapy, thus enhancing the toxic effects of the chemotherapy, and dose reductions were therefore needed [34–38]. These dose reductions resulted in patients being under- or even overdosed, as the pharmacokinetic profile of each individual patient was difficult to predict [46–50]. On the basis of this, we aimed to test the potential inhibitory effects of SCO-201 on common transporters, playing a key role in pharmacokinetics, in order to predict the possibility that SCO-201 would negatively influence the pharmacokinetic profile of co-administered drugs. Specifically, we tested the inhibitory effects of SCO-201 on MDR1/P-gp as well as on several members of the solute carrier (SLC) family involved in drug pharmacokinetics, in accordance with the European Medicines Agency (EMA) Guidance of regulatory requirements for toxicological assessment of small molecules.

MDR1/P-gp and members of the SLC family including the organic anion transporting polypeptides (OATP) OATP1B1, OATP1B3, organic anion transporter (OAT) OAT1 and organic cation transporters (OCT) OCT2 act as major determinants of the absorption, distribution, excretion, and toxicity (ADME-tox) properties of drugs [51,52]. To investigate if SCO-201 inhibits any of the aforementioned transporters, we conducted a cell-based fluorometric drug transporter inhibition assay. We included BCRP as a positive control. The results are presented in Table 2 and show that SCO-201 inhibited BCRP as expected but is not likely an inhibitor of either MDR1/P-gp or any of the tested SLC family members as none of the fluorometric substrates accumulated. In addition, it is seen that the IC_{50} value for BCRP in CHO cells was 1.7 μM, showing that SCO-201 is a potent inhibitor of BCRP (Table 2 and Figure S7).

Table 2. Summary of drug transporter inhibition.

Transport Protein	Cell Line	Substrate	IC_{50} (M)
OCT2	OCT2-CHO	ASP+	NC
BCRP	BCRP-CHO	Hoechst 33342	1.7×10^{-6}
OAT1	OAT-CHO	CF	NC
OAT3	OAT3-CHO	CF	NC
OATP1B1	OATP1B1-CHO	FMTX	NC
OATP1B3	OATP1B3-CHO	FMTX	NC
P-gp (MDR1)	MDR1-MDCK-II	Calcein-AM	NC

NC: not calculable.

To further predict any potential risk of drug–drug interactions, we tested the effect of SCO-201 on key oxidative metabolic drug enzymes of the cytochrome P450 (CYP) family. Specifically, we tested the potential inhibition or induction by SCO-201 on a range of common CYPs playing a key role in determining the pharmacokinetic profile of drugs [53]. We used a standard CYP inhibition assay based on human liver microsomes, and the IC_{50} values of SCO-201 towards CYP1A, CYP2B6, CYP2C8, CYP2C9, CYP2C19, CYP2D6, and CYP3A (with two substrates) were determined in a range of concentrations (from 0.03 to 100 μM). The results are shown in Table 3 and found that no IC_{50} value was less than 100 μM, suggesting that SCO-201 is not likely an inhibitor of these CYP isoforms and may not cause CYP inhibition when its plasma concentration is below 100 μM.

Table 3. Cytochrome P450 (CYP) inhibition.

CYP	Test	Substrate	IC_{50} (M)
CYP1A	Human hepatocytes	Phenacetin substrate	$>1 \times 10^{-4}$
CYP2B6	Human hepatocytes	Bupropion substrate	NC
CYP2C8	Human liver microsomes	Paclitaxel	$>1 \times 10^{-4}$
CYP2C9	Human liver microsomes	Diclofenac	$>1 \times 10^{-4}$
CYP2C19	Human liver microsomes	Omeprazole	NC
CYP2D6	Human liver microsomes	Dextromethorphan	NC
CYP3A	Human liver microsomes	Midazolam	NC
		Testosterone	$>1 \times 10^{-4}$

NC: not calculable.

Inductions of CYP1A2, CYP2B6, and CYP3A4 by SCO-201 were tested at 1, 10, and 100 μM using both enzyme activity and mRNA level changes as the end-points. The results are presented in Table 4. Using enzyme activity as the end-point, the results were all below the cutoff value (40% of positive control), suggesting that SCO-201 is not an inducer for these CYP isoforms. Using mRNA level as the end-point, the results were also below the cutoff values, similarly suggesting that SCO-201 does not induce the CYP isoforms. However, there was a trend in both enzyme and mRNA assays that fold induction decreased with the increase in test concentrations. This trend may have resulted from cytotoxicity toward the hepatocytes.

Table 4. CYP induction.

CYP	Mean Fold Induction of mRNA at 1×10^{-4} M			Mean Fold Enzyme Activity Induction at 1×10^{-4} M		
	Donor 1	Donor 2	Donor 3	Donor 1	Donor 2	Donor 3
CYP1A				1	0.7	0.7
CYP1A2	0.24	0.39	0.26			
CYP2B6	0.17	0.52	0.45	0.8	0.9	0.6
CYP3A				1.3	2.0	0.4
CYP3A	0.25	0.25	0.32			

Fold induction = (activity of test compound treated cells)/(activity of negative control). mRNA fold induction = (mRNA level in test compound treated cells)/(mRNA levels in vehicle treated controls).

In conclusion, our results from these in vitro analyses might imply that SCO-201 does not significantly negatively influence the pharmacokinetic profile of co-administered drugs. This suggest that SCO-201 may be of a new generation of ABC transporter modulators with low risk of increased chemotherapy-mediated toxicity.

4. Discussion

ABC transporter-mediated resistance to multiple anti-cancer drugs is one of the major reasons for cancer treatment failure [1–5]. Overexpression of the transporter BCRP prevents chemotherapeutic agents such as SN-38, mitoxantrone, and fluoruracil from remaining inside cancer cells, and in this way, protects the cancer cells from being killed by these drugs. BCRP expression in cancer cells confers drug resistance in leukemia, and higher levels are reported in solid tumors from the digestive tract, endometrium, lung, and melanoma, although, contrarily, expression is generally low in breast cancer tumours [54]. There is significant association between BCRP expression and tumor response to chemotherapy and progression-free survival [1–4].

In this study, we showed that the pyrazolo-pyrimidine derivative SCO-201 can reverse MDR in vitro by competitively inhibiting the transport function of BCRP. Firstly, we tested the ability of SCO-201 to re-sensitize drug-resistant MDCK-II-BCRP and $HT29_{SN\text{-}38\text{-}RES}$ cells to chemotherapy, and these data demonstrated that SCO-201 can successfully reverse resistance in these cells (Figure 2). To investigate the potential mechanism of action of SCO-201, we conducted dye efflux assay and examined the intracellular accumulation of Hoechst 33,342 in BCRP-overexpressing cells, when treated with SCO-201, by fluorescence microscopy and imaging cytometry (Figure 4). Our results indicated that SCO-201 triggers the accumulation of Hoechst 33,342 in the BCRP-expressing cells, similarly to Ko143. We subsequently performed ATPase assay in order to examine if the effect of SCO-201 was caused by a direct inhibition of the transport function of BCRP. These results showed that SCO-201 competitively inhibits the drug-stimulated activity of BCRP (Figure 5).

To further support these results, we performed molecular docking and molecular dynamics simulations, and found that SCO-201 and SN-38 were predicted to bind in the same binding pocket of BCRP. Both SN-38 and SCO-201 interacted with PHE-439 of the B protein chain through Pi-stacking hydrophobic interactions, and ASN-436 through hydrogen bonds (Figures 6 and 7). From the cryo-EM structure of BCRP (PDB ID: 6ETI), stacking interaction was also seen between the inhibitor and PHE-439, which emphasized the importance of these residues both in transport and in inhibition of BCRP. It further supports SCO-201 being a competitive inhibitor of the BCRP transporter [16].

There are challenges of bringing ABC transporter inhibitors to clinical use, reflected by the fact that after 40 years of research there are still no approved ABC transporter inhibitors for use in the clinical setting [1]. To date, three generations of different MDR1/P-gp inhibitors have been tested and developed pre-clinically and clinically [1,7,9]. The first generation of inhibitors tested in clinical trials were not specifically developed to modulate ABC transporters but were drugs already in clinical use (e.g., verapamil and cyclosporine A). These were weak inhibitors and needed high doses. Such high doses in combination with anti-cancer drugs (e.g., mitoxantrone, daunorubicin, and etoposide) caused toxic side effects and had low therapeutic response [7–10]. Therefore, these were quickly replaced by more potent and specific second-generation inhibitors (e.g., R-verapamil and PSC-833 (Valspodar)) in order to reduce possible primary toxicities. In acute myeloid leukemia (AML) patients, the combination of PSC-833 with anti-cancer drugs seemed to be beneficial for some patients. However, the second-generation inhibitors were also shown to be inhibitors of CYPs and displayed pharmacokinetic interactions leading to increased toxicity [7–10]. Several phase III clinical studies with PSC-833 revealed that the combination with chemotherapeutic agents did not prolong the survival of cancer patients [47,48,50,55]. Third-generation inhibitors (e.g., laniquidar (R101933), ONT-093 (OC14–093), zosuqiodar (LY335979), elacridar (GF120918), and tariquidar (XR9576)) were up to 200-fold more potent and had low pharmacokinetic interaction due to a limited CYP3A inhibition [56]. The third-generation inhibitors are well tolerated in humans, safe to combine with chemotherapy due to less systemic pharmacokinetic interactions than previous MDR1 inhibitors, and were found to cause potent MDR1/P-gp inhibition in humans [57–63]. Furthermore, scanning imaging of tumors for contents of (99m)Tc-sestamibi before and after dosing of third generation inhibitors could possibly be applied to identify subgroups of anti-cancer-resistant cancer patients who may benefit from a combination of inhibitor and anti-cancer drug.

Thus, the development from first to third generation inhibitors has to a large degree abolished the pharmacokinetic interactions and related toxicities with the tested inhibitors and anti-cancer drugs. Even if toxicities should be observed with novel inhibitors and combinations with anti-cancer drugs, this can be taken care of by starting a patient with an ABC transporter inhibitor and reduced dose of chemotherapy. If no severe side effects are noted, the dose of chemotherapy can be increased at the next cycle. It is important to remember that, even with a need for lowering the dose of chemotherapy, a significant anti-tumor effect might be obtained due to the simultaneous inhibition of drug efflux pumps in the cancer cells. Another problem with the clinical studies, which tested the efficacy of ABC transporter inhibitors in combination with chemotherapy, was the general lack of randomization, and in most studies the ABC transporter inhibitor was not combined with the chemotherapy that the patient had developed resistance against. Finally, the clinical studies also lacked the inclusion of predictive biomarkers. In some of the studies, a few of the patients had ABC cassette proteins measured in their tumor tissue, but in none of the studies was this performed on a fresh tumor biopsy, and was instead performed on the primary biopsy obtained at the time of diagnosis and prior to any chemotherapy, which does not necessarily reflect the expression of ABC transporter proteins in the resistant tumor cells.

To our knowledge, no second or third generation BCRP inhibitors have been developed and tested in clinical studies. The BCRP inhibitors tested so far are first generation inhibitors, which are developed to inhibit other targets, and have pharmacokinetics interactions [64]. Some of the mechanisms by which ABC transporter inhibitors could alter the pharmacokinetics of the anti-cancer agent include competition for CYPs, intestinal or liver metabolism, inhibition of ABC transporter-mediated biliary excretion or intestinal transport, or inhibition of renal excretion and elimination [65]. This means that for an inhibitor to succeed, it needs to be non-toxic itself, and have no or low risk of interaction with important pharmacokinetic proteins, such as CYPs.

In this study, in vitro DMPK analyses of SCO-201 demonstrated no inhibition or induction of CYPs or SLCs whatsoever, suggesting a reduced risk of drug–drug interactions with other drugs, such as chemotherapy (Tables 2–4). As mentioned, an obstacle for inhibitors to succeed in clinical development is the fact that these also inhibit ABC transporters found in healthy tissues, which may lead to increased toxic effects of chemotherapy. This is especially a problem with broad-spectrum inhibitors that interact with many different efflux and uptake transporters, such as other ABC transporters or SLCs. However, by applying a specific inhibitor, this will allow the other ABC transporters in healthy tissues to compensate for the inhibition of the specific transporter, thereby protecting the healthy tissue from the toxic effects of the chemotherapy. In contrast, the anti-cancer drug has induced an up-regulation of the specific transporter in the resistant cancer cells, which will therefore be re-sensitized to the toxic effects of the anti-cancer drug. Therefore, it is highly likely that the more specific the inhibitor, the lower is the risk of increased toxicity. The specificity of SCO-201 to BCRP could provide benefits to the safety and tolerability profile in co-medication in cancer treatment compared to application of broad-spectrum inhibitors. Thereby, a BCRP-specific inhibition reduces the risk of potential drug–drug interactions in co-medication, thus decreasing the risk for increased chemotherapy-mediated toxicity.

To our best knowledge, a specific BCRP inhibitor has never been in clinical testing. Future in vivo studies of SCO-201 in combination with BCRP chemotherapy substrates should be conducted to further examine the pharmacology and test for potential increased chemotherapy-mediated toxicity. In such studies, we should utilize all the prior knowledge obtained with ABC transporter inhibitors. This means that we should carefully select patients with acquired drug resistance (a prior benefit to the chemotherapy in question), test for biomarkers such as cancer cell ABCG2 expression, start with a reduced dose of chemotherapy (the chemotherapy that the patient had acquired resistance against, and it should be an ABCG2 substrate drug) in combination with the inhibitor, perform randomization of patients in order to include time-dependent end-points such as progression free survival and overall survival, and perform a post-treatment association study between patient outcome and biomarkers. In vivo pharmacokinetic studies of other pyrazolo-pyrimidine derivatives, such as Reversan [19,34], have indicated that these do not cause increased toxicity of chemotherapy, and therefore it is possible that SCO-201 also will not cause these unwanted toxic effects in vivo.

5. Conclusions

Altogether, our data suggest that SCO-201 is a potential new drug candidate for the reversal of BCRP-mediated resistance in cancer. SCO-201 appears to be a specific and potent inhibitor of BCRP without affecting the CYP450 levels. Additionally, SCO-201 is stable in serum, has a favorable pharmacokinetic, toxicological, and pharmacodynamic profile in mice, and is orally active [33]. We conclude that SCO-201 is a highly promising drug candidate for drug-resistant cancer where overexpression of BCRP is the key mechanism of drug resistance.

Supplementary Materials: Figure S1: Western blot analysis of BCRP expression in SN-38-sensitive and SN-38-resistant HT29 cells. Figure S2: Cell viability assay with HT29 SN38-resistant colon cancer cells. Figure S3: Cell viability assay with mitoxantrone-resistant MDCK-II ATP-binding cassette (ABC)G2 cells. Figure S4: Cell viability assay with HT29 SN38-resistant colon cancer cells. Figure S5: Comparison of ABCG2 (BCRP) inhibition by SCO-201 and Ko143 as determined in the Hoechst 33,342 accumulation assay in MDCK cells. Figure S6: Comparison of SCO-201 and Ko143 as determined in the pheophorbide A accumulation assay in MDCK cells. Figure S7: SCO-201 (OBR-5-340)-mediated inhibition of BCRP. Figure S8: Timeline representation of interaction and contacts between residues in the binding cavity of the BCRP transporter and SCO-201. Figure S9: Timeline representation of interaction and contacts between residues in the binding cavity of the BCRP transporter and SN-38. Table S1: In vitro DMPK analysis of transporter inhibition. Table S2: In vitro DMPK analysis: CYP inhibition. Table S3: In vitro DMPK analysis: CYP induction.

Author Contributions: Conceptualization, J.S. (Jan Stenvang), N.B., S.R., H.W., and S.E.B.A.; methodology, J.S. (Jan Stenvang) and N.B.; validation, S.E.B.A., M.W., S.C.K., L.S., and B.B.; formal analysis, S.E.B.A., J.S. (Joen Svindt), M.W., S.K., X.L.L., M.G., L.S., and B.B.; investigation, S.E.B.A. X.L.L., M.G., L.S., and B.B.; data curation, S.A., S.R., H.W., X.L.L., M.G., L.S., B.B., and J.S. (Joen Svindt); writing—original draft preparation, S.E.B.A.; writing—review and editing, S.R., H.W., N.B., and J.S. (Jan Stenvang); visualization, S.E.B.A., X.L.L., M.G., and L.S.; supervision, J.S. (Jan Stenvang), N.B., S.R., and H.W.; project administration, J.S. (Jan Stenvang); funding acquisition, J.S. (Jan Stenvang) and N.B. All authors have read and agreed to the published version of the manuscript.

Acknowledgments: We would like to thank Signe Lykke Nielsen for her technical support.

References

1. Robey, R.W.; Pluchino, K.M.; Hall, M.D.; Fojo, A.T.; Bates, S.E.; Gottesman, M.M. Revisiting the role of ABC transporters in multidrug-resistant cancer. *Nat. Rev. Cancer* **2018**, *18*, 452–464. [CrossRef]
2. Hammond, W.A.; Swaika, A.; Mody, K. Pharmacologic resistance in colorectal cancer: A review. *Adv. Med. Oncol.* **2016**, *8*, 57–84. [CrossRef]
3. Lage, H. An overview of cancer multidrug resistance: A still unsolved problem. *Cell. Mol. Life Sci.* **2008**, *65*, 3145. [CrossRef] [PubMed]
4. Ren, F.; Shen, J.; Shi, H.; Hornicek, F.J.; Kan, Q.; Duan, Z. Novel mechanisms and approaches to overcome multidrug resistance in the treatment of ovarian cancer. *Biochim. Biophys. Acta Rev. Cancer* **2016**, *1866*, 266–275. [CrossRef] [PubMed]
5. Leonard, G.D. The Role of ABC Transporters in Clinical Practice. *Oncologist* **2003**, *8*, 411–424. [CrossRef] [PubMed]
6. Gottesman, M.M. Mechanisms of Cancer Drug Resistance. *Annu. Rev. Med.* **2002**, *53*, 615–627. [CrossRef] [PubMed]
7. Gottesman, M.M.; Fojo, T.; Bates, S.E. Multidrug resistance in cancer: Role of ATP–dependent transporters. *Nat. Rev. Cancer* **2002**, *2*, 48–58. [CrossRef] [PubMed]
8. Fletcher, J.I.; Haber, M.; Henderson, M.J.; Norris, M.D. ABC transporters in cancer: More than just drug efflux pumps. *Nat. Rev. Cancer* **2010**, *10*, 147–156. [CrossRef]

9. Ambudkar, S.V.; Dey, S.; Hrycyna, C.A.; Ramachandra, M.; Pastan, I.; Gottesman, M.M. Biochemical, Cellular, And Pharmacological Aspects of The Multidrug Transporter. *Annu. Rev. Pharm. Toxicol.* **1999**, *39*, 361–398. [CrossRef]
10. Li, W.; Zhang, H.; Assaraf, Y.G.; Zhao, K.; Xu, X.; Xie, J.; Yang, D.H.; Chen, Z.S. Overcoming ABC transporter-mediated multidrug resistance: Molecular mechanisms and novel therapeutic drug strategies. *Drug Resist. Updates* **2016**, *27*, 14–29. [CrossRef]
11. Sarkadi, B.; Özvegy-Laczka, C.; Német, K.; Váradi, A. ABCG2—A transporter for all seasons. *FEBS Lett.* **2004**, *567*, 116–120. [CrossRef] [PubMed]
12. Doyle, L.; Ross, D.D. Multidrug resistance mediated by the breast cancer resistance protein BCRP (ABCG2). *Oncogene* **2003**, *22*, 7340–7358. [CrossRef] [PubMed]
13. Litman, T.; Brangi, M.; Hudson, E.; Fetsch, P.; Abati, A.; Ross, D.D.; Miyake, K.; Resau, J.H.; Bates, S.E. The multidrug-resistant phenotype associated with overexpression of the new ABC half-transporter, MXR (ABCG2). *J. Cell Sci.* **2000**, *113*, 2011–2021. [PubMed]
14. Robey, R.W.; Polgar, O.; Deeken, J.; To, K.W.; Bates, S.E. ABCG2: Determining its relevance in clinical drug resistance. *Cancer Metastasis Rev.* **2007**, *26*, 39–57. [CrossRef]
15. Özvegy, C.; Litman, T.; Szakács, G.; Nagy, Z.; Bates, S.; Váradi, A.; Sarkadi, B. Functional Characterization of the Human Multidrug Transporter, ABCG2, Expressed in Insect Cells. *Biochem. Biophys. Res. Commun.* **2001**, *285*, 111–117. [CrossRef]
16. Jackson, S.M.; Manolaridis, I.; Kowal, J.; Zechner, M.; Taylor, N.M.I.; Bause, M.; Bauer, S.; Bartholomaeus, R.; Bernhardt, G.; Koenig, B.; et al. Structural basis of small-molecule inhibition of human multidrug transporter ABCG2. *Nat. Struct. Mol. Biol.* **2018**, *25*, 333–340. [CrossRef]
17. Fojo, T.; Bates, S. Strategies for reversing drug resistance. *Oncogene* **2003**, *22*, 7512–7523. [CrossRef]
18. Shukla, S.; Wu, C.-P.; Ambudkar, S.V. Development of inhibitors of ATP-binding cassette drug transporters-present status and challenges. *Expert Opin. Drug Metab. Toxicol.* **2008**, *4*, 205–223. [CrossRef]
19. Falasca, M.; Linton, K.J. Investigational ABC transporter inhibitors. *Expert Opin. Investig. Drugs* **2012**, *21*, 657–666. [CrossRef]
20. Ahmed-Belkacem, A.; Pozza, A.; Macalou, S.; Pérez-Victoria, J.M.; Boumendjel, A.; Di Pietro, A. Inhibitors of cancer cell multidrug resistance mediated by breast cancer resistance protein (BCRP/ABCG2). *Anti-Cancer Drugs* **2006**, *17*, 239–243. [CrossRef]
21. Rabindran, S.K.; He, H.; Singh, M.; Brown, E.; Collins, K.I.; Annable, T.; Greenberger, L.M. Reversal of a Novel Multidrug Resistance Mechanism in Human Colon Carcinoma Cells by Fumitremorgin C. *Cancer Res.* **1998**, *58*, 5850–5858. [PubMed]
22. Allen, J.D.; van Loevezijn, A.; Lakhai, J.M.; van der Valk, M.; van Tellingen, O.; Reid, G.; Schellens, J.H.; Koomen, G.J.; Schinkel, A.H. Potent and specific inhibition of the breast cancer resistance protein multidrug transporter in vitro and in mouse intestine by a novel analogue of fumitremorgin C. *Mol. Cancer* **2002**, *1*, 417–425.
23. Weidner, L.D.; Zoghbi, S.S.; Lu, S.; Shukla, S.; Ambudkar, S.V.; Pike, V.W.; Mulder, J.; Gottesman, M.M.; Innis, R.B.; Hall, M.D. The Inhibitor Ko143 Is Not Specific for ABCG2. *J. Pharm. Exp. Ther.* **2015**, *354*, 384–393. [CrossRef] [PubMed]
24. Stenvang, J.M.; Moreira, J.M.A.; Jensen, N.F.; Nielsen, S.L.; Orntoft, T.; Lassen, U.; Hansen, S.N.; Jandu, H.; Andreasen, M.; Noer, J.B.; et al. DEN-50R-establishment of a novel and unique cell line based drug screening platform for cancer treatment. In Proceedings of the AACR-NCI-EORTC International Conference on Molecular Targets and Cancer Therapeutics, Boston, MA, USA, 5–9 November 2015.
25. Jensen, N.F.; Stenvang, J.; Beck, M.K.; Hanáková, B.; Belling, K.C.; Do, K.N.; Viuff, B.; Nygård, S.B.; Gupta, R.; Rasmussen, M.H.; et al. Establishment and characterization of models of chemotherapy resistance in colorectal cancer: Towards a predictive signature of chemoresistance. *Mol. Oncol.* **2015**, *9*, 1169–1185. [CrossRef] [PubMed]
26. Lin, X.; Stenvang, J.; Rasmussen, M.H.; Zhu, S.; Jensen, N.F.; Tarpgaard, L.S.; Yang, G.; Belling, K.; Andersen, C.L.; Li, J.; et al. The potential role of Alu Y in the development of resistance to SN38 (Irinotecan) or oxaliplatin in colorectal cancer. *BMC Genom.* **2015**, *16*, 404. [CrossRef]
27. Guo, J.; Xu, S.; Huang, X.; Li, L.; Zhang, C.; Pan, Q.; Ren, Z.; Zhou, R.; Ren, Y.; Zi, J.; et al. Drug Resistance in Colorectal Cancer Cell Lines is Partially Associated with Aneuploidy Status in Light of Profiling Gene Expression. *J. Proteome Res.* **2016**, *15*, 4047–4059. [CrossRef]

28. Hansen, S.N.; Westergaard, D.; Thomsen, M.B.; Vistesen, M.; Do, K.N.; Fogh, L.; Belling, K.C.; Wang, J.; Yang, H.; Gupta, R.; et al. Acquisition of docetaxel resistance in breast cancer cells reveals upregulation of ABCB1 expression as a key mediator of resistance accompanied by discrete upregulation of other specific genes and pathways. *Tumour. Biol.* **2015**, *36*, 4327–4338. [CrossRef]
29. Jandu, H.; Aluzaite, K.; Fogh, L.; Thrane, S.W.; Noer, J.B.; Proszek, J.; Do, K.N.; Hansen, S.N.; Damsgaard, B.; Nielsen, S.L.; et al. Molecular characterization of irinotecan (SN-38) resistant human breast cancer cell lines. *BMC Cancer* **2016**, *16*, 34. [CrossRef]
30. Hansen, S.N.; Ehlers, N.S.; Zhu, S.; Thomsen, M.B.; Nielsen, R.L.; Liu, D.; Wang, G.; Hou, Y.; Zhang, X.; Xu, X.; et al. The stepwise evolution of the exome during acquisition of docetaxel resistance in breast cancer cells. *BMC Genom.* **2016**, *17*, 442. [CrossRef]
31. Bates, S.E.; Medina-Pérez, W.Y.; Kohlhagen, G.; Antony, S.; Nadjem, T.; Robey, R.W.; Pommier, Y. ABCG2 Mediates Differential Resistance to SN-38 (7-Ethyl-10-hydroxycamptothecin) and Homocamptothecins. *J. Pharm. Exp.* **2004**, *310*, 836–842. [CrossRef]
32. Braun, H.; Makarov, V.A.; Riabova, O.B.; Komarova, E.S.; Richter, M.; Wutzler, P.; Schmidtke, M. OBR-5-340—A Novel Pyrazolo-Pyrimidine Derivative with Strong Antiviral Activity Against Coxsackievirus B3 In Vitro and In Vivo. *Antivir. Res.* **2011**, *90*, A29. [CrossRef]
33. Makarov, V.A.; Braun, H.; Richter, M.; Riabova, O.B.; Kirchmair, J.; Kazakova, E.S.; Seidel, N.; Wutzler, P.; Schmidtke, M. Pyrazolopyrimidines: Potent Inhibitors Targeting the Capsid of Rhino- and Enteroviruses. *ChemMedChem* **2015**, *10*, 1629–1634. [CrossRef] [PubMed]
34. Burkhart, C.A.; Watt, F.; Murray, J.; Pajic, M.; Prokvolit, A.; Xue, C.; Flemming, C.; Smith, J.; Purmal, A.; Isachenko, N.; et al. Small-molecule multidrug resistance-associated protein 1 inhibitor reversan increases the therapeutic index of chemotherapy in mouse models of neuroblastoma. *Cancer Res.* **2009**, *69*, 6573–6580. [CrossRef] [PubMed]
35. Kim, S.; Chen, J.; Cheng, T.; Gindulyte, A.; He, J.; He, S.; Li, Q.; Shoemaker, B.A.; Thiessen, P.A.; Yu, B.; et al. PubChem 2019 update: Improved access to chemical data. *Nucleic Acids Res.* **2019**, *47*, D1102–D1109. [CrossRef]
36. National Center for Biotechnology Information. PubChem Database. 7-Ethyl-10-hydroxycamptothecin, CID= 104842. Available online: https://pubchem.ncbi.nlm.nih.gov/compound/7-Ethyl-10-hydroxycamptothecin (accessed on 28 January 2020).
37. Pick, A.; Müller, H.; Wiese, M. Structure-activity relationships of new inhibitors of breast cancer resistance protein (ABCG2). *Bioorg. Med. Chem.* **2008**, *16*, 8224–8236. [CrossRef] [PubMed]
38. Müller, M.; Bakos, E.; Welker, E.; Váradi, A.; Germann, U.A.; Gottesman, M.M.; Morse, B.S.; Roninson, I.B.; Sarkadi, B. Altered drug-stimulated ATPase activity in mutants of the human multidrug resistance protein. *J. Biol. Chem.* **1996**, *271*, 1877–1883. [CrossRef]
39. Friesner, R.A.; Murphy, R.B.; Repasky, M.P.; Frye, L.L.; Greenwood, J.R.; Halgren, T.A.; Sanschagrin, P.C.; Mainz, D.T. Extra Precision Glide: Docking and Scoring Incorporating a Model of Hydrophobic Enclosure for Protein–Ligand Complexes. *J. Med. Chem.* **2006**, *49*, 6177–6196. [CrossRef]
40. Halgren, T.A.; Murphy, R.B.; Friesner, R.A.; Beard, H.S.; Frye, L.L.; Pollard, W.T.; Banks, J.L. Glide: A New Approach for Rapid, Accurate Docking and Scoring. 2. Enrichment Factors in Database Screening. *J. Med. Chem.* **2004**, *47*, 1750–1759. [CrossRef]
41. Friesner, R.A.; Banks, J.L.; Murphy, R.B.; Halgren, T.A.; Klicic, J.J.; Mainz, D.T.; Repasky, M.P.; Knoll, E.H.; Shelley, M.; Perry, J.K.; et al. Glide: A New Approach for Rapid, Accurate Docking and Scoring. 1. Method and Assessment of Docking Accuracy. *J. Med. Chem.* **2004**, *47*, 1739–1749. [CrossRef]
42. Sastry, G.M.; Adzhigirey, M.; Day, T.; Annabhimoju, R.; Sherman, W. Protein and ligand preparation: Parameters, protocols, and influence on virtual screening enrichments. *J. Comput. Aided Mol. Des. Des.* **2013**, *27*, 221–234. [CrossRef]
43. Bowers, A.K.J.; Chow, E.; Xu, H.; Dror, R.O.; Eastwood, M.P.; Gregersen, B.A.; Klepeis, J.L.; Kolossvary, I.; Moraes, M.A.; Sacerdoti, F.D.; et al. Scalable algorithms for molecular dynamics simulations on commodity clusters. In Proceedings of the 2006 ACM/IEEE Conference on Supercomputing, Tampa, FL, USA, 11–17 November 2006; p. 84-es.
44. Krapf, M.K.; Gallus, J.; Vahdati, S.; Wiese, M. New Inhibitors of Breast Cancer Resistance Protein (ABCG2) Containing a 2,4-Disubstituted Pyridopyrimidine Scaffold. *J. Med. Chem.* **2018**, *61*, 3389–3408. [CrossRef] [PubMed]

45. Diop, N.K.; Hrycyna, C.A. N-Linked Glycosylation of the Human ABC Transporter ABCG2 on Asparagine 596 Is Not Essential for Expression, Transport Activity, or Trafficking to the Plasma Membrane. *Biochemistry* **2005**, *44*, 5420–5429. [CrossRef] [PubMed]
46. Szakács, G.; Paterson, J.K.; Ludwig, J.A.; Booth-Genthe, C.; Gottesman, M.M. Targeting multidrug resistance in cancer. *Nat. Rev. Drug Discov.* **2006**, *5*, 219–234. [CrossRef] [PubMed]
47. Baer, M.R.; George, S.L.; Dodge, R.K.; O'Loughlin, K.L.; Minderman, H.; Caligiuri, M.A.; Anastasi, J.; Powell, B.L.; Kolitz, J.E.; Schiffer, C.A.; et al. Phase 3 study of the multidrug resistance modulator PSC-833 in previously untreated patients 60 years of age and older with acute myeloid leukemia: Cancer and Leukemia Group B Study 9720. *Blood* **2002**, *100*, 1224–1232. [CrossRef]
48. Lhommé, C.; Joly, F.; Walker, J.L.; Lissoni, A.A.; Nicoletto, M.O.; Manikhas, G.M.; Baekelandt, M.M.O.; Gordon, A.N.; Fracasso, P.M.; Mietlowski, W.L.; et al. Phase III Study of Valspodar (PSC 833) Combined With Paclitaxel and Carboplatin Compared With Paclitaxel and Carboplatin Alone in Patients With Stage IV or Suboptimally Debulked Stage III Epithelial Ovarian Cancer or Primary Peritoneal Cancer. *J. Clin. Oncol.* **2008**, *26*, 2674–2682. [CrossRef]
49. Leonard, G.D.; Polgar, O.; Bates, S.E. ABC transporters and inhibitors: New targets, new agents. *Curr. Opin. Investig. Drugs* **2002**, *3*, 1652–1659.
50. Greenberg, P.L.; Lee, S.J.; Advani, R.; Tallman, M.S.; Sikic, B.I.; Letendre, L.; Dugan, K.; Lum, B.; Chin, D.L.; Dewald, G.; et al. Mitoxantrone, etoposide, and cytarabine with or without valspodar in patients with relapsed or refractory acute myeloid leukemia and high-risk myelodysplastic syndrome: A phase III trial (E2995). *J. Clin. Oncol.* **2004**, *22*, 1078–1086. [CrossRef]
51. Kovacsics, D.; Patik, I.; Özvegy-Laczka, C. The role of organic anion transporting polypeptides in drug absorption, distribution, excretion and drug-drug interactions. *Expert Opin. Drug Metab. Toxicol.* **2017**, *13*, 409–424. [CrossRef]
52. Szakács, G.; Váradi, A.; Özvegy-Laczka, C.; Sarkadi, B. The role of ABC transporters in drug absorption, distribution, metabolism, excretion and toxicity (ADME–Tox). *Drug Discov. Today* **2008**, *13*, 379–393. [CrossRef]
53. Zanger, U.M.; Schwab, M. Cytochrome P450 enzymes in drug metabolism: Regulation of gene expression, enzyme activities, and impact of genetic variation. *Pharmacol. Ther.* **2013**, *138*, 103–141. [CrossRef]
54. Noguchi, K.; Katayama, K.; Sugimoto, Y. Human ABC transporter ABCG2/BCRP expression in chemoresistance: Basic and clinical perspectives for molecular cancer therapeutics. *Pharmgenom. Pers. Med.* **2014**, *7*, 53–64. [CrossRef] [PubMed]
55. Friedenberg, W.R.; Rue, M.; Blood, E.A.; Dalton, W.S.; Shustik, C.; Larson, R.A.; Sonneveld, P.; Greipp, P.R. Phase III study of PSC-833 (valspodar) in combination with vincristine, doxorubicin, and dexamethasone (valspodar/VAD) versus VAD alone in patients with recurring or refractory multiple myeloma (E1A95): A trial of the Eastern Cooperative Oncology Group. *Cancer* **2006**, *106*, 830–838. [CrossRef]
56. Romanov, R.A.; Bystrova, M.F.; Rogachevskaya, O.A.; Sadovnikov, V.B.; Shestopalov, V.I.; Kolesnikov, S.S. The ATP permeability of pannexin 1 channels in a heterologous system and in mammalian taste cells is dispensable. *J. Cell Sci.* **2012**, *125*, 5514. [CrossRef]
57. Kelly, R.J.; Draper, D.; Chen, C.C.; Robey, R.W.; Figg, W.D.; Piekarz, R.L.; Chen, X.; Gardner, E.R.; Balis, F.M.; Venkatesan, A.M.; et al. A pharmacodynamic study of docetaxel in combination with the P-glycoprotein antagonist tariquidar (XR9576) in patients with lung, ovarian, and cervical cancer. *Clin. Cancer Res.* **2011**, *17*, 569–580. [CrossRef] [PubMed]
58. Abraham, J.; Edgerly, M.; Wilson, R.; Chen, C.; Rutt, A.; Bakke, S.; Robey, R.; Dwyer, A.; Goldspiel, B.; Balis, F.; et al. A phase I study of the P-glycoprotein antagonist tariquidar in combination with vinorelbine. *Clin. Cancer Res. Off. J. Am. Assoc. Cancer Res.* **2009**, *15*, 3574–3582. [CrossRef] [PubMed]
59. Pusztai, L.; Wagner, P.; Ibrahim, N.; Rivera, E.; Theriault, R.; Booser, D.; Symmans, F.W.; Wong, F.; Blumenschein, G.; Fleming, D.R.; et al. Phase II study of tariquidar, a selective P-glycoprotein inhibitor, in patients with chemotherapy-resistant, advanced breast carcinoma. *Cancer* **2005**, *104*, 682–691. [CrossRef] [PubMed]
60. Fox, E.; Widemann, B.C.; Pastakia, D.; Chen, C.C.; Yang, S.X.; Cole, D.; Balis, F.M. Pharmacokinetic and pharmacodynamic study of tariquidar (XR9576), a P-glycoprotein inhibitor, in combination with doxorubicin, vinorelbine, or docetaxel in children and adolescents with refractory solid tumors. *Cancer Chemother. Pharm.* **2015**, *76*, 1273–1283. [CrossRef]

61. Ruff, P.; Vorobiof, D.A.; Jordaan, J.P.; Demetriou, G.S.; Moodley, S.D.; Nosworthy, A.L.; Werner, I.D.; Raats, J.; Burgess, L.J. A randomized, placebo-controlled, double-blind phase 2 study of docetaxel compared to docetaxel plus zosuquidar (LY335979) in women with metastatic or locally recurrent breast cancer who have received one prior chemotherapy regimen. *Cancer Chemother. Pharmacol.* **2009**, *64*, 763–768. [CrossRef]
62. Lê, L.H.; Moore, M.J.; Siu, L.L.; Oza, A.M.; MacLean, M.; Fisher, B.; Chaudhary, A.; de Alwis, D.P.; Slapak, C.; Seymour, L.; et al. Phase I study of the multidrug resistance inhibitor zosuquidar administered in combination with vinorelbine in patients with advanced solid tumours. *Cancer Chemother. Pharm.* **2005**, *56*, 154–160. [CrossRef]
63. Fracasso, P.M.; Goldstein, L.J.; de Alwis, D.P.; Rader, J.S.; Arquette, M.A.; Goodner, S.A.; Wright, L.P.; Fears, C.L.; Gazak, R.J.; Andre, V.A.M.; et al. Phase I Study of Docetaxel in Combination with the P-Glycoprotein Inhibitor, Zosuquidar, in Resistant Malignancies. *Clin. Cancer Res.* **2004**, *10*, 7220. [CrossRef]
64. Brackman, D.J.; Giacomini, K.M. Reverse Translational Research of ABCG2 (BCRP) in Human Disease and Drug Response. *Clin. Pharm.* **2018**, *103*, 233–242. [CrossRef] [PubMed]
65. Relling, M.V. Are the Major Effects of P-Glycoprotein Modulators Due to Altered Pharmacokinetics of Anticancer Drugs? *Ther. Drug Monit.* **1996**, *18*, 350–356. [CrossRef] [PubMed]

10

Immunotherapy, Inflammation and Colorectal Cancer

Charles Robert Lichtenstern [1,2], Rachael Katie Ngu [1,2], Shabnam Shalapour [1,2,*] and Michael Karin [1,2,3]

[1] Department of Pharmacology, School of Medicine, University of California, San Diego, La Jolla, CA 92093, USA; karinoffice@health.ucsd.edu
[2] Laboratory of Gene Regulation and Signal Transduction, Department of Pharmacology, School of Medicine, University of California, San Diego, La Jolla, CA 92093, USA
[3] Moores Cancer Center, University of California, San Diego, La Jolla, CA 92093, USA
* Correspondence: sshalapour@health.ucsd.edu

Abstract: Colorectal cancer (CRC) is the third most common cancer type, and third highest in mortality rates among cancer-related deaths in the United States. Originating from intestinal epithelial cells in the colon and rectum, that are impacted by numerous factors including genetics, environment and chronic, lingering inflammation, CRC can be a problematic malignancy to treat when detected at advanced stages. Chemotherapeutic agents serve as the historical first line of defense in the treatment of metastatic CRC. In recent years, however, combinational treatment with targeted therapies, such as vascular endothelial growth factor, or epidermal growth factor receptor inhibitors, has proven to be quite effective in patients with specific CRC subtypes. While scientific and clinical advances have uncovered promising new treatment options, the five-year survival rate for metastatic CRC is still low at about 14%. Current research into the efficacy of immunotherapy, particularly immune checkpoint inhibitor therapy (ICI) in mismatch repair deficient and microsatellite instability high (dMMR–MSI-H) CRC tumors have shown promising results, but its use in other CRC subtypes has been either unsuccessful, or not extensively explored. This Review will focus on the current status of immunotherapies, including ICI, vaccination and adoptive T cell therapy (ATC) in the treatment of CRC and its potential use, not only in dMMR–MSI-H CRC, but also in mismatch repair proficient and microsatellite instability low (pMMR-MSI-L).

Keywords: colorectal cancer; immunotherapy; inflammation; microsatellite instability

---

1. Introduction

Colorectal cancer (CRC) is the third most common cancer type and a leading cause of mortality among cancer-related deaths in the United States [1]. While scientific and clinical advances in early detection and surgery have led to five-year survival rates of 90% and 71% for localized and regionalized CRCs, respectively, the five-year survival rate for metastatic CRC is low, remaining at around 14% [2]. Moreover, 25% of CRC patients display metastasis at diagnosis, and roughly 50% of those treated will eventually develop metastasis during their lifetime [3]. These alarming statistics can most likely be attributed to the ineffectiveness of standard treatment regimens, and thus indicates an urgent need for the development of more effective treatment options. Immunotherapy, a treatment option that takes advantage of the body's own immune system to attack cancer, has shown promise in the treatment of certain cancers [4–7]. Whereas some cancers, such as melanoma and lung cancer, respond well to immune checkpoint inhibitor therapy (ICI), others do not.

More recently, ICIs were found effective in a specific subset of CRC that is mismatch-repair-deficient (dMMR) and microsatellite instability-high (MSI-H) (referred to as dMMR-MSI-H tumors) and ineffective in subsets that are mismatch-repair-proficient (pMMR) and microsatellite instability-low

(MSI-L) (referred to as pMMR-MSI-L tumors) [8]. This Review will serve to discuss recent findings in the effectiveness of immunotherapies in the treatment of CRC, both localized and metastatic, from clinical trials and experimental models, and its potential use in pMMR-MSI-L tumors and other CRC subsets.

2. Origins of CRC

CRC can originate from a multitude of intrinsic and extrinsic factors, including an accumulation of new mutations, pre-existing mutations, and susceptibility alleles associated with family history, or chronic, lingering inflammation, as described in Figure 1. The majority (75%) of CRCs are sporadic, meaning family history is not involved in their pathogenesis [9]. Common mutations in tumor suppressor genes and oncogenes that give rise to CRC include adenomatous polyposis coli (*APC*), tumor protein 53 (*TP53*), and Kirsten rat sarcoma (*KRAS*), which are present in 81%, 60% and 43% of the cases of sporadic CRCs, respectively [10]. The role of these genetic alterations in the pathogenesis of CRC has been extensively reviewed [11–13]. Most CRC-inducing mutations act in a particular order, controlling the adenoma–carcinoma sequence, which describes the progression of a normal intestinal epithelia to an adenoma, invasive carcinoma, and eventual metastatic tumor [14,15].

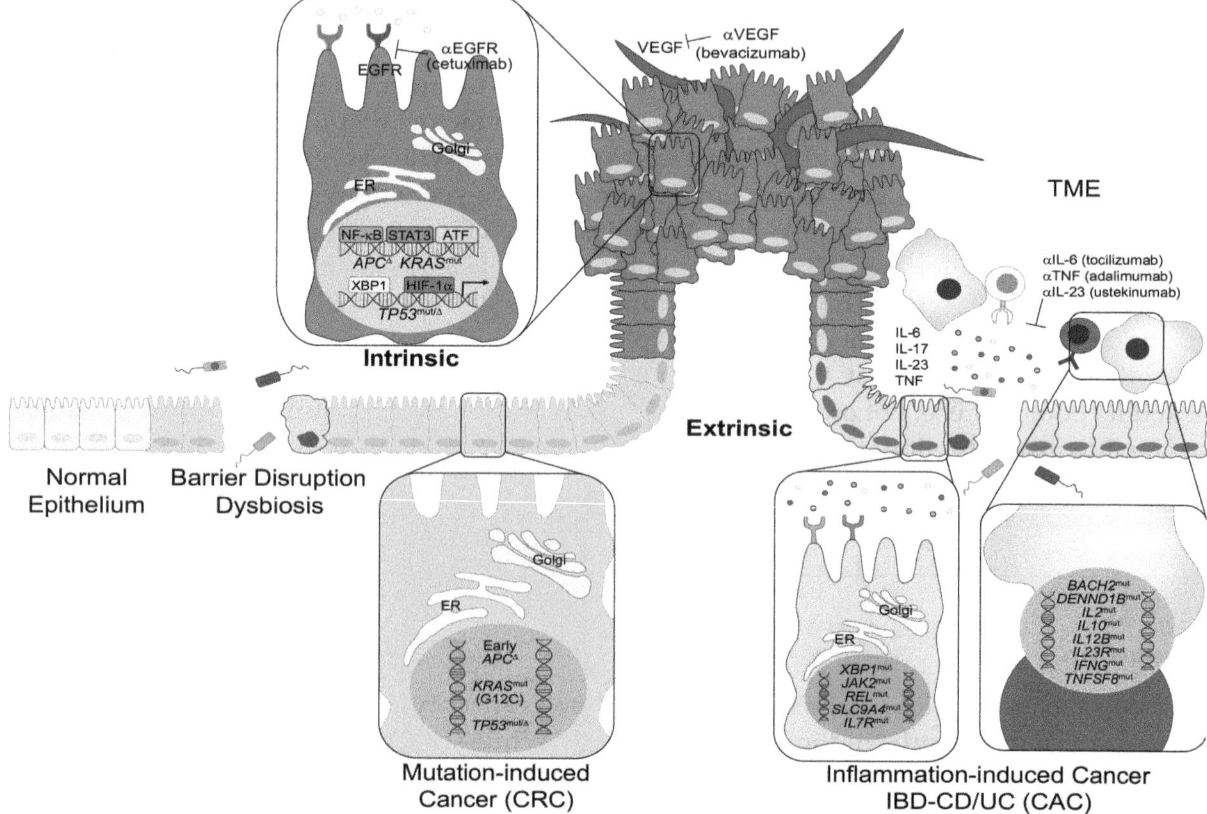

Figure 1. Intrinsic and extrinsic factors contributing to the pathogenesis of colorectal cancer (CRC). CRC can develop from a multitude of both intrinsic and extrinsic factors. Extrinsic factors, including inflammation from hyperactivated immune cells, the release of proinflammatory cytokines, or gut dysbiosis, can lead to an inflammatory and possibly premalignant environment. Intrinsic factors include sporadic mutations, such as those leading to mutation-induced CRC (sporadic CRC). Similarly, precancerous mutations, or mutations induced by prior inflammation, can lead to colitis-associated cancer (CAC), a specific subset of CRC stemming from chronic inflammation caused by inflammatory bowel disease (IBD), specifically ulcerative colitis (UC) or Crohn's disease (CD).

Family history is implicated in approximately 10–30% of CRCs [16,17]. For example, familial adenomatous polyposis (FAP) and hereditary nonpolyposis colorectal cancer (Lynch syndrome) are the most commonly inherited CRC syndromes, and account for 2–4% and 1% of CRC cases, respectively [17].

Although 96% of all CRCs do not develop in the context of pre-existing inflammation, the roles of chronic inflammation, tumor-elicited inflammation, the tumor microenvironment (TME), and partially adaptive immune cells in CRC development, have been established, particularly in the context of their interaction with gut dysbiosis [18–23]. Colitis-associated cancer (CAC) is a specific subset of CRC characterized by its implication with inflammation that accounts for 1%–2% of all CRCs [24]. CAC, originating from either the chronic inflammation in both the colon and the small intestine, or solely the colon, as is the case of Crohn's disease (CD) or ulcerative colitis (UC), respectively, is classified by the excessive activation and recruitment of immune cells that produce inflammatory cytokines, such as TNF, IL-17, IL-23 and IL-6, that lead to the propagation of an inflammatory and possibly premalignant environment [25]. Mutations involved in inflammatory bowel disease (IBD) development include genes that regulate immune activation and the subsequent response, such as *IL12B, IL2, IFNG, IL10, TNFSF8, TNFSF15, IL7R, DENND1B, JAK2* and those that also regulate ER stress, glucose, bile salt transfer and organic ion transporter, including *XBP1, SLC9A4, SLC22A5* and *SCL11A1*, as shown in Figure 1 [26]. Both CRC and CAC exhibit inflammatory microenvironments, but the order in which inflammation and tumorigenesis occur seems to be different. In CRC, inflammation follows tumorigenesis. Mutations due to environmental factors initiate tumor development in CRCs, and the subsequent activation of inflammatory cells can induce further DNA damage through the production of reactive oxygen species (ROS) and reactive nitrogen intermediates (RNIs) [25,27]. On the other hand, inflammation precedes tumorigenesis in CAC. Inflammation induced by the activation of immune cells and their release of proinflammatory cytokines can induce DNA damage and mutations in CAC [25]. Correspondingly, both CRC and CAC may entail similar mutations, but the timing and order of these mutations are different, as displayed by early *APC* and late *TP53* mutations in CRC, and early *TP53* and late *APC* mutations in CAC [28–30]. Another important contributor to CRC emergence is so-called tumor-elicited inflammation driven by the loss of normal barrier function as a result of *APC* inactivation [18].

3. Mismatch Repair Deficiency and Microsatellite Instability in CRC

dMMR or MSI-H exists in about 15% of all cases of CRC, but only in 4% of metastatic CRC, as opposed to pMMR or MSI-L, which is present in roughly 85% of all cases of CRC. MSI occurs in both spontaneous CRC and IBD-induced CAC, although the rates and timing at which MSI occurs are similar in both malignancies [31].

Microsatellites are repetitive DNA sequences that can experience a sudden and prolonged change in size, due to errors during DNA replication, such as the formation of small loops in the DNA strands, leading to MSI-H [32]. These errors are combated by the mismatch repair (MMR) system, an ancient mechanism used to correct insertions, deletions, or mismatched bases that are generated by the erroneous loops that form during DNA replication [32–34]. However, if there is a dysfunction or mutation in the MMR system, referred to as dMMR, these errors are left uncorrected, allowing them to be integrated into the DNA permanently [32]. Thus, MSI-H tumors have varied lengths of microsatellites (compared to MSI-L) due to errors in the MMR system, as shown in Figure 2.

The MMR system relies on the DNA repair genes *MLH1, MSH2, PMS1, MSH6, PMS2* and *MSH3*, all of which are involved in correcting mismatched or wrongly inserted or deleted bases in DNA [32,35]. Loss, inactivation, or the silencing of any one of these genes, classifies a patient as dMMR. More importantly, errors in this repair system lead to a high mutational profile, which explains why dMMR tumors have an average mutational profile of 1782, compared to 73 for pMMR tumors [36].

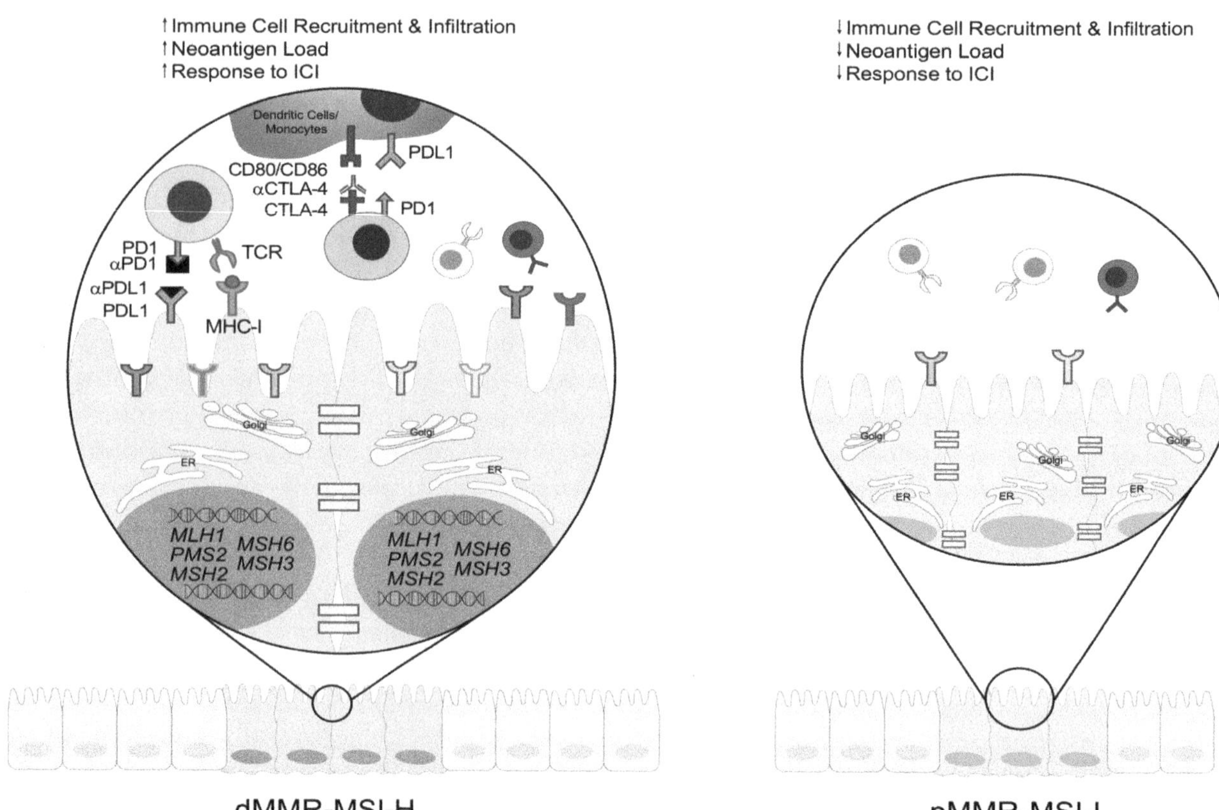

Figure 2. Immuno-landscape of dMMR-MSI-H and pMMR-MSI-L CRC. CRC can be classified into two subsets based on its MMR/MSI status. The DNA MMR system relies on key genes, such as MLH1, MSH2, MSH6, PMS2, or MSH3, that correct mismatched or wrongly inserted or deleted bases in the DNA. If this machinery fails due to defects in one or more of the repair genes, these errors are free to be integrated into the DNA permanently, forming microsatellites. Thus, dMMR-MSI-H tumors are those that have a defect in one of the major DNA repair genes (dMMR), resulting in high levels of microsatellites (MSI-H). On the other hand, pMMR-MSI-L tumors have a functional MMR system (pMMR), resulting in low or stable levels of microsatellites (MSI-L). The result of this damaged repair system in dMMR-MSI-H tumors is a higher mutational burden, which correlates with a higher expression of neoantigens on MHC-I molecules.

As the identification and classification of CRCs is necessary and crucial for proper diagnoses and treatments, methods have been practiced in order to detect MSI. Current methods include the amplification and examination of polymerase chain reaction (PCR) products from commonly affected microsatellite markers in tumors [34,37,38]. These markers include two mononucleotide repeat markers (BAT-25 and BAT-26) and three dinucleotide repeat markers (D2S123, D5S346, and D17S250) [37]. MSI-H status is classified if instability is present in two or more of the markers, whereas the MSI-L status is classified if instability is only detected in one of the markers. More recently, however, are methods that use DNA-sequencing technology for MSI detection and classification on the same markers [33,39,40]. Regardless of the screening method, albeit some more efficient and accurate than others, classification of MSI status in regard to the CRC subtype is of the upmost importance for proper treatment planning, and should be one of the primary steps when diagnosing patients.

4. Classical Treatment Options

CRC treatment can be divided into two main treatment categories: neoadjuvant and adjuvant. Neoadjuvant therapy refers to therapeutics that are given before the main cancer treatment, usually surgery, whereas adjuvant refers to that which is given after or in combination with the main cancer treatment. Neoadjuvant therapy offers many clinical benefits, in that it can potentially lessen the severity of the malignancy, through eliminating early metastatic tumors, preventing complications during surgery, and allowing for a more accurate plan for adjuvant therapy (if necessary), based on the subsequent response to neoadjuvant therapy [41–43]. Most studies have shown that neoadjuvant chemotherapy may improve overall survival, depending on the severity and stage of the disease [41,44–46].

Chemotherapy is usually the first line of defense in the treatment of CRC. 5-fluorouracil (5-FU), the most common of the chemotherapeutic agents for CRC, acts through inhibition of thymidylate synthase, which converts deoxyuridine monophosphate (dUMP) to deoxythymidine monophosphate (dTMP), causing DNA damage [47]. While it is relatively effective in early disease stages, response rates in metastatic CRC are only 10–15% [47,48]. On the other hand, combinatorial chemotherapeutic regimens consisting of 5-FU, in combination with oxaliplatin (FOLFOX) or irinotecan (FOLFIRI), have heightened response rates to 40–50% [47]. Studies into the usefulness of using MMR/MSI status as a predictor of responsiveness to chemotherapy have shown mixed results, depending on the stage of the disease and the specific type of chemotherapy, thus explaining the necessity for a more reliable and dependable treatment option for these CRC subsets [49–53].

More recently introduced are the targeted therapies, including monoclonal antibodies against epidermal growth factor receptor (EGFR) and vascular endothelial growth factor (VEGF), which inhibit cancer cell proliferation and angiogenesis, respectively. Bevacizumab, a monoclonal antibody against VEGF, was shown to improve the survival of patients with metastatic CRC in combination with 5-FU [54] and oxaliplatin-based therapies [55]. Moreover, patients with irinotecan- [56] and fluoropyrimidine- and oxaliplatin-resistant [57] CRCs were shown to have improved response rates when treated with cetuximab, a monoclonal antibody against EGFR, alone or in combination with irinotecan. Extensive research has shown *KRAS* mutational status to be a predictor of non-responsiveness to EGFR inhibitors [58–60]. It was found that patients with pMMR tumors that had mutations in *BRAF* or *KRAS*, had worse survival rates than patients with pMMR tumors free of these mutations, and patients with dMMR tumors [61]. Despite major scientific and clinical research into targeted therapies, patients that do respond to EGFR inhibitors only show improvements for 3–12 months before disease progression, suggesting that this specific therapy is not conducive to long term survival and remission [56,58,62,63]. This obstacle has paved the way for research into the efficacy of immunotherapy in the treatment of CRCs.

5. Role of Immune Cells and Tumor Microenvironment in the Classification of CRC

A positive correlation is seen between tumoral $CD3^+$ and $CD8^+$ T cell densities and the risk of recurrence, disease-free survival rate, and the overall survival rate in patients with different stages of CRC [64]. This is in accordance and supports evidence which shows that increased amounts of tumor-infiltrating lymphocytes correlate with an improved clinical outcome and prognosis [65–68]. Both dMMR-MSI-H and pMMR-MSI-L tumors have distinctly different TME makeups and distributions of immune cell populations, contributing to the variation in response rates to therapy, treatment targets and clinical prognoses [69–71]. Comparison of the makeup of the TME shows a higher expression of cytotoxic, Th1, Th2, $CD8^+$ T and follicular helper (Tfh) cell markers, in addition to macrophages and B cells in dMMR-MSI-H tumors than pMMR-MSI-L tumors [69,72]. Some of these immune cells can mediate antitumor immune responses, thus explaining why dMMR-MSI-H tumors have better response rates and clinical outcomes [73]. Higher mutational load in dMMR-MSI-H tumors correlates with the higher expression of neoantigens on major histocompatibility complex (MHC)-I molecules, thus recruiting more cytotoxic $CD8^+$ T cells for the subsequent immune response and tumor destruction, which follows the notion that frameshift mutations positively correlate with $CD8^+$ T cell infiltration in CRCs [74,75].

Since T cell infiltration is representative of a better clinical outcome in CRC patients, it is clear why dMMR-MSI-H tumors respond well to ICI, and pMMR-MSI-L tumors do not [76,77].

In addition to the wide variety of immune cells distributed throughout the TME, there are also many cytokines and other molecules secreted by these cells that have specific roles in inflammation, immunity and CRC development. These cytokines can have both antitumorigenic properties, such as interferon-gamma (IFN-γ) and granulysin, or pro-tumorigenic properties, such as IL-6, IL-23 and IL-17. IFN-γ [78] and granulysin [79] bolster and induce MHC-I antigen processing and presentation machinery, and they also recruit antigen presenting cells to stimulate tumor destruction, thus showcasing their antitumorigenic functions, and as so, are overexpressed in dMMR-MSI-H tumors [69]. Induction of proinflammatory cytokines originates as a result of NF-κB and STAT3 activation in epithelial cells, and serves an important role in supporting colorectal tumorigenesis [80–82]. IL-6 is overexpressed in CRC [83–85], and serves a pro-tumorigenic function through multiple processes, including bolstering angiogenesis through an enhanced expression of VEGF [86], protecting both healthy and malignant intestinal epithelial cells (IECs) from damage-associated molecular patterns (DAMPS), and pathogen-associated molecular patterns (PAMPS), by supporting their growth and survival [87–91], along with bolstering defects in the DNA MMR system [92]. Ablation of IL-6 in the dextran sodium sulfate/azoxymethane (DSS/AOM) mouse model of CRC resulted in diminished tumorigenesis, thus confirming its pro-tumorigenic properties [87]. Both IL-23 and IL-17 have also been implicated in the pathogenesis of CRC in human and murine models. An upregulation of IL-17 and IL-23 expression was found in tumors excised from the CPC-APC mouse model of CRC [18]. IL-23 enhances the production of IL-17, and IL-17 activates NF-κB which stimulates the proliferation and survival of IECs, resulting in accelerated colorectal tumorigenesis [18,19,80]. Correspondingly, the elevated expression of IL-6, IL-23 and IL-17 in CRC correlates with a worse prognosis and clinical outcome [93]. The role of other immunomodulatory cytokines involved in CRC has also been discussed [81,82,94]. The presence of a wide variety of immune cells and other cytokines and signaling molecules in the TME provide important topics for future research, but most importantly can serve as new possible targets for immunotherapy.

Moreover, CAC presents a different immuno-profile compared to CRC, which may increase the responsiveness to immunotherapy. However, it may also increase the risk for immunopathological side effects.

6. Why Immunotherapy?

Immunotherapy, particularly ICI, has revolutionized cancer treatment, and although response rates rarely exceed 20%, those who do respond show a durable response [95–97]. The responsiveness to ICI was suggested to depend on several key factors, including mutational load (high levels of tumor neoantigens), tumor-infiltrating lymphocytes and regulatory checkpoint receptors. ICI, a specific type of immunotherapy, functions through inhibiting negative regulatory receptors, such as cytotoxic T lymphocyte antigen 4 (CTLA4) and programmed cell death 1 (PD-1), on T cells, and thereby boosts antitumor immune responses [98–101]. T cells enable the immune system to recognize foreign antigens through an interaction between their T cell receptors (TCR) and peptide epitopes presented by MHC-I molecules on tumor cells [102,103]. Thus, it was suggested that cancers that are characterized by high mutational profiles can produce and present more neoantigens via their MHC-I molecules, and thereby lead to recognition, T cell activation and eventual self-destruction [8,104,105]. However, these effector T cells can become exhausted due to prolonged antigen stimulation, or through an interaction between their surface PD-1 with PD-L1 expressed by immune cells or tumor cells, or their surface CTLA-4 with CD80/CD86 expressed by dendritic cells, which are professional antigen-presenting cells (DC-APC) [101]. Inhibition of these interactions has been observed to partially reactivate exhausted T cells and induce tumor regression [106]. Higher response rates in non-small cell lung cancer (NSCLC) [104,107] and melanoma [108–110] have been attributed to the higher mutational loads in these tumor types [111].

However, for some tumors with lower inflammation and T cell infiltration, which could be due to defects on priming or the absence of high affinity T cells, vaccinations or more specific approaches like adoptive T cell therapy (ATC), which are specific for a particular mutated antigen, may prove favorable options in combination with ICI.

Therapeutic cancer vaccines can induce an immune response through a direct stimulation of the immune system by delivering antigens to DC-APC, which prime and activate $CD4^+$ and $CD8^+$ T cells to initiate tumor destruction [112]. Therapeutic cancer vaccines can target tumor-associated antigens (TAAs) or tumor-specific antigens (TSAs). TAAs are self-antigens expressed in both tumor and normal cells, however T cells that bind to these self-antigens can be removed from the immune system through immunotolerance mechanisms [113]. On the other hand, TSAs are unique to tumor cells, and can strongly induce an immune response through the binding and activation of T cells [113]. However, cancer vaccines comprising TSAs present a noticeable limitation, the necessity for a personalized vaccine specific to the individual's particular tumor neoantigen.

Moreover, ATC provides tumor-antigen-specific approaches that have been shown to have promising results, and may be useful when the neoantigen load is lower, or if information regarding this neoantigen load is unavailable [114]. For example, CD8 T cells targeting mutant KRAS [115] or TP53 "Hotspot" Mutations [116] have been identified. Moreover, circulating PD-1^+ lymphocytes have recently been shown to recognize human gastrointestinal cancer neoantigens [117].

7. Is There a Place for Immunotherapy in CRC?

Initially, ICI was not considered a viable treatment option for CRC. An initial phase II study assessed the efficacy of tremelimumab, a monoclonal antibody against CTLA4, in patients with previous treatment-refractory CRC, which resulted in no improvement post-treatment [118]. Furthermore, two phase I studies of anti-PD-1 [119] and anti-PD-L1 [120] antibodies in previously-treated CRC patients produced no responses. Unfortunately, the MMR/MSI status of the patients in both of these studies was unknown, compromising the interpretation of the results. Indeed, a subsequent phase I clinical trial of an anti-PD-1 antibody (MDX-1106) in patients with a variety of treatment-resistant tumors, including one patient with CRC, culminated in the patient achieving a durable complete response [121]. In accordance with the understanding that the response to ICI may correlate with mutational burden, Le et al. postulated that CRC tumors that are characterized by high mutational burdens due to mismatch–repair deficiencies may respond to ICI [36]. The results of the study showed that patients with dMMR-MSI-H tumors had a 40% objective response rate when treated with pembrolizumab, as compared to 0% for patients with pMMR-MSI-L tumors, and also exhibited 78% immune-related progression-free survival [36]. Importantly, these results suggested that the MMR/MSI status can be an accurate predictor of responsiveness to ICI using pembrolizumab.

Currently, a plethora of clinical trials aim to further examine ICIs in combination with a variety of other therapeutics in the treatment of CRC. Progress has led to United States Food and Drug Administration (FDA) approval of pembrolizumab and nivolumab in patients with dMMR-MSI-H CRC. Approval of pembrolizumab followed the results of the aforementioned study, being the first FDA approval based on a genetic biomarker of a particular tumor type [36]. Approval of nivolumab in patients with dMMR-MSI-H CRC followed the results of CheckMate-142, which showed a 31% objective response rate and 73% twelve month overall survival rate in treatment-resistant dMMR-MSI-H CRC [122]. This same trial also examined the efficacy of the combination of nivolumab and ipilimumab in treatment-resistant dMMR-MSI-H CRC, resulting in a 55% objective response rate and 85% twelve month overall survival rate [123]. The results of this study paved the way for FDA approval of that ICI combination in treatment-resistant dMMR-MSI-H CRC.

As the responsiveness to immunotherapy is generally associated with mutational load, as discussed previously, and dMMR-MSI-H patients comprise high mutational profiles, vaccinations targeting individuals' unique neoantigens may prove to be effective, specifically in dMMR-MSI-H patients. In a murine model of induced dMMR by knockout of MLH1, vaccination extended overall survival and reduced the tumor burden, proving that vaccination can be a viable option for treatment in mouse models of dMMR [124].

Similarly, human clinical trials of therapeutic cancer vaccines have shown promising results depending on MSI status [125,126]. Ultimately, the main question to be determined is whether the combination of ICI and vaccination may prove to be more efficacious than ICI alone in dMMR-MSI-H CRC, or have the ability to elicit a response in pMMR-MSI-L CRC, which is unresponsive to ICI alone.

8. ICI-Resistance in pMMR-MSI-L CRC

Despite its effectiveness in dMMR-MSI-H CRC, ICI is not effective in pMMR-MSI-L CRC. The lack of response of pMMR-MSI-L tumors to ICI has been suggested to trace back to the diminished antitumor immune response, due to the inability for recognition by immune cells as a result of the low mutational profile of these tumors. This lack of response was also shown to be consistent in mouse models, as mice injected with MSI-H CRC experienced greater tumor regression and T cell infiltration than MSI-L or MSI-intermediate CRC when treated with anti-PD-1 therapy [127].

Although MSI-L tumors do not respond to ICI, higher T cell infiltration in MSI-L CRC is correlated with better disease free survival, indicating that some of these tumors can be recognized by T cells [64]. Thus, the main question to be discussed is whether MSI-L CRC utilizes other mechanisms to escape immunorecognition. Perhaps those patients with higher T cell infiltration can be selected for responsiveness to ICI.

One phase 3 trial examined the combination of cobimetinib, an MEK inhibitor, with atezolizumab, an anti-PD-L1 monoclonal antibody, in patients with metastatic CRC [128]. MEK inhibition resulted in increased amounts of tumor-infiltrating $CD8^+$ T cells, and the combination with anti-PD-L1 treatment potentiated tumor regression in mouse models [129]. Despite the promising data in mouse models, the phase 3 trial failed to reach improved response or survival [128], leading to the conclusion that even when combined with MEK inhibitors, anti-PD-(L)1 is not effective in low immunoscore tumors, such as pMMR-MSI-L.

9. Conclusion: Thoughts, Obstacles, and Future Possibilities

CRC is a highly multifaceted and complex disease with an extensive mutational signature and an intricate TME. Just as complex as the disease itself, are the therapies used to combat it. Despite ICI's initial effectiveness in patients exhibiting dMMR-MSI-H tumors, not all dMMR-MSI-H responds to ICI, and as of yet, no response is seen in pMMR-MSI-L. This has led to the necessity for new combinatorial targets that can be used to further bolster the response or lack of response to ICI in these two CRC subsets, as described in Figure 3. Recent advances in the development of new CRC therapeutics include AMG 510, a KRAS(G12C) inhibitor [130]. Analysis of AMG 510 in mouse models with $KRAS^{G12C}$-injected tumors resulted in tumor regression, and combining this molecule with chemotherapy (carboplatin) or ICI (anti-PD-1) resulted in a further increase in tumor regression [130]. Analysis of these tumors showcased increased amounts of $CD8^+$ T cells, macrophages and DC-APC in both the AMG 510 alone, and combination with anti-PD-1 treatment groups [130]. Clinical trials with AMG 510 in four patients with NSCLC resulted in objective partial responses and stable disease in two patients each [130]. The two partial responders were unresponsive to previous chemotherapy and ICI treatment, but exhibited tumor reduction of 34% and 67% when treated with AMG 510 [130]. Overall, this data suggests that AMG 510 may have the ability to induce T cell recruitment, and thus potentiate antitumor immunity. Whether AMG 510 can be combined with ICI in the treatment of CRC remains to be seen.

Cancer vaccines are a rapidly expanding immunotherapeutic approach that also seeks to exploit the body's immune system to fight cancer. Therapeutic cancer vaccines can stimulate and activate T cells to initiate an immune response through the detection of TAAs or TSAs specific to the individuals' tumors. Cancer vaccinations have shown mixed results in different stages of CRC, and more research is needed to truly uncover benefits [131–133]. Moreover, studies have shown that vaccinations may be efficacious in dMMR-MSI-H tumors, but not pMMR-MSI-L [126]. More interestingly, recent studies suggest that the combination of both ICI and cancer vaccinations may result in an improved response in some cancers, but not others [134–144]. Expanding on the possible immunotherapeutic options available, ATC may also provide a possible route in treating specific pMMR-MSI-L CRCs comprising KRAS mutations [145]. However, more research is warranted to determine its effectiveness in CRC, particularly dMMR-MSI-H and pMMR-MSI-L CRC in combination with ICIs. Just as CRC followed melanoma and NSCLC in its application in ICI therapy, CRC may be the next poster boy for vaccination and ICI combination-based therapy.

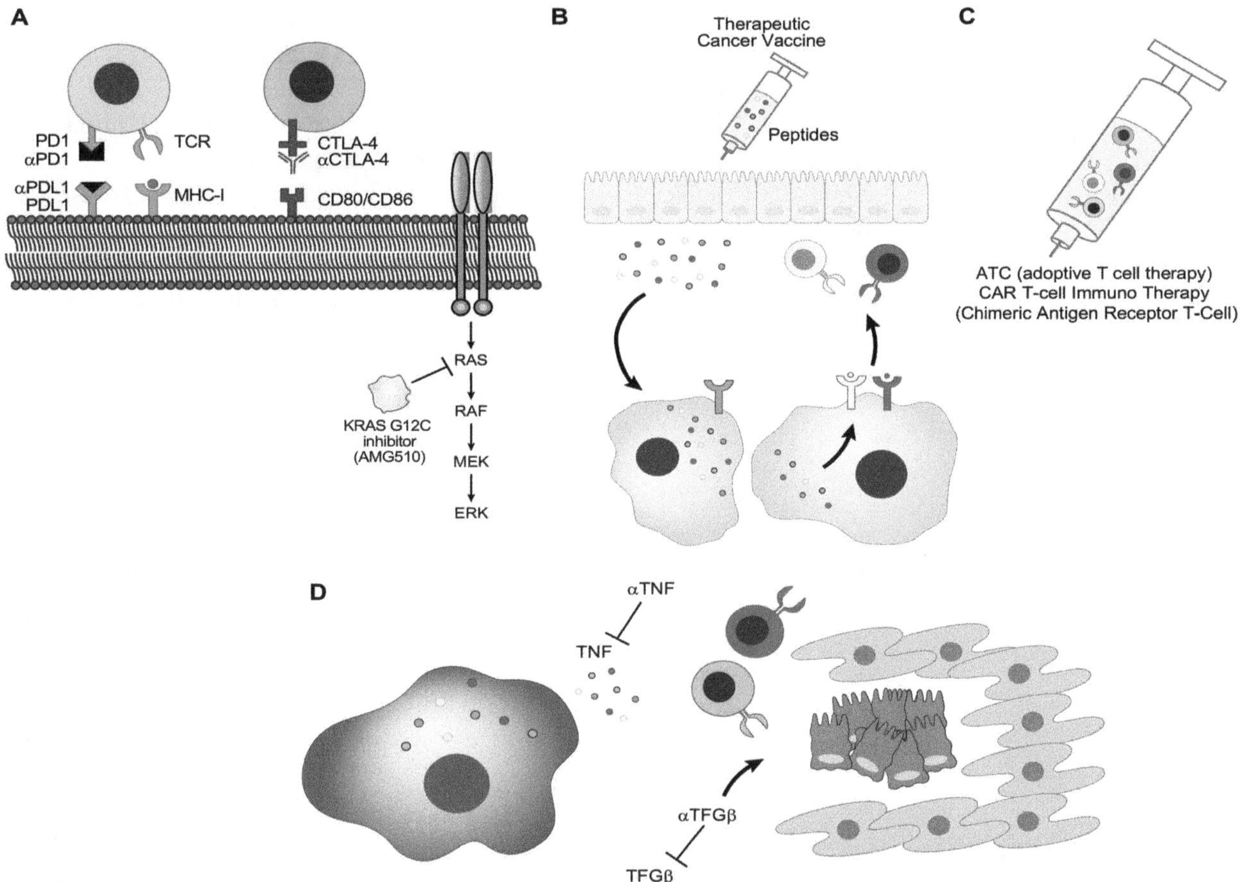

Figure 3. The future of CRC therapy: combinatorial agents. The current status of the use of inhibitor therapy (ICI) in the treatment of CRC has shown promising results, despite the lack of a complete response in dMMR-MSI-H tumors, and no response in pMMR-MSI-L. This obstacle has paved the way for insight and research into plausible combinatorial agents that can overcome this scientific impediment. (**A**) ICI in combination with AMG 510, a KRAS (G12C) inhibitor, or (**B**) therapeutic cancer vaccines, or (**C**) adoptive T cell therapy, or (**D**) TNF and TGFβ inhibitors may serve as the next candidates for combinatorial therapy with ICI.

There are also a number of other factors that can modulate the response to ICI. The gut microbiome has been implicated in variations in response rates to ICI. The presence of particular microbiota seems to be correlated with a heightened response to ICI, depending on the strain and cancer type [146–150].

A possible adverse side effect common with ICI is immune-related colitis, which is often treated with antitumor necrosis factor α (TNF) antibodies. Such treatment in combination with ICI has been shown to improve antitumor immune responses and the severity of colitis in mouse models [151,152].

Furthermore, transforming growth factor β (TGFβ) signaling has been shown to cause resistance to ICI, and inhibition of TGFβ signaling in combination with ICI led to greater tumor regression, as opposed to ICI alone in mouse models, by inhibiting the cancer-associated fibroblast, and increasing the accessibility of cancer cells to T cells [153,154] (Figure 3D). These are just three further examples of possible factors that may be utilized to produce a better response to ICI in CRC.

Immunotherapy serves as a groundbreaking step towards new and more rational treatment options, and lay the groundwork for new combinatorial agents. Further research should be conducted to investigate new combinations of treatments that can be used to produce an improved response to ICI in dMMR-MSI-H CRC, and furthermore, a response that has not yet been obtained in pMMR-MSI-L CRC.

References

1. Siegel, R.; DeSantis, C.; Jemal, A. Colorectal cancer statistics, 2014. *Cancer J. Clin.* **2014**, *64*, 104–117. [CrossRef]
2. American Cancer Society. Cancer Facts & Figures, American Cancer Society, Atlanta, Georgia, 2019. Available online: https://www.cancer.org/content/dam/cancer-org/research/cancer-facts-and-statistics/annual-cancer-facts-and-figures/2019/cancer-facts-and-figures-2019.pdf (accessed on 4 January 2020).
3. Vatandoust, S.; Price, T.J.; Karapetis, C.S. Colorectal cancer: Metastases to a single organ. *World J. Gastroenterol.* **2015**, *21*, 11767–11776. [CrossRef]
4. Eggermont, A.M.M.; Blank, C.U.; Mandala, M.; Long, G.V.; Atkinson, V.; Dalle, S.; Haydon, A.; Lichinitser, M.; Khattak, A.; Carlino, M.S.; et al. Adjuvant Pembrolizumab versus Placebo in Resected Stage III Melanoma. *N. Engl. J. Med.* **2018**, *378*, 1789–1801. [CrossRef]
5. Gandhi, L.; Rodríguez-Abreu, D.; Gadgeel, S.; Esteban, E.; Felip, E.; De Angelis, F.; Domine, M.; Clingan, P.; Hochmair, M.J.; Powell, S.F.; et al. Pembrolizumab plus Chemotherapy in Metastatic Non-Small-Cell Lung Cancer. *N. Engl. J. Med.* **2018**, *378*, 2078–2092. [CrossRef]
6. Hugo, W.; Zaretsky, J.M.; Sun, L.; Song, C.; Moreno, B.H.; Hu-Lieskovan, S.; Berent-Maoz, B.; Pang, J.; Chmielowski, B.; Cherry, G.; et al. Genomic and Transcriptomic Features of Response to Anti-PD-1 Therapy in Metastatic Melanoma. *Cell* **2016**, *165*, 35–44. [CrossRef]
7. Schachter, J.; Ribas, A.; Long, G.V.; Arance, A.; Grob, J.-J.; Mortier, L.; Daud, A.; Carlino, M.S.; McNeil, C.; Lotem, M.; et al. Pembrolizumab versus ipilimumab for advanced melanoma: Final overall survival results of a multicentre, randomised, open-label phase 3 study (KEYNOTE-006). *Lancet* **2017**, *390*, 1853–1862. [CrossRef]
8. Ganesh, K.; Stadler, Z.K.; Cercek, A.; Mendelsohn, R.B.; Shia, J.; Segal, N.H.; Diaz, L.A. Immunotherapy in colorectal cancer: Rationale, challenges and potential. *Nat. Rev. Gastroenterol Hepatol.* **2019**, *16*, 361–375. [CrossRef]
9. Yamagishi, H.; Kuroda, H.; Imai, Y.; Hiraishi, H. Molecular pathogenesis of sporadic colorectal cancers. *Chin. J. Cancer* **2016**, *35*, 4. [CrossRef]
10. Robles, A.I.; Traverso, G.; Zhang, M.; Roberts, N.J.; Khan, M.A.; Joseph, C.; Lauwers, G.Y.; Selaru, F.M.; Popoli, M.; Pittman, M.E.; et al. Whole-Exome Sequencing Analyses of Inflammatory Bowel Disease-Associated Colorectal Cancers. *Gastroenterology* **2016**, *150*, 931–943. [CrossRef]
11. Schell, M.J.; Yang, M.; Teer, J.K.; Lo, F.Y.; Madan, A.; Coppola, D.; Monteiro, A.N.A.; Nebozhyn, M.V.; Yue, B.; Loboda, A.; et al. A multigene mutation classification of 468 colorectal cancers reveals a prognostic role for APC. *Nat. Commun.* **2016**, *7*, 1–12. [CrossRef]
12. Pandurangan, A.k.; Divya, T.; Kumar, K.; Dineshbabu, V.; Velavan, B.; Sudhandiran, G. Colorectal carcinogenesis: Insights into the cell death and signal transduction pathways: A review. *World J. Gastrointest Oncol.* **2018**, *10*, 244–259. [CrossRef] [PubMed]
13. Fearon, E.R. Molecular Genetics of Colorectal Cancer. *Annu. Rev. Pathol. Mech. Dis.* **2011**, *6*, 479–507. [CrossRef]
14. Leslie, A.; Carey, F.A.; Pratt, N.R.; Steele, R.J.C. The colorectal adenoma–carcinoma sequence. *Br. J. Surg.* **2002**, *89*, 845–860. [CrossRef]
15. Taylor, D.P.; Burt, R.W.; Williams, M.S.; Haug, P.J.; Cannon-Albright, L.A. Population-based family history-specific risks for colorectal cancer: A constellation approach. *Gastroenterology* **2010**, *138*, 877–885. [CrossRef]
16. Kerber, R.A.; Neklason, D.W.; Samowitz, W.S.; Burt, R.W. Frequency of Familial Colon Cancer and Hereditary Nonpolyposis Colorectal Cancer (Lynch Syndrome) in a Large Population Database. *Familial. Cancer* **2005**, *4*, 239–244. [CrossRef]

17. Stoffel, E.M.; Kastrinos, F. Familial colorectal cancer, beyond Lynch syndrome. *Clin. Gastroenterol. Hepatol.* **2014**, *12*, 1059–1068. [CrossRef]
18. Grivennikov, S.I.; Wang, K.; Mucida, D.; Stewart, C.A.; Schnabl, B.; Jauch, D.; Taniguchi, K.; Yu, G.-Y.; Österreicher, C.H.; Hung, K.E.; et al. Adenoma-linked barrier defects and microbial products drive IL-23/IL-17-mediated tumour growth. *Nature* **2012**, *491*, 254–258. [CrossRef]
19. Wang, K.; Kim, M.K.; Di Caro, G.; Wong, J.; Shalapour, S.; Wan, J.; Zhang, W.; Zhong, Z.; Sanchez-Lopez, E.; Wu, L.-W.; et al. Interleukin-17 Receptor A Signaling in Transformed Enterocytes Promotes Early Colorectal Tumorigenesis. *Immunity* **2014**, *41*, 1052–1063. [CrossRef]
20. Dmitrieva-Posocco, O.; Dzutsev, A.; Posocco, D.F.; Hou, V.; Yuan, W.; Thovarai, V.; Mufazalov, I.A.; Gunzer, M.; Shilovskiy, I.P.; Khaitov, M.R.; et al. Cell-Type-Specific Responses to Interleukin-1 Control Microbial Invasion and Tumor-Elicited Inflammation in Colorectal Cancer. *Immunity* **2019**, *50*, 166–180.e7. [CrossRef]
21. Greten, F.R.; Grivennikov, S.I. Inflammation and Cancer: Triggers, Mechanisms, and Consequences. *Immunity* **2019**, *51*, 27–41. [CrossRef]
22. Ziegler, P.K.; Bollrath, J.; Pallangyo, C.K.; Matsutani, T.; Canli, Ö.; De Oliveira, T.; Diamanti, M.A.; Müller, N.; Gamrekelashvili, J.; Putoczki, T.; et al. Mitophagy in Intestinal Epithelial Cells Triggers Adaptive Immunity during Tumorigenesis. *Cell* **2018**, *174*, 88–101.e16. [CrossRef] [PubMed]
23. Goldszmid, R.S.; Dzutsev, A.; Viaud, S.; Zitvogel, L.; Restifo, N.P.; Trinchieri, G. Microbiota modulation of myeloid cells in cancer therapy. *Cancer Immunol. Res.* **2015**, *3*, 103–109. [CrossRef] [PubMed]
24. Zhen, Y.; Luo, C.; Zhang, H. Early detection of ulcerative colitis-associated colorectal cancer. *Gastroenterol. Rep. (Oxf.)* **2018**, *6*, 83–92. [CrossRef]
25. Terzić, J.; Grivennikov, S.; Karin, E.; Karin, M. Inflammation and Colon Cancer. *Gastroenterology* **2010**, *138*, 2101–2114.e5. [CrossRef]
26. Khor, B.; Gardet, A.; Xavier, R.J. Genetics and pathogenesis of inflammatory bowel disease. *Nature* **2011**, *474*, 307–317. [CrossRef]
27. Shaked, H.; Hofseth, L.J.; Chumanevich, A.; Chumanevich, A.A.; Wang, J.; Wang, Y.; Taniguchi, K.; Guma, M.; Shenouda, S.; Clevers, H.; et al. Chronic epithelial NF- B activation accelerates APC loss and intestinal tumor initiation through iNOS up-regulation. *PNAS* **2012**, *109*, 14007–14012. [CrossRef]
28. Levin, B.; Lieberman, D.A.; McFarland, B.; Andrews, K.S.; Brooks, D.; Bond, J.; Dash, C.; Giardiello, F.M.; Glick, S.; Johnson, D.; et al. Screening and Surveillance for the Early Detection of Colorectal Cancer and Adenomatous Polyps, 2008: A Joint Guideline From the American Cancer Society, the US Multi-Society Task Force on Colorectal Cancer, and the American College of Radiology. *Gastroenterology* **2008**, *134*, 1570–1595. [CrossRef]
29. Carethers, J.M.; Jung, B.H. Genetics and Genetic Biomarkers in Sporadic Colorectal Cancer. *Gastroenterology* **2015**, *149*, 1177–1190.e3. [CrossRef]
30. Kameyama, H.; Nagahashi, M.; Shimada, Y.; Tajima, Y.; Ichikawa, H.; Nakano, M.; Sakata, J.; Kobayashi, T.; Narayanan, S.; Takabe, K.; et al. Genomic characterization of colitis-associated colorectal cancer. *World J. Surg. Oncol.* **2018**, *16*. [CrossRef]
31. Fleisher, A.S.; Esteller, M.; Harpaz, N.; Leytin, A.; Rashid, A.; Xu, Y.; Liang, J.; Stine, O.C.; Yin, J.; Zou, T.-T.; et al. Microsatellite Instability in Inflammatory Bowel Disease-associated Neoplastic Lesions Is Associated with Hypermethylation and Diminished Expression of the DNA Mismatch Repair Gene, hMLH1. *Cancer Res.* **2000**, *60*, 4864–4868. [PubMed]
32. Wheeler, J.M.D.; Bodmer, W.F.; Wheeler, J.M.D.; Mortensen, N.J.M. DNA mismatch repair genes and colorectal cancer. *Gut* **2000**, *47*, 148–153. [CrossRef] [PubMed]
33. Hause, R.J.; Pritchard, C.C.; Shendure, J.; Salipante, S.J. Classification and characterization of microsatellite instability across 18 cancer types. *Nat. Med.* **2016**, *22*, 1342–1350. [CrossRef] [PubMed]
34. De la Chapelle, A.; Hampel, H. Clinical relevance of microsatellite instability in colorectal cancer. *J. Clin. Oncol.* **2010**, *28*, 3380–3387. [CrossRef] [PubMed]
35. Chen, W.; Swanson, B.J.; Frankel, W.L. Molecular genetics of microsatellite-unstable colorectal cancer for pathologists. *Diagn. Pathol.* **2017**, *12*. [CrossRef]
36. Le, D.T.; Uram, J.N.; Wang, H.; Bartlett, B.R.; Kemberling, H.; Eyring, A.D.; Skora, A.D.; Luber, B.S.; Azad, N.S.; Laheru, D.; et al. PD-1 Blockade in Tumors with Mismatch-Repair Deficiency. *N. Engl. J. Med.* **2015**, *372*, 2509–2520. [CrossRef]

37. Boland, C.R.; Thibodeau, S.N.; Hamilton, S.R.; Sidransky, D.; Eshleman, J.R.; Burt, R.W.; Meltzer, S.J.; Rodriguez-Bigas, M.A.; Fodde, R.; Ranzani, G.N.; et al. A National Cancer Institute Workshop on Microsatellite Instability for Cancer Detection and Familial Predisposition: Development of International Criteria for the Determination of Microsatellite Instability in Colorectal Cancer. *Cancer Res.* **1998**, *58*, 5248. [PubMed]
38. Bacher, J.W.; Flanagan, L.A.; Smalley, R.L.; Nassif, N.A.; Burgart, L.J.; Halberg, R.B.; Megid, W.M.A.; Thibodeau, S.N. Development of a fluorescent multiplex assay for detection of MSI-High tumors. *Dis. Markers* **2004**, *20*, 237–250. [CrossRef]
39. Lu, Y.; Soong, T.D.; Elemento, O. A novel approach for characterizing microsatellite instability in cancer cells. *PLoS ONE* **2013**, *8*, e63056. [CrossRef]
40. Huang, M.N.; McPherson, J.R.; Cutcutache, I.; Teh, B.T.; Tan, P.; Rozen, S.G. MSIseq: Software for Assessing Microsatellite Instability from Catalogs of Somatic Mutations. *Sci. Rep.* **2015**, *5*, 13321. [CrossRef]
41. Dehal, A.; Graff-Baker, A.N.; Vuong, B.; Fischer, T.; Klempner, S.J.; Chang, S.-C.; Grunkemeier, G.L.; Bilchik, A.J.; Goldfarb, M. Neoadjuvant Chemotherapy Improves Survival in Patients with Clinical T4b Colon Cancer. *J. Gastrointest Surg.* **2018**, *22*, 242–249. [CrossRef]
42. Denoya, P.; Wang, H.; Sands, D.; Nogueras, J.; Weiss, E.; Wexner, S.D. Short-term outcomes of laparoscopic total mesorectal excision following neoadjuvant chemoradiotherapy. *Surg. Endosc.* **2010**, *24*, 933–938. [CrossRef] [PubMed]
43. Sauer, R.; Becker, H.; Hohenberger, W.; Rödel, C.; Wittekind, C.; Fietkau, R.; Martus, P.; Tschmelitsch, J.; Hager, E.; Hess, C.F.; et al. Preoperative versus Postoperative Chemoradiotherapy for Rectal Cancer. *N. Engl. J. Med.* **2004**, *351*, 1731–1740. [CrossRef] [PubMed]
44. Seymour, M.T.; Morton, D. FOxTROT: An international randomised controlled trial in 1052 patients (pts) evaluating neoadjuvant chemotherapy (NAC) for colon cancer. *J. Clin. Oncol.* **2019**, *37*, 3504. [CrossRef]
45. De Gooyer, J.-M.; Verstegen, M.G.; 't Lam-Boer, J.; Radema, S.A.; Verhoeven, R.H.A.; Verhoef, C.; Schreinemakers, J.M.J.; de Wilt, J.H.W. Neoadjuvant Chemotherapy for Locally Advanced T4 Colon Cancer: A Nationwide Propensity-Score Matched Cohort Analysis. *Dig. Surg.* **2019**, 1–10. [CrossRef] [PubMed]
46. Miyamoto, R.; Kikuchi, K.; Uchida, A.; Ozawa, M.; Sano, N.; Tadano, S.; Inagawa, S.; Oda, T.; Ohkohchi, N. Pathological complete response after preoperative chemotherapy including FOLFOX plus bevacizumab for locally advanced rectal cancer: A case report and literature review. *Int. J. Surg. Case. Rep.* **2019**, *62*, 85–88. [CrossRef] [PubMed]
47. Longley, D.B.; Harkin, D.P.; Johnston, P.G. 5-Fluorouracil: Mechanisms of action and clinical strategies. *Nat. Rev. Cancer* **2003**, *3*, 330–338. [CrossRef] [PubMed]
48. Giacchetti, S.; Perpoint, B.; Zidani, R.; Le Bail, N.; Faggiuolo, R.; Focan, C.; Chollet, P.; Llory, J.f.; Letourneau, Y.; Coudert, B.; et al. Phase III Multicenter Randomized Trial of Oxaliplatin Added to Chronomodulated Fluorouracil–Leucovorin as First-Line Treatment of Metastatic Colorectal Cancer. *J. Clin. Oncol.* **2000**, *18*, 136. [CrossRef] [PubMed]
49. Ribic, C.M.; Sargent, D.J.; Moore, M.J.; Thibodeau, S.N.; French, A.J.; Goldberg, R.M.; Hamilton, S.R.; Laurent-Puig, P.; Gryfe, R.; Shepherd, L.E.; et al. Tumor Microsatellite-Instability Status as a Predictor of Benefit from Fluorouracil-Based Adjuvant Chemotherapy for Colon Cancer. *N. Engl. J. Med.* **2003**, *349*, 247–257. [CrossRef] [PubMed]
50. Vilar, E.; Gruber, S.B. Microsatellite instability in colorectal cancer—The stable evidence. *Nat. Rev. Clin. Oncol.* **2010**, *7*, 153–162. [CrossRef] [PubMed]
51. Sinicrope, F.A.; Foster, N.R.; Thibodeau, S.N.; Marsoni, S.; Monges, G.; Labianca, R.; Yothers, G.; Allegra, C.; Moore, M.J.; Gallinger, S.; et al. DNA Mismatch Repair Status and Colon Cancer Recurrence and Survival in Clinical Trials of 5-Fluorouracil-Based Adjuvant Therapy. *J. Natl. Cancer Inst.* **2011**, *103*, 863–875. [CrossRef] [PubMed]
52. Jover, R.; Zapater, P.; Castells, A.; Llor, X.; Andreu, M.; Cubiella, J.; Piñol, V.; Xicola, R.M.; Bujanda, L.; Reñé, J.M.; et al. Mismatch repair status in the prediction of benefit from adjuvant fluorouracil chemotherapy in colorectal cancer. *Gut* **2006**, *55*, 848–855. [CrossRef] [PubMed]

53. Bertagnolli, M.M.; Niedzwiecki, D.; Compton, C.C.; Hahn, H.P.; Hall, M.; Damas, B.; Jewell, S.D.; Mayer, R.J.; Goldberg, R.M.; Saltz, L.B.; et al. Microsatellite Instability Predicts Improved Response to Adjuvant Therapy With Irinotecan, Fluorouracil, and Leucovorin in Stage III Colon Cancer: Cancer and Leukemia Group B Protocol 89803. *J. Clin. Oncol.* **2009**, *27*, 1814–1821. [CrossRef]
54. Hurwitz, H.; Fehrenbacher, L.; Novotny, W.; Cartwright, T.; Hainsworth, J.; Heim, W.; Berlin, J.; Baron, A.; Griffing, S.; Holmgren, E.; et al. Bevacizumab plus Irinotecan, Fluorouracil, and Leucovorin for Metastatic Colorectal Cancer. *N. Engl. J. Med.* **2004**, *350*, 2335–2342. [CrossRef]
55. Saltz, L.B.; Clarke, S.; Díaz-Rubio, E.; Scheithauer, W.; Figer, A.; Wong, R.; Koski, S.; Lichinitser, M.; Yang, T.-S.; Rivera, F.; et al. Bevacizumab in combination with oxaliplatin-based chemotherapy as first-line therapy in metastatic colorectal cancer: A randomized phase III study. *J. Clin. Oncol.* **2008**, *26*, 2013–2019. [CrossRef]
56. Cunningham, D.; Humblet, Y.; Siena, S.; Khayat, D.; Bleiberg, H.; Santoro, A.; Bets, D.; Mueser, M.; Harstrick, A.; Verslype, C.; et al. Cetuximab Monotherapy and Cetuximab plus Irinotecan in Irinotecan-Refractory Metastatic Colorectal Cancer. *N. Engl. J. Med.* **2004**, *351*, 337–345. [CrossRef]
57. Sobrero, A.F.; Maurel, J.; Fehrenbacher, L.; Scheithauer, W.; Abubakr, Y.A.; Lutz, M.P.; Vega-Villegas, M.E.; Eng, C.; Steinhauer, E.U.; Prausova, J.; et al. EPIC: Phase III Trial of Cetuximab Plus Irinotecan After Fluoropyrimidine and Oxaliplatin Failure in Patients With Metastatic Colorectal Cancer. *J. Clin. Oncol.* **2008**, *26*, 2311–2319. [CrossRef]
58. Lièvre, A.; Bachet, J.-B.; Corre, D.L.; Boige, V.; Landi, B.; Emile, J.-F.; Côté, J.-F.; Tomasic, G.; Penna, C.; Ducreux, M.; et al. KRAS Mutation Status Is Predictive of Response to Cetuximab Therapy in Colorectal Cancer. *Cancer Res.* **2006**, *66*, 3992–3995. [CrossRef]
59. Cunningham, D.; Atkin, W.; Lenz, H.-J.; Lynch, H.T.; Minsky, B.; Nordlinger, B.; Starling, N. Colorectal cancer. *Lancet* **2010**, *375*, 1030–1047. [CrossRef]
60. Misale, S.; Yaeger, R.; Hobor, S.; Scala, E.; Janakiraman, M.; Liska, D.; Valtorta, E.; Schiavo, R.; Buscarino, M.; Siravegna, G.; et al. Emergence of KRAS mutations and acquired resistance to anti-EGFR therapy in colorectal cancer. *Nature* **2012**, *486*, 532–536. [CrossRef] [PubMed]
61. Sinicrope, F.A.; Shi, Q.; Smyrk, T.C.; Thibodeau, S.N.; Dienstmann, R.; Guinney, J.; Bot, B.M.; Tejpar, S.; Delorenzi, M.; Goldberg, R.M.; et al. Molecular markers identify subtypes of stage III colon cancer associated with patient outcomes. *Gastroenterology* **2015**, *148*, 88–99. [CrossRef] [PubMed]
62. Van Emburgh, B.O.; Sartore-Bianchi, A.; Di Nicolantonio, F.; Siena, S.; Bardelli, A. Acquired resistance to EGFR-targeted therapies in colorectal cancer. *Mol. Oncol.* **2014**, *8*, 1084–1094. [CrossRef] [PubMed]
63. Van Cutsem, E.; Peeters, M.; Siena, S.; Humblet, Y.; Hendlisz, A.; Neyns, B.; Canon, J.-L.; Van Laethem, J.-L.; Maurel, J.; Richardson, G.; et al. Open-Label Phase III Trial of Panitumumab Plus Best Supportive Care Compared With Best Supportive Care Alone in Patients With Chemotherapy-Refractory Metastatic Colorectal Cancer. *J. Clin. Oncol.* **2007**, *25*, 1658–1664. [CrossRef] [PubMed]
64. Pagès, F.; Mlecnik, B.; Marliot, F.; Bindea, G.; Ou, F.-S.; Bifulco, C.; Lugli, A.; Zlobec, I.; Rau, T.T.; Berger, M.D.; et al. International validation of the consensus Immunoscore for the classification of colon cancer: A prognostic and accuracy study. *Lancet* **2018**, *391*, 2128–2139. [CrossRef]
65. Galon, J.; Costes, A.; Sanchez-Cabo, F.; Kirilovsky, A.; Mlecnik, B.; Lagorce-Pagès, C.; Tosolini, M.; Camus, M.; Berger, A.; Wind, P.; et al. Type, Density, and Location of Immune Cells Within Human Colorectal Tumors Predict Clinical Outcome. *Science* **2006**, *313*, 1960–1964. [CrossRef]
66. Mlecnik, B.; Tosolini, M.; Kirilovsky, A.; Berger, A.; Bindea, G.; Meatchi, T.; Bruneval, P.; Trajanoski, Z.; Fridman, W.-H.; Pagès, F.; et al. Histopathologic-Based Prognostic Factors of Colorectal Cancers Are Associated With the State of the Local Immune Reaction. *J. Clin. Oncol.* **2011**, *29*, 610–618. [CrossRef]
67. Bindea, G.; Mlecnik, B.; Tosolini, M.; Kirilovsky, A.; Waldner, M.; Obenauf, A.C.; Angell, H.; Fredriksen, T.; Lafontaine, L.; Berger, A.; et al. Spatiotemporal Dynamics of Intratumoral Immune Cells Reveal the Immune Landscape in Human Cancer. *Immunity* **2013**, *39*, 782–795. [CrossRef]
68. Galon, J.; Angell, H.K.; Bedognetti, D.; Marincola, F.M. The continuum of cancer immunosurveillance: Prognostic, predictive, and mechanistic signatures. *Immunity* **2013**, *39*, 11–26. [CrossRef]
69. Mlecnik, B.; Bindea, G.; Angell, H.K.; Maby, P.; Angelova, M.; Tougeron, D.; Church, S.E.; Lafontaine, L.; Fischer, M.; Fredriksen, T.; et al. Integrative Analyses of Colorectal Cancer Show Immunoscore Is a Stronger Predictor of Patient Survival Than Microsatellite Instability. *Immunity* **2016**, *44*, 698–711. [CrossRef]

70. Ogino, S.; Nosho, K.; Irahara, N.; Meyerhardt, J.A.; Baba, Y.; Shima, K.; Glickman, J.N.; Ferrone, C.R.; Mino-Kenudson, M.; Tanaka, N.; et al. Lymphocytic Reaction to Colorectal Cancer is Associated with Longer Survival, Independent of Lymph Node Count, MSI and CpG Island Methylator Phenotype. *Clin. Cancer Res.* **2009**, *15*, 6412–6420. [CrossRef]
71. Popat, S.; Hubner, R.; Houlston, R.S. Systematic Review of Microsatellite Instability and Colorectal Cancer Prognosis. *J. Clin. Oncol.* **2005**, *23*, 609–618. [CrossRef]
72. Narayanan, S.; Kawaguchi, T.; Peng, X.; Qi, Q.; Liu, S.; Yan, L.; Takabe, K. Tumor Infiltrating Lymphocytes and Macrophages Improve Survival in Microsatellite Unstable Colorectal Cancer. *Sci. Rep.* **2019**, *9*, 1–10. [CrossRef] [PubMed]
73. Tosolini, M.; Kirilovsky, A.; Mlecnik, B.; Fredriksen, T.; Mauger, S.; Bindea, G.; Berger, A.; Bruneval, P.; Fridman, W.-H.; Pagès, F.; et al. Clinical Impact of Different Classes of Infiltrating T Cytotoxic and Helper Cells (Th1, Th2, Treg, Th17) in Patients with Colorectal Cancer. *Cancer Res.* **2011**, *71*, 1263–1271. [CrossRef] [PubMed]
74. Maby, P.; Tougeron, D.; Hamieh, M.; Mlecnik, B.; Kora, H.; Bindea, G.; Angell, H.K.; Fredriksen, T.; Elie, N.; Fauquembergue, E.; et al. Correlation between Density of CD8+ T-cell Infiltrate in Microsatellite Unstable Colorectal Cancers and Frameshift Mutations: A Rationale for Personalized Immunotherapy. *Cancer Res.* **2015**, *75*, 3446–3455. [CrossRef]
75. Zhao, P.; Li, L.; Jiang, X.; Li, Q. Mismatch repair deficiency/microsatellite instability-high as a predictor for anti-PD-1/PD-L1 immunotherapy efficacy. *J. Hematol. Oncol.* **2019**, *12*, 54. [CrossRef]
76. Pagès, F.; Berger, A.; Camus, M.; Sanchez-Cabo, F.; Costes, A.; Molidor, R.; Mlecnik, B.; Kirilovsky, A.; Nilsson, M.; Damotte, D.; et al. Effector memory T cells, early metastasis, and survival in colorectal cancer. *N. Engl. J. Med.* **2005**, *353*, 2654–2666. [CrossRef]
77. Tang, H.; Wang, Y.; Chlewicki, L.K.; Zhang, Y.; Guo, J.; Liang, W.; Wang, J.; Wang, X.; Fu, Y.-X. Facilitating T cell infiltration in tumor microenvironment overcomes resistance to PD-L1 blockade. *Cancer Cell* **2016**, *29*, 285–296. [CrossRef]
78. Zhou, F. Molecular Mechanisms of IFN-γ to Up-Regulate MHC Class I Antigen Processing and Presentation. *Int. Rev. Immunol.* **2009**, *28*, 239–260. [CrossRef] [PubMed]
79. Tewary, P.; Yang, D.; de la Rosa, G.; Li, Y.; Finn, M.W.; Krensky, A.M.; Clayberger, C.; Oppenheim, J.J. Granulysin activates antigen-presenting cells through TLR4 and acts as an immune alarmin. *Blood* **2010**, *116*, 3465–3474. [CrossRef]
80. Taniguchi, K.; Karin, M. NF-κB, inflammation, immunity and cancer: Coming of age. *Nat. Rev. Immunol.* **2018**, *18*, 309–324. [CrossRef]
81. Lasry, A.; Zinger, A.; Ben-Neriah, Y. Inflammatory networks underlying colorectal cancer. *Nat. Immunol.* **2016**, *17*, 230–240. [CrossRef] [PubMed]
82. West, N.R.; McCuaig, S.; Franchini, F.; Powrie, F. Emerging cytokine networks in colorectal cancer. *Nat. Rev. Immunol.* **2015**, *15*, 615–629. [CrossRef]
83. Zeng, J.; Tang, Z.-H.; Liu, S.; Guo, S.-S. Clinicopathological significance of overexpression of interleukin-6 in colorectal cancer. *World J. Gastroenterol.* **2017**, *23*, 1780–1786. [CrossRef]
84. Chung, Y.-C.; Chang, Y.-F. Serum interleukin-6 levels reflect the disease status of colorectal cancer. *J. Surg. Oncol.* **2003**, *83*, 222–226. [CrossRef] [PubMed]
85. Knüpfer, H.; Preiss, R. Serum interleukin-6 levels in colorectal cancer patients—A summary of published results. *Int. J. Colorectal. Dis.* **2010**, *25*, 135–140. [CrossRef] [PubMed]
86. Nagasaki, T.; Hara, M.; Nakanishi, H.; Takahashi, H.; Sato, M.; Takeyama, H. Interleukin-6 released by colon cancer-associated fibroblasts is critical for tumour angiogenesis: Anti-interleukin-6 receptor antibody suppressed angiogenesis and inhibited tumour–stroma interaction. *Br. J. Cancer* **2014**, *110*, 469–478. [CrossRef] [PubMed]
87. Grivennikov, S.; Karin, E.; Terzic, J.; Mucida, D.; Yu, G.-Y.; Vallabhapurapu, S.; Scheller, J.; Rose-John, S.; Cheroutre, H.; Eckmann, L.; et al. IL-6 and Stat3 Are Required for Survival of Intestinal Epithelial Cells and Development of Colitis-Associated Cancer. *Cancer Cell* **2009**, *15*, 103–113. [CrossRef] [PubMed]
88. Corvinus, F.M.; Orth, C.; Moriggl, R.; Tsareva, S.A.; Wagner, S.; Pfitzner, E.B.; Baus, D.; Kaufmann, R.; Huber, L.A.; Zatloukal, K.; et al. Persistent STAT3 activation in colon cancer is associated with enhanced cell proliferation and tumor growth. *Neoplasia* **2005**, *7*, 545–555. [CrossRef] [PubMed]

89. Bollrath, J.; Phesse, T.J.; von Burstin, V.A.; Putoczki, T.; Bennecke, M.; Bateman, T.; Nebelsiek, T.; Lundgren-May, T.; Canli, Ö.; Schwitalla, S.; et al. gp130-Mediated Stat3 Activation in Enterocytes Regulates Cell Survival and Cell-Cycle Progression during Colitis-Associated Tumorigenesis. *Cancer Cell* **2009**, *15*, 91–102. [CrossRef] [PubMed]
90. Taniguchi, K.; Wu, L.-W.; Grivennikov, S.I.; de Jong, P.R.; Lian, I.; Yu, F.-X.; Wang, K.; Ho, S.B.; Boland, B.S.; Chang, J.T.; et al. A gp130–Src–YAP module links inflammation to epithelial regeneration. *Nature* **2015**, *519*, 57–62. [CrossRef]
91. Taniguchi, K.; Karin, M. IL-6 and related cytokines as the critical lynchpins between inflammation and cancer. *Semin. Immunol.* **2014**, *26*, 54–74. [CrossRef]
92. Tseng-Rogenski, S.; Hamaya, Y.; Choi, D.Y.; Carethers, J.M. Interleukin 6 Alters Localization of hMSH3, Leading to DNA Mismatch Repair Defects in Colorectal Cancer Cells. *Gastroenterology* **2015**, *148*, 579–589. [CrossRef] [PubMed]
93. Schetter, A.J.; Nguyen, G.H.; Bowman, E.D.; Mathé, E.A.; Yuen, S.T.; Hawkes, J.E.; Croce, C.M.; Leung, S.Y.; Harris, C.C. Association of Inflammation-Related and microRNA Gene Expression with Cancer-Specific Mortality of Colon Adenocarcinoma. *Clin. Cancer Res.* **2009**, *15*, 5878–5887. [CrossRef] [PubMed]
94. Wang, K.; Karin, M. Chapter Five—Tumor-Elicited Inflammation and Colorectal Cancer. In *Advances in Cancer Research*; Wang, X.-Y., Fisher, P.B., Eds.; Academic Press: Cambridge, MA, USA, 2015; Volume 128, pp. 173–196, ISBN 0065-230X.
95. Couzin-Frankel, J. Cancer Immunotherapy. *Science* **2013**, *342*, 1432–1433. [CrossRef] [PubMed]
96. Zugazagoitia, J.; Guedes, C.; Ponce, S.; Ferrer, I.; Molina-Pinelo, S.; Paz-Ares, L. Current Challenges in Cancer Treatment. *Clinical. Therapeutics* **2016**, *38*, 1551–1566. [CrossRef] [PubMed]
97. Franke, A.J.; Skelton, W.P., IV; Starr, J.S.; Parekh, H.; Lee, J.J.; Overman, M.J.; Allegra, C.; George, T.J. Immunotherapy for Colorectal Cancer: A Review of Current and Novel Therapeutic Approaches. *J. Natl. Cancer Inst.* **2019**, *111*, 1131–1141. [CrossRef]
98. Sharma, P.; Allison, J.P. The future of immune checkpoint therapy. *Science* **2015**, *348*, 56–61. [CrossRef]
99. Topalian, S.L.; Drake, C.G.; Pardoll, D.M. Immune Checkpoint Blockade: A Common Denominator Approach to Cancer Therapy. *Cancer Cell* **2015**, *27*, 450–461. [CrossRef]
100. Pardoll, D.M. The blockade of immune checkpoints in cancer immunotherapy. *Nat. Rev. Cancer* **2012**, *12*, 252–264. [CrossRef]
101. Wei, S.C.; Duffy, C.R.; Allison, J.P. Fundamental Mechanisms of Immune Checkpoint Blockade Therapy. *Cancer Discov.* **2018**, *8*, 1069–1086. [CrossRef]
102. Khalil, D.N.; Smith, E.L.; Brentjens, R.J.; Wolchok, J.D. The future of cancer treatment: Immunomodulation, CARs and combination immunotherapy. *Nat. Rev. Clin. Oncol.* **2016**, *13*, 273–290. [CrossRef]
103. Khalil, D.N.; Budhu, S.; Gasmi, B.; Zappasodi, R.; Hirschhorn-Cymerman, D.; Plitt, T.; De Henau, O.; Zamarin, D.; Holmgaard, R.B.; Murphy, J.T.; et al. Chapter One—The New Era of Cancer Immunotherapy: Manipulating T-Cell Activity to Overcome Malignancy. In *Advances in Cancer Research*; Wang, X.-Y., Fisher, P.B., Eds.; Academic Press: Cambridge, MA, USA, 2015; Volume 128, pp. 1–68. ISBN 0065-230X.
104. Rizvi, N.A.; Hellmann, M.D.; Snyder, A.; Kvistborg, P.; Makarov, V.; Havel, J.J.; Lee, W.; Yuan, J.; Wong, P.; Ho, T.S.; et al. Cancer immunology. Mutational landscape determines sensitivity to PD-1 blockade in non-small cell lung cancer. *Science* **2015**, *348*, 124–128. [CrossRef] [PubMed]
105. Schumacher, T.N.; Schreiber, R.D. Neoantigens in cancer immunotherapy. *Science* **2015**, *348*, 69–74. [CrossRef] [PubMed]
106. Keir, M.E.; Butte, M.J.; Freeman, G.J.; Sharpe, A.H. PD-1 and Its Ligands in Tolerance and Immunity. *Annu. Rev. Immunol.* **2008**, *26*, 677–704. [CrossRef] [PubMed]
107. Garon, E.B.; Rizvi, N.A.; Hui, R.; Leighl, N.; Balmanoukian, A.S.; Eder, J.P.; Patnaik, A.; Aggarwal, C.; Gubens, M.; Horn, L.; et al. Pembrolizumab for the Treatment of Non-Small-Cell Lung Cancer. *N. Engl. J. Med.* **2015**, *372*, 2018–2028. [CrossRef]
108. Snyder, A.; Makarov, V.; Merghoub, T.; Yuan, J.; Zaretsky, J.M.; Desrichard, A.; Walsh, L.A.; Postow, M.A.; Wong, P.; Ho, T.S.; et al. Genetic Basis for Clinical Response to CTLA-4 Blockade in Melanoma. *N. Engl. J. Med.* **2014**, *371*, 2189–2199. [CrossRef]
109. Van Allen, E.M.; Miao, D.; Schilling, B.; Shukla, S.A.; Blank, C.; Zimmer, L.; Sucker, A.; Hillen, U.; Geukes Foppen, M.H.; Goldinger, S.M.; et al. Genomic correlates of response to CTLA-4 blockade in metastatic melanoma. *Science* **2015**, *350*, 207. [CrossRef]

110. Hodi, F.S.; O'Day, S.J.; McDermott, D.F.; Weber, R.W.; Sosman, J.A.; Haanen, J.B.; Gonzalez, R.; Robert, C.; Schadendorf, D.; Hassel, J.C.; et al. Improved Survival with Ipilimumab in Patients with Metastatic Melanoma. *N. Engl. J. Med.* **2010**, *363*, 711–723. [CrossRef]
111. Alexandrov, L.B.; Nik-Zainal, S.; Wedge, D.C.; Aparicio, S.A.J.R.; Behjati, S.; Biankin, A.V.; Bignell, G.R.; Bolli, N.; Borg, A.; Børresen-Dale, A.-L.; et al. Signatures of mutational processes in human cancer. *Nature* **2013**, *500*, 415–421. [CrossRef]
112. Sahin, U.; Türeci, Ö. Personalized vaccines for cancer immunotherapy. *Science* **2018**, *359*, 1355. [CrossRef]
113. Hollingsworth, R.E.; Jansen, K. Turning the corner on therapeutic cancer vaccines. *NPJ Vaccines* **2019**, *4*, 7. [CrossRef]
114. Blankenstein, T.; Leisegang, M.; Uckert, W.; Schreiber, H. Targeting cancer-specific mutations by T cell receptor gene therapy. *Curr. Opin. Immunol.* **2015**, *33*, 112–119. [CrossRef] [PubMed]
115. Tran, E.; Robbins, P.F.; Lu, Y.-C.; Prickett, T.D.; Gartner, J.J.; Jia, L.; Pasetto, A.; Zheng, Z.; Ray, S.; Groh, E.M.; et al. T-Cell Transfer Therapy Targeting Mutant KRAS in Cancer. *N. Engl. J. Med.* **2016**, *375*, 2255–2262. [CrossRef] [PubMed]
116. Malekzadeh, P.; Pasetto, A.; Robbins, P.F.; Parkhurst, M.R.; Paria, B.C.; Jia, L.; Gartner, J.J.; Hill, V.; Yu, Z.; Restifo, N.P.; et al. Neoantigen screening identifies broad TP53 mutant immunogenicity in patients with epithelial cancers. *J. Clin. Invest.* **2019**, *129*, 1109–1114. [CrossRef] [PubMed]
117. Gros, A.; Tran, E.; Parkhurst, M.R.; Ilyas, S.; Pasetto, A.; Groh, E.M.; Robbins, P.F.; Yossef, R.; Garcia-Garijo, A.; Fajardo, C.A.; et al. Recognition of human gastrointestinal cancer neoantigens by circulating PD-1+ lymphocytes. *J. Clin. Invest.* **2019**, *129*, 4992–5004. [CrossRef] [PubMed]
118. Chung, K.Y.; Gore, I.; Fong, L.; Venook, A.; Beck, S.B.; Dorazio, P.; Criscitiello, P.J.; Healey, D.I.; Huang, B.; Gomez-Navarro, J.; et al. Phase II Study of the Anti-Cytotoxic T-Lymphocyte–Associated Antigen 4 Monoclonal Antibody, Tremelimumab, in Patients With Refractory Metastatic Colorectal Cancer. *J. Clin. Oncol.* **2010**, *28*, 3485–3490. [CrossRef] [PubMed]
119. Topalian, S.L.; Hodi, F.S.; Brahmer, J.R.; Gettinger, S.N.; Smith, D.C.; McDermott, D.F.; Powderly, J.D.; Carvajal, R.D.; Sosman, J.A.; Atkins, M.B.; et al. Safety, Activity, and Immune Correlates of Anti–PD-1 Antibody in Cancer. *N. Engl. J. Med.* **2012**, *366*, 2443–2454. [CrossRef]
120. Brahmer, J.R.; Tykodi, S.S.; Chow, L.Q.M.; Hwu, W.-J.; Topalian, S.L.; Hwu, P.; Drake, C.G.; Camacho, L.H.; Kauh, J.; Odunsi, K.; et al. Safety and Activity of Anti–PD-L1 Antibody in Patients with Advanced Cancer. *N. Engl. J. Med.* **2012**, *366*, 2455–2465. [CrossRef]
121. Brahmer, J.R.; Drake, C.G.; Wollner, I.; Powderly, J.D.; Picus, J.; Sharfman, W.H.; Stankevich, E.; Pons, A.; Salay, T.M.; McMiller, T.L.; et al. Phase I study of single-agent anti-programmed death-1 (MDX-1106) in refractory solid tumors: Safety, clinical activity, pharmacodynamics, and immunologic correlates. *J. Clin. Oncol.* **2010**, *28*, 3167–3175. [CrossRef]
122. Overman, M.J.; McDermott, R.; Leach, J.L.; Lonardi, S.; Lenz, H.-J.; Morse, M.A.; Desai, J.; Hill, A.; Axelson, M.; Moss, R.A.; et al. Nivolumab in patients with metastatic DNA mismatch repair-deficient or microsatellite instability-high colorectal cancer (CheckMate 142): An open-label, multicentre, phase 2 study. *Lancet Oncol.* **2017**, *18*, 1182–1191. [CrossRef]
123. Overman, M.J.; Lonardi, S.; Wong, K.Y.M.; Lenz, H.-J.; Gelsomino, F.; Aglietta, M.; Morse, M.A.; Van Cutsem, E.; McDermott, R.; Hill, A.; et al. Durable Clinical Benefit With Nivolumab Plus Ipilimumab in DNA Mismatch Repair-Deficient/Microsatellite Instability-High Metastatic Colorectal Cancer. *J. Clin. Oncol.* **2018**, *36*, 773–779. [CrossRef]
124. Maletzki, C.; Gladbach, Y.S.; Hamed, M.; Fuellen, G.; Semmler, M.-L.; Stenzel, J.; Linnebacher, M. Cellular vaccination of MLH1(-/-) mice—An immunotherapeutic proof of concept study. *Oncoimmunology* **2017**, *7*, e1408748. [CrossRef] [PubMed]
125. Kloor, M.; Reuschenbach, M.; Karbach, J.; Rafiyan, M.; Al-Batran, S.-E.; Pauligk, C.; Jaeger, E.; von Knebel Doeberitz, M. Vaccination of MSI-H colorectal cancer patients with frameshift peptide antigens: A phase I/IIa clinical trial. *J. Clin. Oncol.* **2015**, *33*, 3020. [CrossRef]
126. De Weger, V.A.; Turksma, A.W.; Voorham, Q.J.M.; Euler, Z.; Bril, H.; van den Eertwegh, A.J.; Bloemena, E.; Pinedo, H.M.; Vermorken, J.B.; van Tinteren, H.; et al. Clinical effects of adjuvant active specific immunotherapy differ between patients with microsatellite-stable and microsatellite-instable colon cancer. *Clin. Cancer Res.* **2012**, *18*, 882–889. [CrossRef]

127. Mandal, R.; Samstein, R.M.; Lee, K.-W.; Havel, J.J.; Wang, H.; Krishna, C.; Sabio, E.Y.; Makarov, V.; Kuo, F.; Blecua, P.; et al. Genetic diversity of tumors with mismatch repair deficiency influences anti-PD-1 immunotherapy response. *Science* **2019**, *364*, 485. [CrossRef]
128. Eng, C.; Kim, T.W.; Bendell, J.; Argilés, G.; Tebbutt, N.C.; Di Bartolomeo, M.; Falcone, A.; Fakih, M.; Kozloff, M.; Segal, N.H.; et al. Atezolizumab with or without cobimetinib versus regorafenib in previously treated metastatic colorectal cancer (IMblaze370): A multicentre, open-label, phase 3, randomised, controlled trial. *Lancet Oncol.* **2019**, *20*, 849–861. [CrossRef]
129. Ebert, P.J.R.; Cheung, J.; Yang, Y.; McNamara, E.; Hong, R.; Moskalenko, M.; Gould, S.E.; Maecker, H.; Irving, B.A.; Kim, J.M.; et al. MAP Kinase Inhibition Promotes T Cell and Anti-tumor Activity in Combination with PD-L1 Checkpoint Blockade. *Immunity* **2016**, *44*, 609–621. [CrossRef]
130. Canon, J.; Rex, K.; Saiki, A.Y.; Mohr, C.; Cooke, K.; Bagal, D.; Gaida, K.; Holt, T.; Knutson, C.G.; Koppada, N.; et al. The clinical KRAS(G12C) inhibitor AMG 510 drives anti-tumour immunity. *Nature* **2019**, *575*, 217–223. [CrossRef]
131. Hanna, M.G.; Hoover, H.C.; Vermorken, J.B.; Harris, J.E.; Pinedo, H.M. Adjuvant active specific immunotherapy of stage II and stage III colon cancer with an autologous tumor cell vaccine: First randomized phase III trials show promise. *Vaccine* **2001**, *19*, 2576–2582. [CrossRef]
132. Harris, J.E.; Ryan, L.; Hoover, H.C.; Stuart, R.K.; Oken, M.M.; Benson, A.B.; Mansour, E.; Haller, D.G.; Manola, J.; Hanna, M.G. Adjuvant active specific immunotherapy for stage II and III colon cancer with an autologous tumor cell vaccine: Eastern Cooperative Oncology Group Study E5283. *J. Clin. Oncol.* **2000**, *18*, 148–157. [CrossRef]
133. Ockert, D.; Schirrmacher, V.; Beck, N.; Stoelben, E.; Ahlert, T.; Flechtenmacher, J.; Hagmüller, E.; Buchcik, R.; Nagel, M.; Saeger, H.D. Newcastle disease virus-infected intact autologous tumor cell vaccine for adjuvant active specific immunotherapy of resected colorectal carcinoma. *Clin. Cancer Res.* **1996**, *2*, 21–28. [PubMed]
134. Puzanov, I.; Milhem, M.M.; Minor, D.; Hamid, O.; Li, A.; Chen, L.; Chastain, M.; Gorski, K.S.; Anderson, A.; Chou, J.; et al. Talimogene Laherparepvec in Combination With Ipilimumab in Previously Untreated, Unresectable Stage IIIB-IV Melanoma. *J. Clin. Oncol.* **2016**, *34*, 2619–2626. [CrossRef] [PubMed]
135. Chesney, J.; Puzanov, I.; Collichio, F.; Singh, P.; Milhem, M.M.; Glaspy, J.; Hamid, O.; Ross, M.; Friedlander, P.; Garbe, C.; et al. Randomized, Open-Label Phase II Study Evaluating the Efficacy and Safety of Talimogene Laherparepvec in Combination With Ipilimumab Versus Ipilimumab Alone in Patients With Advanced, Unresectable Melanoma. *J. Clin. Oncol.* **2018**, *36*, 1658–1667. [CrossRef] [PubMed]
136. Scholz, M.; Yep, S.; Chancey, M.; Kelly, C.; Chau, K.; Turner, J.; Lam, R.; Drake, C.G. Phase I clinical trial of sipuleucel-T combined with escalating doses of ipilimumab in progressive metastatic castrate-resistant prostate cancer. *Immunotargets Ther.* **2017**, *6*, 11–16. [CrossRef] [PubMed]
137. Ku, J.; Wilenius, K.; Larsen, C.; De Guzman, K.; Yoshinaga, S.; Turner, J.S.; Lam, R.Y.; Scholz, M.C. Survival after sipuleucel-T (SIP-T) and low-dose ipilimumab (IPI) in men with metastatic, progressive, castrate-resistant prostate cancer (M-CRPC). *J. Clin. Oncol.* **2018**, *36*, 368. [CrossRef]
138. Singh, H.; Madan, R.A.; Dahut, W.L.; O'Sullivan Coyne, G.H.; Rauckhorst, M.; McMahon, S.; Heery, C.R.; Schlom, J.; Gulley, J.L. Combining active immunotherapy and immune checkpoint inhibitors in prostate cancer. *J. Clin. Oncol.* **2015**, *33*, e14008. [CrossRef]
139. Jochems, C.; Tucker, J.A.; Tsang, K.-Y.; Madan, R.A.; Dahut, W.L.; Liewehr, D.J.; Steinberg, S.M.; Gulley, J.L.; Schlom, J. A combination trial of vaccine plus ipilimumab in metastatic castration-resistant prostate cancer patients: Immune correlates. *Cancer Immunol. Immunother.* **2014**, *63*, 407–418. [CrossRef]
140. Long, G.V.; Dummer, R.; Ribas, A.; Puzanov, I.; Michielin, O.; VanderWalde, A.; Andtbacka, R.H.; Cebon, J.; Fernandez, E.; Malvehy, J.; et al. A Phase I/III, multicenter, open-label trial of talimogene laherparepvec (T-VEC) in combination with pembrolizumab for the treatment of unresected, stage IIIb-IV melanoma (MASTERKEY-265). *J. Immuno. Ther. Cancer* **2015**, *3*, P181. [CrossRef]
141. Ribas, A.; Dummer, R.; Puzanov, I.; VanderWalde, A.; Andtbacka, R.H.I.; Michielin, O.; Olszanski, A.J.; Malvehy, J.; Cebon, J.; Fernandez, E.; et al. Oncolytic Virotherapy Promotes Intratumoral T Cell Infiltration and Improves Anti-PD-1 Immunotherapy. *Cell* **2017**, *170*, 1109–1119.e10. [CrossRef]
142. Weber, J.S.; Kudchadkar, R.R.; Yu, B.; Gallenstein, D.; Horak, C.E.; Inzunza, H.D.; Zhao, X.; Martinez, A.J.; Wang, W.; Gibney, G.; et al. Safety, efficacy, and biomarkers of nivolumab with vaccine in ipilimumab-refractory or -naive melanoma. *J. Clin. Oncol.* **2013**, *31*, 4311–4318. [CrossRef]

143. Gibney, G.T.; Kudchadkar, R.R.; DeConti, R.C.; Thebeau, M.S.; Czupryn, M.P.; Tetteh, L.; Eysmans, C.; Richards, A.; Schell, M.J.; Fisher, K.J.; et al. Safety, correlative markers, and clinical results of adjuvant nivolumab in combination with vaccine in resected high-risk metastatic melanoma. *Clin. Cancer Res.* **2015**, *21*, 712–720. [CrossRef]
144. Ribas, A.; Medina, T.; Kummar, S.; Amin, A.; Kalbasi, A.; Drabick, J.J.; Barve, M.; Daniels, G.A.; Wong, D.J.; Schmidt, E.V.; et al. SD-101 in Combination with Pembrolizumab in Advanced Melanoma: Results of a Phase Ib, Multicenter Study. *Cancer Discov.* **2018**, *8*, 1250–1257. [CrossRef] [PubMed]
145. Chatani, P.D.; Yang, J.C. Mutated RAS: Targeting the "Untargetable" with T-cells. *Clin. Cancer Res.* **2019**. [CrossRef] [PubMed]
146. Gopalakrishnan, V.; Spencer, C.N.; Nezi, L.; Reuben, A.; Andrews, M.C.; Karpinets, T.V.; Prieto, P.A.; Vicente, D.; Hoffman, K.; Wei, S.C.; et al. Gut microbiome modulates response to anti-PD-1 immunotherapy in melanoma patients. *Science* **2018**, *359*, 97–103. [CrossRef] [PubMed]
147. Chaput, N.; Lepage, P.; Coutzac, C.; Soularue, E.; Le Roux, K.; Monot, C.; Boselli, L.; Routier, E.; Cassard, L.; Collins, M.; et al. Baseline gut microbiota predicts clinical response and colitis in metastatic melanoma patients treated with ipilimumab. *Ann. Oncol.* **2017**, *28*, 1368–1379. [CrossRef]
148. Routy, B.; Chatelier, E.L.; Derosa, L.; Duong, C.P.M.; Alou, M.T.; Daillère, R.; Fluckiger, A.; Messaoudene, M.; Rauber, C.; Roberti, M.P.; et al. Gut microbiome influences efficacy of PD-1-based immunotherapy against epithelial tumors. *Science* **2018**, *359*, 91–97. [CrossRef]
149. Matson, V.; Fessler, J.; Bao, R.; Chongsuwat, T.; Zha, Y.; Alegre, M.-L.; Luke, J.J.; Gajewski, T.F. The commensal microbiome is associated with anti-PD-1 efficacy in metastatic melanoma patients. *Science* **2018**, *359*, 104–108. [CrossRef]
150. Routy, B.; Gopalakrishnan, V.; Daillère, R.; Zitvogel, L.; Wargo, J.A.; Kroemer, G. The gut microbiota influences anticancer immunosurveillance and general health. *Nat. Rev. Clin. Oncol.* **2018**, *15*, 382–396. [CrossRef]
151. Bertrand, F.; Montfort, A.; Marcheteau, E.; Imbert, C.; Gilhodes, J.; Filleron, T.; Rochaix, P.; Andrieu-Abadie, N.; Levade, T.; Meyer, N.; et al. TNFα blockade overcomes resistance to anti-PD-1 in experimental melanoma. *Nat. Commun.* **2017**, *8*, 2256. [CrossRef] [PubMed]
152. Perez-Ruiz, E.; Minute, L.; Otano, I.; Alvarez, M.; Ochoa, M.C.; Belsue, V.; de Andrea, C.; Rodriguez-Ruiz, M.E.; Perez-Gracia, J.L.; Marquez-Rodas, I.; et al. Prophylactic TNF blockade uncouples efficacy and toxicity in dual CTLA-4 and PD-1 immunotherapy. *Nature* **2019**, *569*, 428–432. [CrossRef]
153. Mariathasan, S.; Turley, S.J.; Nickles, D.; Castiglioni, A.; Yuen, K.; Wang, Y.; Kadel, E.E., III; Koeppen, H.; Astarita, J.L.; Cubas, R.; et al. TGFβ attenuates tumour response to PD-L1 blockade by contributing to exclusion of T cells. *Nature* **2018**, *554*, 544–548. [CrossRef]
154. Tauriello, D.V.F.; Palomo-Ponce, S.; Stork, D.; Berenguer-Llergo, A.; Badia-Ramentol, J.; Iglesias, M.; Sevillano, M.; Ibiza, S.; Cañellas, A.; Hernando-Momblona, X.; et al. TGFβ drives immune evasion in genetically reconstituted colon cancer metastasis. *Nature* **2018**, *554*, 538–543. [CrossRef] [PubMed]

11

Targeting the NPL4 Adaptor of p97/VCP Segregase by Disulfiram as an Emerging Cancer Vulnerability Evokes Replication Stress and DNA Damage while Silencing the ATR Pathway

Dusana Majera [1,†], Zdenek Skrott [1,†], Katarina Chroma [1], Joanna Maria Merchut-Maya [2], Martin Mistrik [1,*] and Jiri Bartek [1,2,3,*]

1 Laboratory of Genome Integrity, Institute of Molecular and Translational Medicine, Faculty of Medicine and Dentistry, Palacky University, 77 147 Olomouc, Czech Republic; dusana.majera@upol.cz (D.M.); zdenek.skrott@upol.cz (Z.S.); katarina.chroma@upol.cz (K.C.)

2 Danish Cancer Society Research Center, 2100 Copenhagen, Denmark; jomema@cancer.dk

3 Division of Genome Biology, Department of Medical Biochemistry and Biophysics, Science for Life Laboratory, Karolinska Institute, 171 77 Stockholm, Sweden

* Correspondence: martin.mistrik@upol.cz (M.M.); jb@cancer.dk (J.B.)

† These authors contributed equally to this work.

Abstract: Research on repurposing the old alcohol-aversion drug disulfiram (DSF) for cancer treatment has identified inhibition of NPL4, an adaptor of the p97/VCP segregase essential for turnover of proteins involved in multiple pathways, as an unsuspected cancer cell vulnerability. While we reported that NPL4 is targeted by the anticancer metabolite of DSF, the bis-diethyldithiocarbamate-copper complex (CuET), the exact, apparently multifaceted mechanism(s) through which the CuET-induced aggregation of NPL4 kills cancer cells remains to be fully elucidated. Given the pronounced sensitivity to CuET in tumor cell lines lacking the genome integrity caretaker proteins BRCA1 and BRCA2, here we investigated the impact of NPL4 targeting by CuET on DNA replication dynamics and DNA damage response pathways in human cancer cell models. Our results show that CuET treatment interferes with DNA replication, slows down replication fork progression and causes accumulation of single-stranded DNA (ssDNA). Such a replication stress (RS) scenario is associated with DNA damage, preferentially in the S phase, and activates the homologous recombination (HR) DNA repair pathway. At the same time, we find that cellular responses to the CuET-triggered RS are seriously impaired due to concomitant malfunction of the ATRIP-ATR-CHK1 signaling pathway that reflects an unorthodox checkpoint silencing mode through ATR (Ataxia telangiectasia and Rad3 related) kinase sequestration within the CuET-evoked NPL4 protein aggregates.

Keywords: targeted cancer therapy; disulfiram; NPL4; replication stress; DNA damage; BRCA1; BRCA2; ATR pathway

---

1. Introduction

Recent advances in understanding of the altered wiring of cancer cell regulatory pathways, and hence vulnerabilities and dependencies of tumor cells have led to discoveries of new molecular targets potentially exploitable in cancer therapy. As the development of a new drug is time-consuming, very expensive, and prone to frequent failure, drug repurposing as a possible alternative approach to cancer treatment is currently undergoing serious consideration [1]. One of the candidate drugs for repurposing in oncology is disulfiram (tetraethylthiuram disulfide, DSF, commercially known as Antabuse), a cheap and well-tolerated generic drug that has been used for decades to treat alcohol dependency. DSF has shown anticancer activity in preclinical models, and multiple clinical trials to treat various types of human malignancies by DSF are currently underway [2]. We have recently published that DSF is metabolized in vivo into the bis-diethyldithiocarbamate-copper complex (CuET), in a process that requires copper ions, and demonstrated that CuET represents the ultimate anticancer metabolite of DSF in-vivo [3]. Furthermore, our nationwide epidemiological study in Denmark yielded results consistent with the emerging anticancer effects of DSF, documenting a lower risk of death from cancer in those cancer patients who were treated by DSF after their cancer diagnosis [3]. Mechanistically, we reported that CuET causes aggregation and thereby immobilization and dysfunction of NPL4, an essential cofactor of the p97/VCP segregase. This otherwise highly mobile protein complex is involved in the regulation of protein turnover upstream of the proteasome, with important roles in a wide range of cellular processes including fundamental pro-survival stress-tolerance pathways [3].

In a follow-up study devoted to target validation and further mechanistic insights into CuET effects [4], we explored the reported exceptional sensitivity to DSF of human cancer cell lines defective in BRCA1 or BRCA2 tumor suppressors, key components of the genome integrity maintenance machinery [4,5]. We found that CuET spontaneously forms from DSF and available copper ions also in cell culture media, and our experiments confirmed NPL4 as the molecular target while excluding the proposed inhibition of aldehyde dehydrogenase (ALDH) [5] and accumulation of toxic acetaldehydes causing DNA-protein and DNA interstrand cross-links [6], as the potential mechanistic explanation for the reported sensitivity of BRCA-defective tumors [4]. In addition to ALDH, we also excluded the proteasome, another previously suggested candidate target of DSF's anticancer effects, as a valid target. Indeed, we showed that the observed 'proteasome-inhibition-like features' triggered by DSF/CuET turned out to be fully attributable to the disabled NPL4 acting upstream of the proteasome [3]. Collectively, these mechanistic studies identified and validated NPL4 as the genuine, and possibly the only or dominant direct molecular target of DSF/CuET responsible for the widely appreciated tumor-inhibitory effects of DSF [3,4]. Indeed, the available evidence in the field now points to CuET-induced aggregation of NPL4 as the key anticancer mechanism of DSF under both in vitro and in vivo conditions, and a promising cancer vulnerability.

Relevant to the present study and the sensitivity of the BRCA-defective cancers to DSF/CuET, we and others previously discovered enhanced replication stress and endogenous DNA damage as a candidate hallmark of cancer [7–10], thereby pioneering the concept of the ATM-Chk2- and ATR-Chk1-mediated DNA damage response (DDR) checkpoints as important cell-intrinsic barriers against oncogene activation and tumor progression [10–12]. Currently, replication stress is recognized to play a prominent role in driving genomic instability and tumorigenesis, while further drug-mediated enhancement of replication stress or inhibition of replication stress-tolerance pathways such as ATR-Chk1 signaling may provide additional targetable vulnerabilities of cancer [13,14]. The main mechanistic consequence of replication stress is the accumulation of ssDNA and stalling of replication forks [15]. The ssDNA stretches become rapidly coated with replication protein A (RPA), thereby facilitating activation of the ATR-Chk1 signaling module and subsequent phosphorylation of hundreds of cellular proteins as substrates of ATR and Chk1 kinases [15,16]. These phosphorylation cascades also involve BRCA1 and BRCA2 and help to stabilize the stalled forks, thereby preventing fork collapse, while in parallel limiting the cellular entry into mitosis by activation of the S-M checkpoint [17]. Under inhibition or genetic deficiency of ATR, stalled replication forks tend to collapse, leading to a generation of DNA double-strand breaks (DSBs), which, if unrepaired or misrepaired, can cause chromosomal instability, severe pathologies or cell death [14,18].

With the above-mentioned knowledge as the starting point, here we examined potential mechanistic links between cancer-associated replication stress, DNA damage checkpoint signaling and the functional impact of DSF/CuET treatment on DNA replication and genome integrity maintenance, searching for possible explanations of the overall sensitivity of tumor cells, and the observed preferential sensitivity of cancer cells lacking BRCA1 and BRCA2, to treatment with DSF/CuET.

2. Materials and Methods

2.1. Cell Culture

Human non-small cell lung carcinoma H1299 cells expressing a doxycycline (DOX)-inducible BRCA1 and BRCA2 shRNAs, U2OS, MDA-MB-231, MDA-MB-436, U2OS cells expressing NPL4-GFP, U2OS expressing DOX-inducible MUT-NPL4-GFP [3] and U2OS cells expressing ATR-GFP [19] were cultured and maintained in DMEM (Dulbecco's Modified Eagle Medium, Lonza, Basel, Switzerland), supplemented with 10% fetal bovine serum (Thermo Fisher Scientific, Waltham, MA, USA) and 1% penicillin/streptomycin (Sigma-Aldrich, St. Louis, MO, USA). CAPAN-1 cells were grown in DMEM medium, supplemented with 20% fetal bovine serum and 1% penicillin/streptomycin. H1299 expressing a DOX-inducible BRCA1 and BRCA2 shRNA were kindly provided [5]. For efficient BRCA1 and BRCA2 knockdown cells were cultivated in the presence of 2 μg/mL DOX for at least three days.

2.2. Immunoblotting

Equal amounts of cell lysates were separated by SDS-PAGE on hand casted gels and then transferred onto the nitrocellulose membrane. The membrane was blocked in Tris-buffered saline containing 5% milk and 0.1% Tween 20 for 1 h at room temperature and then incubated 1 h at room temperature with primary antibodies, followed by detection with secondary antibodies. Secondary antibodies were visualized by ELC detection reagent (Thermo Fisher Scientific, Waltham, MA, USA).

2.3. Immunofluorescence

Cells were seeded on plastic inserts in 12-well dishes. The next day, cells were treated with compounds at indicated concentrations and subsequently either pre-extracted (0.1% Triton X 100 in Phosphate-Buffered Saline(PBS) for 2 min or fixed with formaldehyde for 15 min at room temperature, washed with PBS and permeabilized with 0.5% Triton X-100 in PBS for 5 min. After PBS washes, the cells on the plastic inserts were immunostained with primary antibody for 1 h at room temperature, followed by PBS washes and staining with fluorescently-conjugated secondary antibody for 60 min at room temperature. Nuclei were visualized by 4′,6-diamidino-2-phenylindole (DAPI, 1 μg/mL) staining at room temperature for 2 min. For NPL4 staining, the cells were pre-extracted (0.1% Triton X 100 in PBS, for 2 min) and fixed with −20 °C methanol for 15 min at room temperature, washed with PBS and permeabilized with 0.5% Triton X-100 in PBS for 5 min. After PBS washes, the cells on the plastic inserts were immunostained with primary antibody for 120 min at room temperature, followed by PBS washes and staining with fluorescently-conjugated secondary antibody for 60 min at room temperature. Dried plastic inserts with cells were mounted using Vectashield mounting medium (Vector Laboratories, Burlingame, CA, USA), and images were acquired using the Zeiss Axioimager Z.1 platform.

2.4. Ethynyldeoxyuridine (EdU) and Bromodeoxyuridine (BrdU) Incorporation and Detection

To detect active DNA replication, cells were incubated with 10 μM EdU (Life Technologies, Carlsbad, CA, USA) for 30 min, fixed, permeabilized and stained using Click-iT reaction (100 mM Tris pH 8.5, 1 mM copper sulfate, 100 μM ascorbic acid, 1 μM azide Alexa fluor 488 (Life Technologies, Carlsbad, CA, USA) for 30 min at room temperature. To detect ssDNA, cells were incubated with 10 μM BrdU (Sigma) for 24 h, then BrdU was washed out, and cells were incubated with the tested compounds as indicated. After pre-extraction and fixation in buffered formol, the incorporated BrdU was detected by an anti-BrdU antibody (BD Biosciences, San Jose, CA, USA) without denaturation.

2.5. Image Quantification

Images were acquired using the Olympus IX81 fluorescence microscope and ScanR Acquisition software. The scans were quantified in automated image and data analysis software ScanR Analysis.

The data was further analyzed in the STATISTICA 13 software tool (Dell Software, Round Rock, TX, USA).

2.6. DNA Combing

H1299 cells were treated with 125 nM CuET for 5 h and subsequently pulsed with 5-Iodo-2′-deoxyuridine (IdU, 20 μM) for 30 min, washed and pulsed with 5-Chloro-2′-deoxyuridine (CIdU, 200 μM) for additional 30 min. DNA replication was stopped by ice-cold PBS. Cells were collected and embedded in 0,5% insert agarose plugs. The plugs were incubated for 32 h in buffer containing proteinase K at 50 °C. Plugs were then washed with TE buffer and melted at 68 °C. The obtained solution was further digested overnight with Agarase I at 42 °C. The next day, the concentration of DNA was measured on nanodrop and combed on silanized cover glasses (Matsunami, Japan) with a speed of 0,3 mm/s. The cover glasses with combed DNA were baked at 60 °C, dehydrated with 70%, 90%, and 100% ethanol series for 3 min each. DNA was denatured at 75 °C in 2xSSC, 50% formamide for 2 min. Next, the cover glasses were dehydrated with a 70%, 90% and 100% ice-cold ethanol series for 5 min each, air dried, blocked using 1% BSA in PBS-Tween for 1 h at 37 °C and subsequently incubated with primary antibodies, mouse anti-BrdU for IdU detection (1:5) and rat anti-BrdU for CIdU detection (1:25) for 1 h at 37 °C. After several washes with PBS-Tween, cover glasses were incubated with secondary antibodies goat anti-mouse A488 (1:100) and goat anti-rat A549 (1:100) for 30 min at 37 °C. After several washes with PBS-Tween, cover glasses were air-dried, mounted, and images of DNA fibers were acquired using the Zeiss Axioimager Z.1 platform.

2.7. Estimation of DNA Replication Origin Density

After the treatment by tested compounds, cells were pulsed with EdU (10 μM) for 20 min, then harvested and resuspended in cold PBS (1 million of cells per 1 mL). 2 μL of cell suspension was applied on glass slides (Superfrost Plus, Thermo Fisher) and allowed to partially evaporate for 5 min, then mixed with a lysis buffer (50 mM EDTA and 0.5% SDS in 200 mM Tris-HCl, pH 7.5) and incubated for 2 min. Slides were tilted to 15° to allow the spreading of fibers. After drying, the samples were fixed in methanol/acetic acid solution for 15 min and thoroughly washed. EdU was detected by click reaction using Alexafluor 488 azide. The signal was further enhanced by anti-Alexa fluor 488 antibody (A-11094, Thermo Fisher) and secondary antibody. DNA was visualized by YOYO-1 (Molecular Probes) staining (1 μM for 20 min). Fiber images were acquired using the Zeiss Axioimager Z.1 platform, and the number of DNA replication origins was calculated on single well-stretched DNA fibers. A conversion factor of 2.59 kb/μm was used in calculations [20].

2.8. Cell Fractionation for Triton X Insoluble Pellets

Cells were treated as indicated, washed in cold PBS and lysed in lysis buffer (50 mM Tris-HCl, pH 7.5, 150 mM NaCl, 2 mM MgCl2, 10% glycerol, 0.5% Triton-X100, protease inhibitor cocktail by Roche) for 2 min, under gentle agitation at 4 °C. Then, cells were scraped to Eppendorf tubes and kept for another 10 min on ice with vortex steps. Next, the lysate was centrifuged at 20,000× *g* for 10 min at 4 °C. Insoluble fraction and supernatant were re-suspended in Laemmli Sample Buffer (1X final concentration; 10% glycerol, 60 mM Tris-HCl, pH 6.8, 2% SDS, 0.01% bromophenol blue, 50 mM dithiothreitol).

2.9. Laser Micro-Irradiation

U2OS cells stably expressing GFP-ATR were seeded into 24-well plates with a glass-bottom (Cellvis) 24 h before laser micro-irradiation in a density of 6 × 105 cells/mL. After seeding the cells into the 24 well plates, the specimen was first placed on an equilibrated bench for 20 min at room temperature (RT) to ensure equal cell distribution and then placed into an incubator. CuET was added to cells 5 h before micro-irradiation in final concentrations of 250 nM and 500 nM. Twenty minutes before laser micro-irradiation, cells were pre-sensitized towards UV-A wavelength by 20 μM 8-Methoxypsoralen

(8-MOP) and placed inside Zeiss Axioimager Z.1 inverted microscope combined with the LSM 780 confocal module. Laser micro-irradiation was performed at 37 °C via X 40 water immersion objective (Zeiss C-Apo 403/1.2WDICIII), using a 355 nm 65 mW laser set on 100% power to induce the DNA damage. The total laser dose that can be further manipulated by the number of irradiation cycles was empirically set to two irradiation cycles. Subsequent immunofluorescence detection and quantitative analysis of the striation pattern in photo-manipulated samples were essentially performed as described previously [21].

2.10. Antibodies and Chemicals

The following antibodies were used for immunoblotting: BRCA1 antibody (Santa Cruz Biotechnology, Dallas, TX, USA, D-9), rabbit polyclonal antibody against BRCA2 (Bethyl, Montgomery, TX, USA, A300-005A) antibody and mouse monoclonal antibody against β-actin (Santa Cruz Biotechnology, C4), lamin B (Santa Cruz Biotechnology, sc-6217), α-Tubulin (Santa Cruz Biotechnology, sc-5286), anti-ubiquitin lys48-specific (Merck Millipore, Burlington, MA, USA, clone Apu2) Chk1 (Santa Cruz, Biotechnology, sc-8404), phospho-Chk1 S317 (Cell Signalling, Danvers, MA, USA, 2344), phospho-Chk1 S345 (Cell Signalling, 2348), RPA (Abcam, ab16855, Cambridge, UK), phospho-RPA S33 (Bethyl, A300-246A), ATR (Santa Cruz Biotechnology, N-19). For immunofluorescence were used the following antibodies: γH2AX (Merck Millipore, 05-636), cyclin A (Santa Cruz Biotechnology, H-3, Santa Cruz Biotechnology, sc-239), RPA (Abcam, ab16855), Rad51 (Abcam, ab63801), NPL4 (Santa Cruz Biotechnology, D-1), p97 (Abcam, ab11433), ATR (Santa Cruz Biotechnology, N-19). For DNA combing assay following antibodies were used: anti-BrdU (BD Biosciences, Franklin Lakes, NJ, USA, BD 347580) and rat anti-BrdU (Abcam ab6323).

Chemicals used in this study were as follows: CuET (bis-diethyldithiocarbamate-copper complex, TCI chemicals), disulfiram (Sigma, St. Louis, MO, USA), bortezomib (Velcade, Janssen-Cilag International N.V.), bathocuproinedisulfonic acid (Sigma, St. Louis, MO, USA), CB-5083 (Selleckchem, Houston, TX, USA), hydroxyurea (Sigma, St. Louis, MO, USA), AZD6738 (AstraZeneca, London, UK).

2.11. Field Inversion Gel Electrophoresis (FIGE)

Treated cells, as indicated in the main text, were trypsinized and melted into 1.0% InCert-Agarose inserts. Subsequently, agarose inserts were digested in a mixture of 10 mM Tris-HCl pH 7.5, 50 mM EDTA, 1% N-laurylsarcosyl, and proteinase K (2 mg/mL) at 50 °C for 24 hr and washed five times in Tris-EDTA (TE buffer, 10 mM Tris-HCl pH 8.0, 100 mM EDTA). The inserts were loaded onto a separation gel 1.0% agarose mixed with GelRed® solution (10,000x). Run conditions for the DNA fragments separation were: 110 V, 7.5 V/cm, 16 h, forward pulse 11 s, reverse pulse 5 s in 1X Tris-acetic acid-EDTA (TAE buffer 40 mM Tris, 20 mM acetic acid, 1 mM EDTA).

2.12. Alkaline Comet Assay

The alkaline comet assay was performed essentially as described in [22]. Briefly, CAPAN-1 and MDA-MB-436 cells were treated with 250 nM CuET or 2 mM hydroxyurea (HU) for 5 h, collected and resuspended in PBS (7500 cells/μL). Cells (75000) were then mixed with 37 °C low melting point agarose (Lonza, Basel, Switzerland), spotted on the normal melting point agarose (Invitrogen, Waltham, MA, USA) pre-coated slides and left to sit for 10 min at 4 °C. Slides were then immersed in the cold alkaline lysis buffer for 2 h at 4 °C. Slides were washed three times with the cold alkaline electrophoresis buffer and electrophoresis was performed (25 min, 4 °C, 0.6 V/cm). Slides were then washed with cold PBS and ddH_2O, dehydrated in cold graded ethanol, air-dried and stored at room temperature. For staining, slides were rehydrated with ddH_2O, stained with Sybr Gold (1:4000 in TE buffer; Thermo

Fisher Scientific, Waltham, MA, USA), washed with PBS and mounted with Mowiol (Sigma-Aldrich, St. Louis, MO, USA). Images were acquired using a fluorescent microscope (Carl Zeiss, Oberkochen, Germany), a 20x air immersion objective (Carl Zeiss, Oberkochen, Germany) and Comet Assay IV software (Perceptive Instruments, Haverhill, UK). Presented results are from the technical duplicate. Alkaline lysis buffer: 1.2 M NaCl, 100 mM Na_2EDTA, 0.1% sodium lauryl sarcosinate, 0.26 M NaOH (pH > 13, 4 °C, prepared fresh); alkaline electrophoresis buffer: 0.03 M NaOH, 2 mM Na_2EDTA (pH 12.3, 4 °C).

3. Results

3.1. CuET Causes DNA Damage Preferentially Detectable in S/G2-Phase Cells

To initiate our current study, we first wished to assess the impact of CuET on DNA damage in cultured human cancer cells, including isogenic cell pairs with experimentally altered components of the DDR machinery. To this end, we employed the established H1299 lung cancer model allowing for DOX-inducible shRNA-mediated depletion of BRCA1 or BRCA2 [4,5]. Indeed, treatment of these cell lines with CuET resulted in an increased formation of γH2AX foci as well as enhanced overall γH2AX signal intensity, established surrogate markers for chromatin response to DSBs and overall DNA damage signaling by the upstream DDR kinases, respectively (Figure 1A,B; Supplementary Figure S1A,B). Notably, the CuET-evoked increase of γH2AX was more pronounced in the BRCA1- and BRCA2-depleted cells compared with their BRCA-proficient counterpart H1299 cells (unexposed to DOX) (Figure 1A,B; Supplementary Figure S1B). To clarify whether such DNA damage could also be caused by DSF itself, we treated the BRCA2-depleted H1299 cells with DSF in cell culture settings where the cells were first pre-treated by the copper chelator bathocuproinedisulfonic acid (BCDS), a manipulation that we previously reported prevents the otherwise spontaneous and rapid formation of CuET from DSF and copper in cell culture media [4]. As expected, when used alone, DSF caused a similar increase in DNA damage formation as CuET, however when DSF was combined with the copper chelator BCDS pre-treatment step, the γH2AX-inducing effect of DSF was completely abrogated (Figure 1E). These results showed that the DNA damage observed after the treatment with DSF depends on the copper-dependent spontaneous formation of CuET in the culture media, thereby establishing that analogous to the anticancer effects, the active DNA damage-inducing compound is the CuET metabolite, rather than DSF itself.

Next, we pursued our observation that the increase of γH2AX was apparent only in a subset of cells in a given exponentially growing cell population, suggesting that the DNA damage could be cell cycle-dependent. To examine this possibility, we again treated the above mentioned H1299 cells with CuET, yet in the subsequent immunofluorescence analysis, we double stained the cells for γH2AX and cyclin A, an approach commonly used to distinguish cells in G1 phase (cyclin A negative) from those in S/G2 phases (cyclin A positive). Notably, the CuET-induced γH2AX was preferentially seen in cyclin A positive cells, and this cell-cycle effect was even more pronounced in the BRCA1- and BRCA2-depleted cells (Figure 1C,D, Supplementary Figure S1C). The preference of elevated γH2AX intensity in cyclin A positive cells was also confirmed in additional human cancer cell lines (Supplementary Figure S1D,E), thereby excluding a possibility that such genotoxic effects of CuET could be restricted to the H1299 cell model.

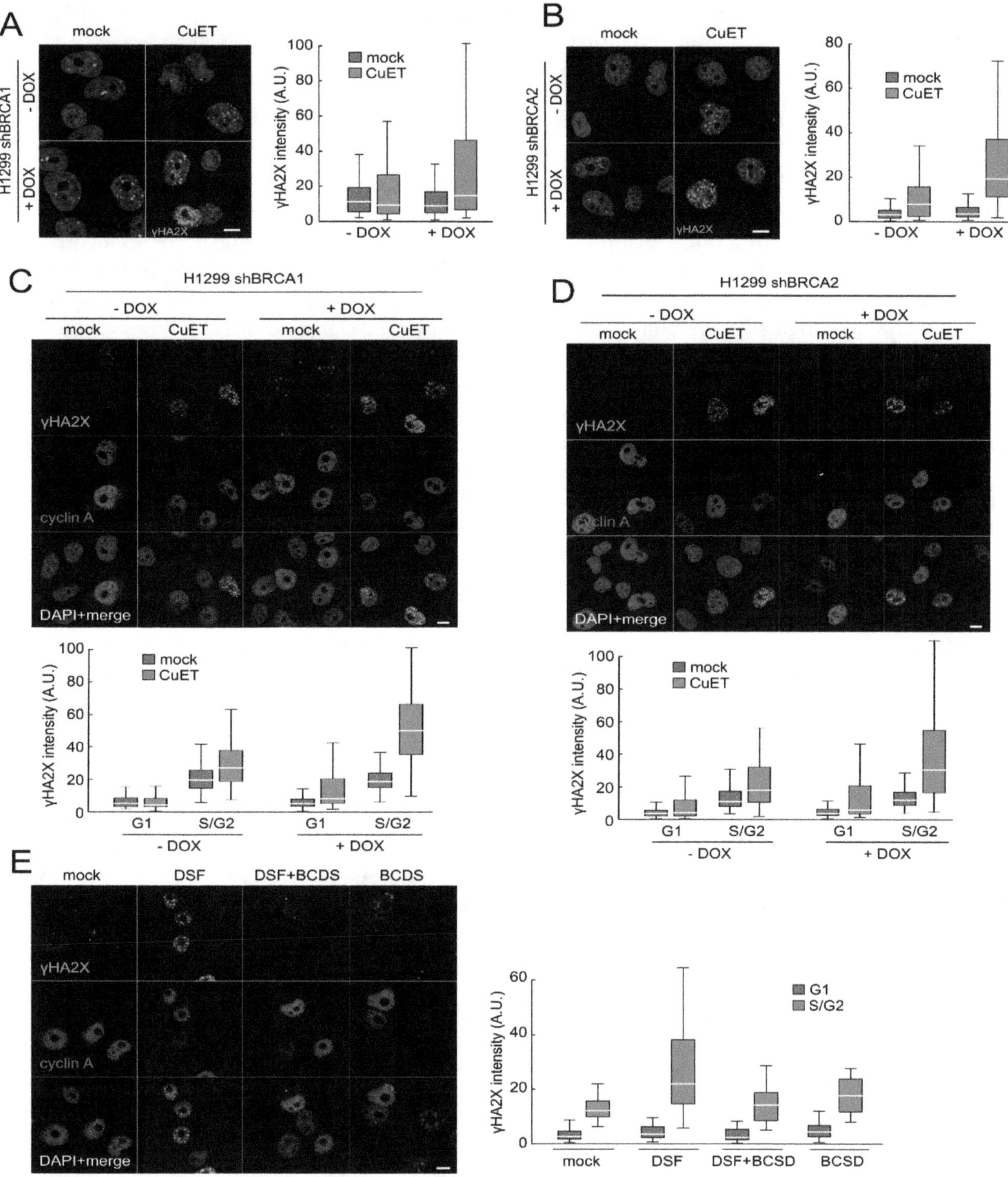

Figure 1. Disulfiram's metabolite bis-diethyldithiocarbamate-copper complex (CuET) causes DNA damage preferentially in S/G2 cells deficient for BRCA1 or BRCA2 proteins. H1299 cells expressing (doxycycline-) DOX-inducible shBRCA1 (**A**) or shBRCA2 (**B**) were cultivated for at least three days in DOX-containing media and then treated with CuET (250 nM) for 5 h, and γH2AX intensity was analyzed by quantitative microscopy. (**C**) H1229 shBRCA1 cells or (**D**) H1299 shBRCA2 cells were treated as in (A) a γH2AX intensity was quantified with respect to cyclin A positivity defining S/G2 phase. (**E**) H1229 shBRCA2 cells pre-incubated with DOX were treated with disulfram (DSF) (500 nM), bathocuproinedisulfonic acid (BCDS) (50 μM), or their combination for 5 h and γH2AX intensity was quantified. Box plot represents 25–75 quartiles, median, and whiskers non-outlier range. Scale bars = 10 μm.

Overall, we conclude from these results that the DNA damage-inducing effects of DSF are attributable to its CuET metabolite, include both elevated γH2AX foci formation and overall γH2AX signal intensity, and occur preferentially in cells traversing S/G2 phases.

3.2. CuET Treatment Decreases DNA Replication Fork Velocity and Increases the Number of Active Replication Origins

Since the CuET-induced DNA damage was more apparent in S/G2 cells, we argued that CuET might preferentially interfere with DNA replication. To examine this possibility, we pre-treated H1299 cells with CuET, followed by a pulse-treatment with the thymine analog EdU that becomes incorporated into newly synthesized DNA, allowing visualization of the rate of ongoing DNA replication using fluorescence readouts. Using this approach, we could indeed confirm severe impairment of DNA replication in CuET treated cells, manifested as a decreased EdU signal in H1299 cells (Figure 2A) and also other cell lines, such as human breast cancer MDA-MB-231 and osteosarcoma U2OS cells (Supplementary Figure S2A,B). DNA replication can be halted by the presence of DNA damage [23] and vice versa; replication interference can be the source of DNA damage [13,14]. To address what is the cause and consequence in this scenario, we performed a kinetic study showing that the decrease of EdU incorporation is an early event, preceding the γH2AX foci formation (Figure 2B). This result indicated that the observed DNA damage most likely results from the CuET-induced impairment of DNA replication. To gain more detailed insights into the observed replication interference phenomenon, we employed DNA combing as an assay enabling us to directly assess the effect of CuET on DNA replication fork velocity. H1299 cells were first pre-treated with a rather low concentration of CuET and then pulsed with IdU and CIdU thymine analogs to detect actively replicating DNA, the length of which can be evaluated by fluorescence microscopy-based measurements [24]. Our analysis of the obtained DNA fibers revealed a robust reduction of DNA replication fork velocity after CuET treatment (Figure 2C). Since such decreased DNA replication fork speed is known to trigger firing of dormant replication origins, we next tested the density of active origins using an established DNA fiber assay [22,25]. We quantified the number of origins per 1 Mb of DNA. Indeed, CuET treatment increased the number of active origins compared to untreated cells, similarly to treatment with the ATR kinase inhibitor AZD6738 (Figure 2D), a known activator of latent replication origin firing used here as a positive control [26].

We interpret these results as documenting a previously unsuspected negative impact of CuET on DNA replication, slowing down the fork velocity and concurrently leading to the firing of more dormant origins.

3.3. CuET-Induced Replication Stress Leads to DNA Damage that Triggers Homologous Recombination Repair Pathway

As replication stress is associated with accumulation of ssDNA stretches detectable by RPA32 protein foci or by staining for DNA-incorporated BrdU under non-denaturating conditions [18,27,28], we next assessed these parameters in human cells treated with CuET. Consistent with the CuET-impaired replication forks (see above), we found enhanced RPA32 foci in several cancer cell lines treated with CuET (Figure 3A,B) and also detected incorporated BrdU under non-denaturing conditions (Figure 3C,D). These data suggest that in CuET-treated cells, DNA helicase becomes uncoupled from DNA polymerases, generating stretches of ssDNA in a manner broadly analogous with effects of the replication stress-inducing drugs such as hydroxyurea or aphidicolin [28]. The RPA-coated ssDNA is known to recruit and activate the ATRIP-ATR-CHK1 signaling pathway [29] to stabilize the stalled replication structures, thereby avoiding fork collapse and formation of DSBs [30]. Importantly, these DNA lesions typically require repair by the homologous recombination (HR) repair pathway that encompasses, among other factors, also BRCA1 and BRCA2, the latter being critical for loading of the Rad51 HR repair protein [31–33]. To test whether Rad51 is involved in the repair process of lesions caused by the CuET treatment, we stained the cells for Rad51 and searched for the typical

DNA-associated Rad51 foci that form within the DSB-flanking chromatin regions under ongoing DNA repair. Indeed, in multiple tested cell lines, the CuET treatment increased the number of Rad51 foci (Figure 3E,F) except for the BRCA2-depleted cells, which are principally incapable of loading Rad51 both after CuET treatment and gamma-irradiation (here used as a positive control) (Figure 3G). The presence of DNA breaks in CuET treated cells was confirmed also by direct physical methods including Field Inversion Gel Electrophoresis (FIGE, detecting largely DSBs) (Figure 3H, Supplementary Figure S3D) and comet assay (Supplementary 3A,B,C, detecting a mixture of single-stranded and double stranded DNA breaks) in BRCA-deficient human cell lines derived from carcinomas of the breast (MDA-MB-436), lung (the H1299 series) and pancreas (CAPAN1), the latter reported by us previously as very sensitive to CuET treatment [3].

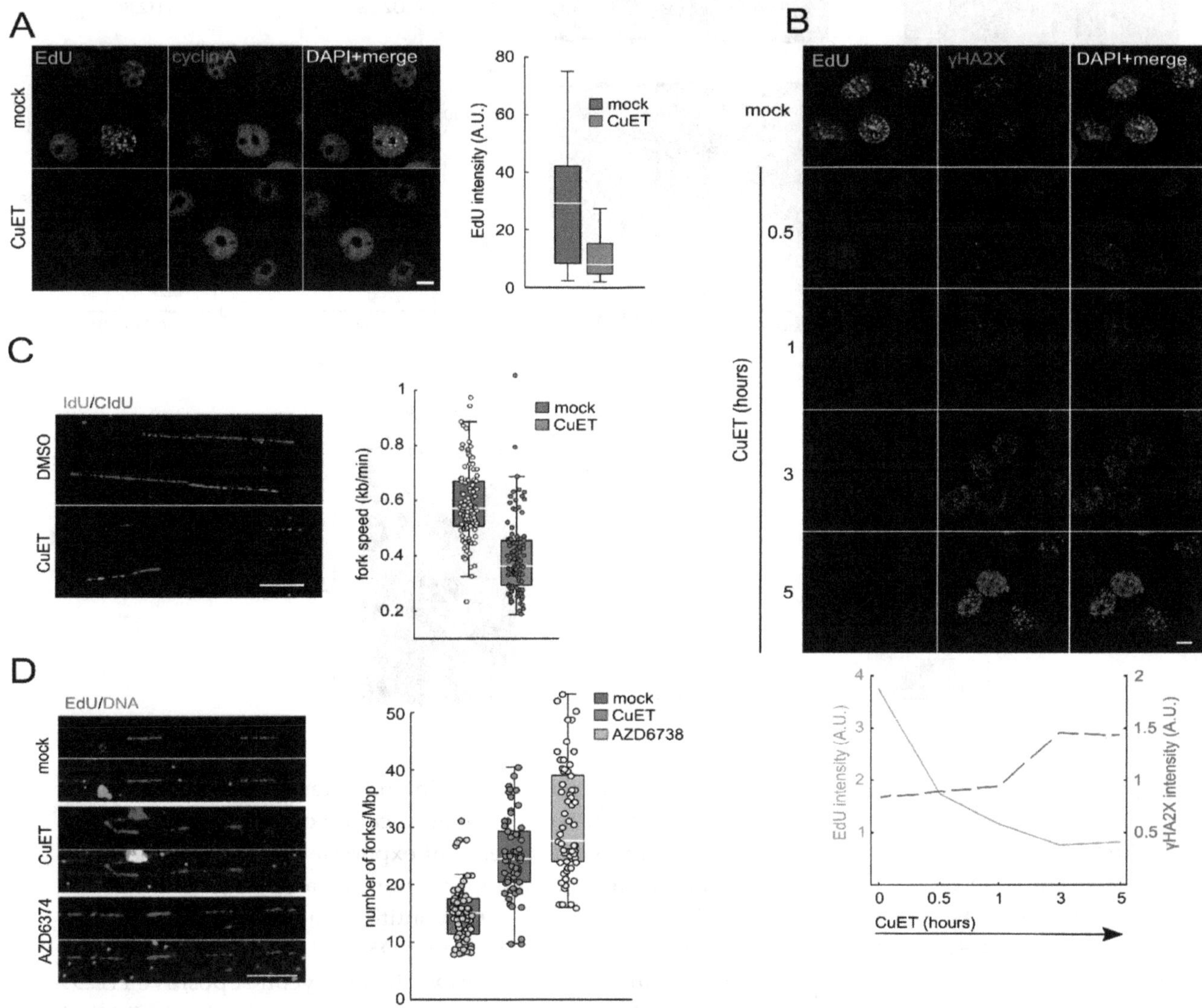

Figure 2. CuET impairs DNA replication. (**A**) H1299 cells were treated with CuET (250 nM) for 3 h, and ethynyldeoxyuridine (EdU) intensity was analyzed in cells positive for cyclin A. (**B**) H1299 cells were treated with CuET (250 nM) for different time points, and EdU and γH2AX intensities were quantified. (**C**) H1299 cells were treated with CuET (125 nM) for 5 h, then pulse-labeled with5-Iodo-2′-deoxyuridine (IdU) and 5-Chloro-2′-deoxyuridine (CIdU) and processed for DNA combing. (**D**) H1299 cells were treated with CuET (250 nM) or AZD6372 (10 μM) for 3 h and then pulsed with EdU and processed for DNA fiber assay. Box plot represents 25–75 quartiles, median, and whiskers non-outlier range. Scale bars = 10 μm.

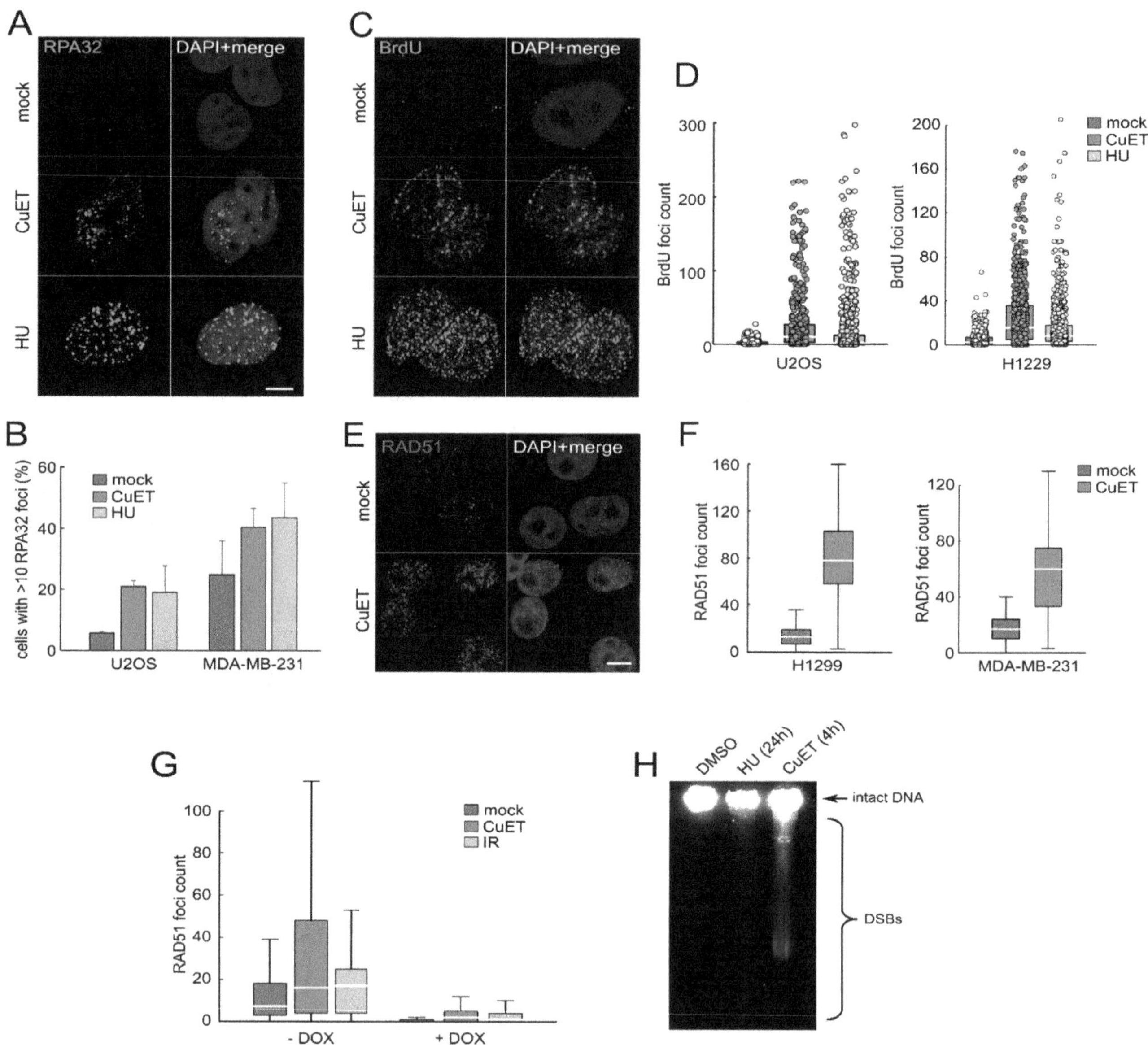

Figure 3. CuET induces replication stress. (**A**) RPA32 foci detection in pre-extracted U2OS cells treated with CuET (250 nM) or hydroxyurea (HU, 2 mM) for 5 h. (**B**) Quantification of cells with more than 10 RPA32 foci treated as in (A) (mean, SD from three independent experiments). (**C**) Formation of single-stranded DNA (ssDNA) visualized by BrdU detected under non-denaturating conditions in U2OS cells treated by CuET (250 nM) and HU (2 mM) for 5 h. (**D**) Quantification of bromodeoxyuridine (BrdU) foci in U2OS and H1299 cells treated as in C. (**E**) Detection of RAD51 foci in pre-extracted H1299 cells treated by CuET (250 nM) for 5 h. (**F**) Quantification of RAD51 foci in cyclin A positive H1299 and MDA-MB-231 cells treated by CuET (250 nM) for 5 h. (**G**) Quantification of Rad51 foci in BRCA2 proficient and deficient H1299 cells after 5-h treatment with 250 nM CuET or 4 Gray (Gy) irradiation. (**H**) FIGE analysis of DSBs in H1299 cells exposed to CuET or HU.Box plot represents 25–75 quartiles, median, and whiskers non-outlier range. Scale bars = 10 μm.

Collectively, these results are consistent with CuET inducing replication stress-associated DNA damage that requires HR repair, including Rad51, a process that is defective in the absence of BRCA1 and BRCA2. Consequently, such DNA damage cannot be properly processed in cells lacking the BRCA factors, which explains the higher amount of DNA damage that contributes to the preferential sensitivity of BRCA-deficient cells to DSF [5] and CuET [4].

3.4. The ATR Signaling Pathway is Compromised in CuET-Treated Cells

In the context of the results obtained so far, we were intrigued by the fact that CuET treatment resulted in DNA breaks relatively quickly within 3–4 h. However, stalled or slowed replication forks should be rather stable for many more hours before turning into DSBs as reported in the U2OS cell line after HU treatment [31] (see also Supplementary Figure S3D). As the prominent role in the stabilization and protection of the stalled forks reflects the function of the RPA-ATRIP-ATR-Chk1 signaling pathway [29,30], we performed immunoblot analysis of extracts from various cell lines treated with CuET, to assess the status of the ATR signaling. In contrast to HU treatment which was used as a positive control, the RPA-ATRIP-ATR-Chk1 signaling pathway was not activated in response to CuET, as manifested by the absence of the ATR-mediated phosphorylations of the effector kinase Chk1: Chk1 S317 and Chk1 S345 (Figure 4A). This result was rather surprising as ssDNA is obviously present in the CuET treated cells (see Figure 3A–D) and also coated by the upstream factor RPA, thereby setting the initial stage for ATR activation and phosphorylation of ATR targets including Chk1. To further investigate whether CuET indeed impairs the RPA-ATRIP-ATR-CHk1 signaling, we treated cells with CuET in the presence of HU. While treatment with HU alone efficiently induced phosphorylation of Chk1 S317 and Ckh1 S345, as expected, the combined treatment with CuET and HU revealed the lack of such Chk1 phosphorylations again, indicating that CuET exerted a dominant effect in suppressing the ATR pathway activity (Figure 4B). These unexpected results were then corroborated by the lack of Serine 33 phosphorylation of yet another ATR substrate, the replication stress marker RPA32, an event seen in the HU-treated control but not in CuET- or combined CuET- and HU-treated cells (Figure 4C).

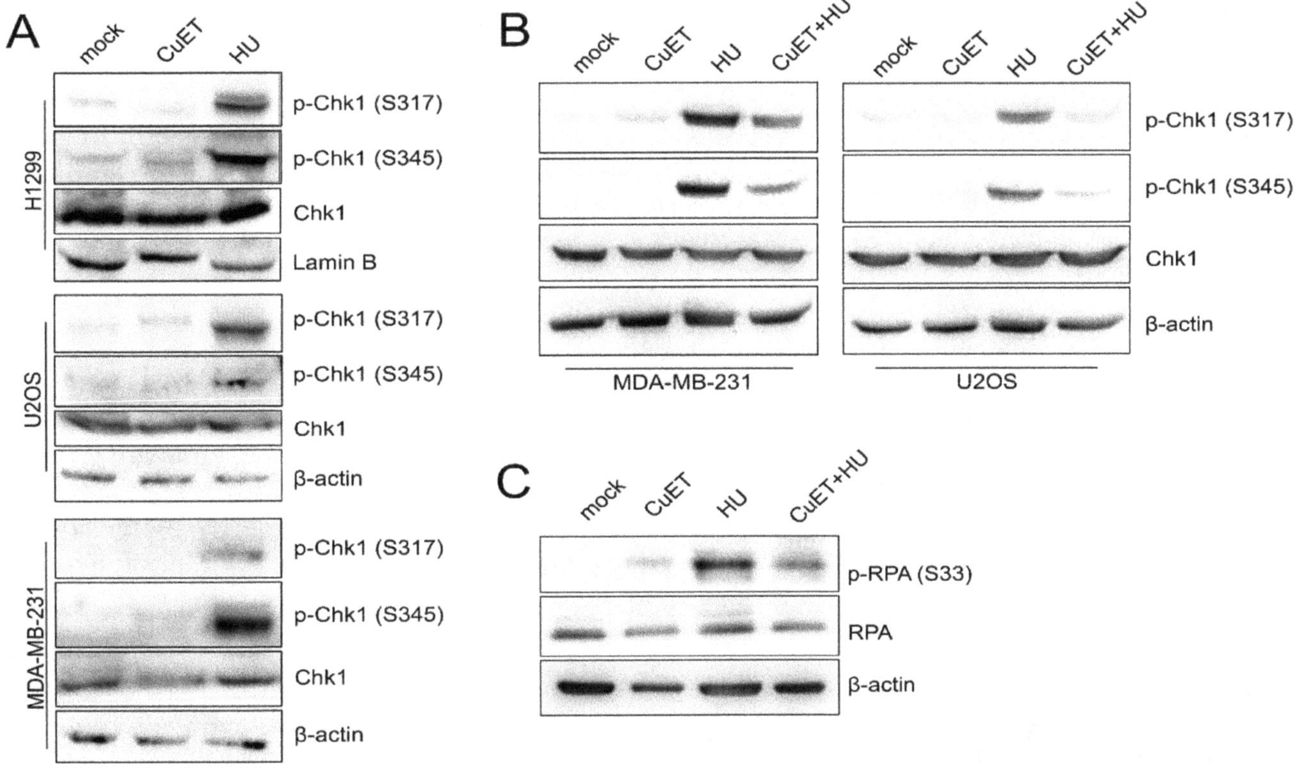

Figure 4. ATR signaling is compromised by CuET. (**A**) Western blotanalysis of phosphorylated forms of Chk1 in various cell lines treated by CuET (250 nM) or HU (2 mM) for 5 h. (**B**) WB analysis of Chk1 phosphorylation in U2OS and MDA-MB-231 cells pre-treated by dimethylsulfoxide (DMSO, mock) or CuET (250 nM) for 2 h and then exposed to HU (2 mM) for additional 3 h. (**C**) WB detection of RPA32 phosphorylation in U2OS cells treated as in B.

Together these results suggest that CuET treatment not only causes replication stress by slowing down and/or stalling replication fork progression but at the same time, it also interferes with the activation of the RPA-ATRIP-ATR-Chk1 signaling cascade that is critical for proper cellular responses to replication stress.

3.5. The ATR Signaling Pathway is Compromised in CuET-Treated Cells

The fact that ATR kinase signaling was suppressed after CuET treatment despite ongoing robust replication stress that also included the formation of ssDNA inspired us to focus directly on the ATR protein and its behavior in response to CuET. As a general readout for analysis of ATR abundance, subcellular localization and function we employed the reporter U2OS cells expressing GFP-labeled ATR (U2OS ATR-GFP) that allowed us to directly assess also recruitment of the ATR protein to acutely inflicted DNA lesions induced by laser microirradiation of psoralen pre-sensitized cell nuclei [19,21]. While in control mock-treated cells, the ATR-GFP protein rapidly formed the expected pattern of fluorescent stripes matching the laser tracks, such recruitment of ATR was markedly impaired after CuET exposure (Figure 5A and Supplementary Figure S4). Moreover, we noticed that in CuET-treated cells without any laser exposure, the otherwise pan-nuclear and generally diffuse ATR-GFP fluorescence signal became altered, forming a pattern that was reminiscent of protein aggregates previously reported by us for the NPL4 protein after CuET treatment [3] (Figure 5B). Indeed, further immunofluorescence analysis confirmed co-localization of ATR-GFP with the NPL4/p97 aggregates formed after CuET treatment (Figure 5C) and general immobilization of the ATR protein was then confirmed by two additional complementary approaches: quantitative microscopy on cultured and pre-extracted U2OS ATR-GFP cells (Figure 5D), and immunoblotting identification of protein translocation from the mobile into the immobile (pre-extraction resistant) protein fraction. Notably, unlike the aggregated immobile ATR protein, the downstream component of the ATR cascade, namely the effector kinase Chk1 was not immobilized after CuET treatment (Figure 5E). To distinguish whether or not ATR immobilization was caused by CuET independently of CuET's key reported target, the NPL4 protein [3], we employed our U2OS cell model conditionally expressing a mutated form of NPL4-GFP, a protein which tends to aggregate spontaneously when expressed in cells due to the point mutation in the putative zinc-finger domain involved in the interaction with CuET [3]. We have already shown that such spontaneous aggregation of the NPL4-MUT protein mimics multiple aspects of CuET treatment including association and immobilization of various cellular stress-response proteins including HSP70, p97, SUMO, polyUb, and TDP43 with the NPL4 aggregates [3]. Indeed, using this model, we found the association and immobilization of ATR-GFP within the spontaneously formed NPL4-MUT aggregates (Figure 5F,H).

In summary, these experiments identified NPL4 aggregation, induced by either CuET in the case of wild-type NPL4, or mutation-caused conformational change of the NPL4-MUT protein in the absence of any added CuET, as the primary event and a pre-requisite for the subsequent sequestration of ATR in such NPL4 aggregates, with the ensuing signaling defect of the ATR-Chk1 signaling pathway.

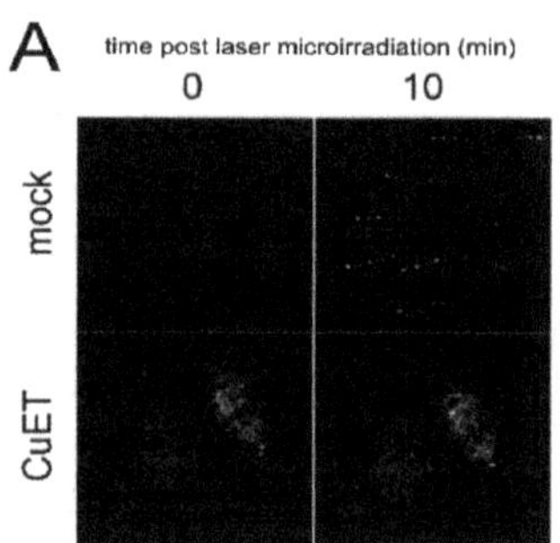

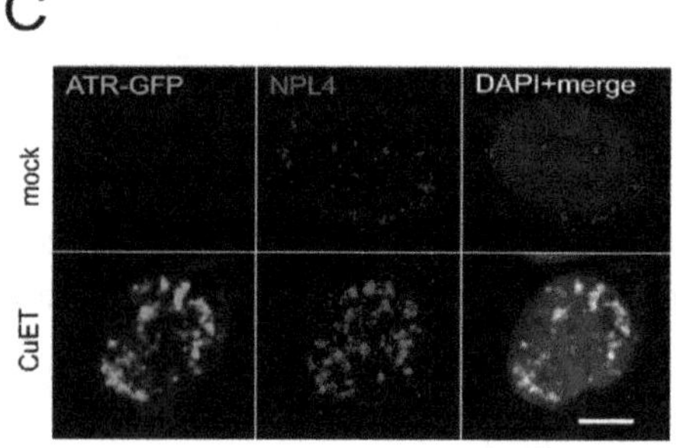

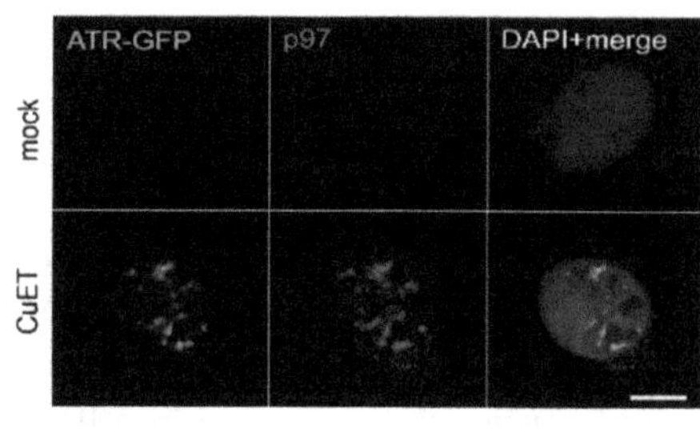

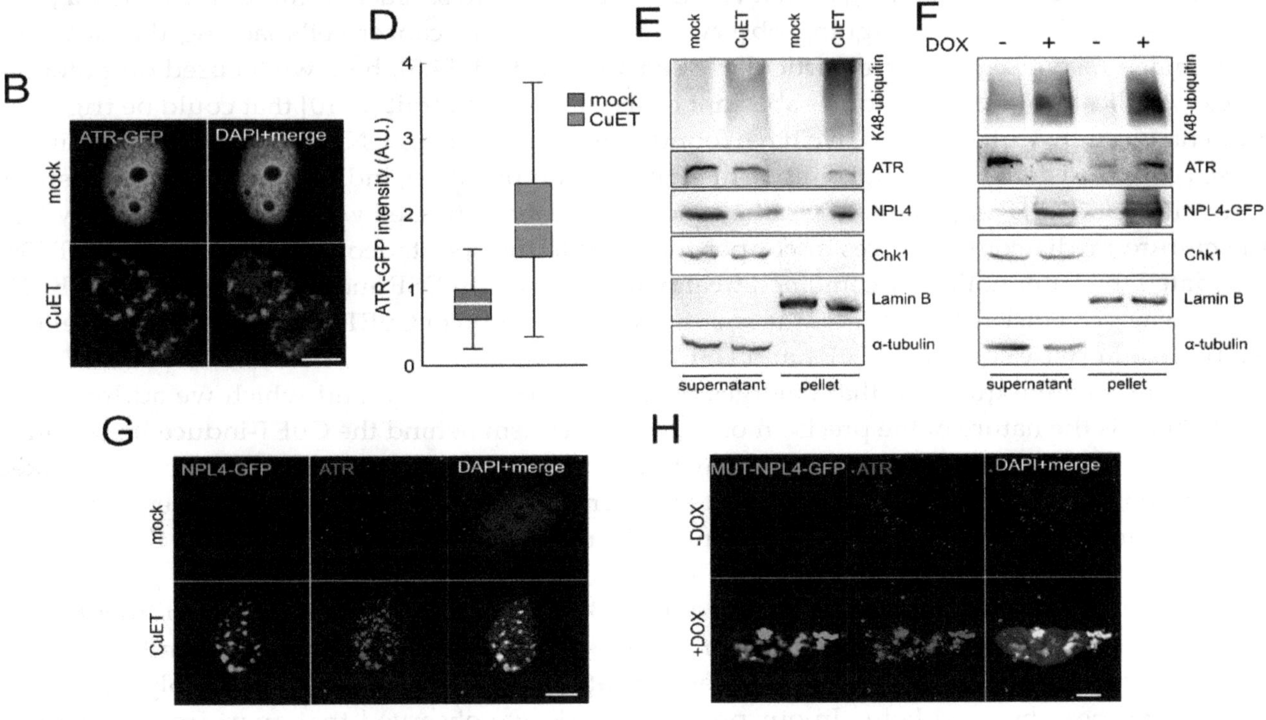

Figure 5. CuET induces immobilization of ATR and its localization to NPL4 aggregates. (**A**) ATR recruitment to sites of damage caused by laser-microirradiation is impaired after CuET treatment (250 nM for 5 h). (**B**) ATR-GFP forms typical nuclear clusters after CuET treatment (250 nM for 5 h). (**C**) Microscopic analysis of co-localization of ATR-GFP with NPL4 and p97 after CuET treatment (250 nM, 3 h) in pre-extracted U2OS cells. (**D**) Quantitative microscopic analysis of pre-extraction resistant ATR-GFP protein in U2OS cells in control and CuET treated cells (250 nM, 5 h). (**E**) WB analysis of immobilized ATR, K48 ubiquitinated proteins, and NPL4 in extracts of CuET-treated (250 nM, 3 h) U2OS cells. (**F**) WB analysis of immobilized ATR, K48 ubiquitinated proteins, and NPL4 in MUT-NPL4-GFP expressing U2OS (Doxycycline induction for 18 h). (**G**) Microscopic analysis of co-localization of NPL4-GFP with ATR after CuET treatment (250 nM, 3 h) in pre-extracted U2OS cells. (**H**) Microscopic analysis of co-localization of MUT-NPL4-GFP with ATR after 18 h doxycycline induction in pre-extracted U2OS cells. Scale bars = 10 μm.

4. Discussion

The major advance provided by the results from our present study is the identification of a new mode of cancer cell cytotoxicity evoked by diethyldithiocarbamate-copper complex, CuET [3,4], the anticancer metabolite of the alcohol aversion drug DSF that is currently tested in clinical trials for repurposing in oncology. Indeed, after years of convoluted efforts to understand the tumor-inhibitory effects of DSF, the field has been aided by our discovery of CuET as the ultimate cancer-killing compound that rapidly forms as DSF becomes metabolized under both in vivo [3], and cell culture [4,34] conditions. At the mechanistic level, we found that CuET impairs the cellular protein degradation machinery upstream of the proteasome, by inducing aggregation and immobilization of NPL4, an essential cofactor of the p97/VCP segregase complex [3]. This mechanism helps explain the observed preferential toxicity in cancer cells experiencing high levels of proteotoxic stress, such as multiple myeloma [3].

Inspired by the recent intriguing observation that human cancer cells lacking the BRCA1/2 DNA damage response genes are particularly sensitive to DSF [4,5], here we focused on potential genotoxic/replication stress as another aberrant cancer-associated trait [7–10] that could be triggered and/or enhanced by CuET. Indeed, we have found that CuET induces DNA damage preferentially in S-phase cells consistent with robust impairment of DNA replication, induction of replication stress, and impairment of ATR signaling. The same effects can be recapitulated with replacing CuET by DSF, as the culture media contain traces of copper that enable the spontaneous formation of CuET [34]. We validated the latter notion by combined treatment of cells with DSF and the copper chelator BCDS (Figure 1E), which efficiently precludes the spontaneous formation of CuET [4] and thereby the cellular phenotypes otherwise shared by CuET and DSF.

The fundamental question that emerges from our present study, and which we address only partially here, is the nature of the precise molecular mechanism behind the CuET-induced replication stress. As CuET impairs the p97/NPL4 pathway that is directly implicated in several processes linked to DNA repair and replication [35], it remains to be seen whether the replication interference could be explained by impacting such processes, including DNA replication, translesion synthesis, DNA-protein crosslinks repair, or termination of replication [36], possibly in a combination. Moreover, p97, together with diverse cofactors, is also directly involved in DSB repair, contributing to the recruitment of the 53BP1 repair factor [37] and also other DDR proteins [38–40]. On the other hand, also indirect effects of NPL4 aggregation, for example, the triggered heat-shock response, could plausibly contribute to the phenotypes observed here. In our previous work, we observed that apart from NPL4/p97, the CuET-induced aggregates contain several proteotoxic stress-related proteins, including HSP70, SUMO2/3, polyubiquitin chains, and TDP-43 [3]. Here, we have surprisingly found that also ATR kinase, a key factor required for proper cellular response to replication stress, is trapped and sequestered in the NPL4 aggregates, thus explaining the dysfunction of ATR signaling in CuET-treated cells. Conceptually, given that ATR dysfunction is known to trigger replication stress, a feature we see also after CuET treatment, one could argue that ATR aggregation could represent the primary and/or major cause of the CuET-induced replication stress. On the other hand, our time-course analysis suggests that DNA replication becomes impaired very quickly upon CuET addition, as judged from the EdU staining (Figure 2B), in fact preceding any detectable ATR aggregation. Therefore, we currently believe that the two processes, replication fork stalling, and ATR aggregation are possibly initiated independent of each other and act rather in a complementary manner to cause the observed robust replication stress phenotype. A related emerging question for future work is what brings ATR to the vicinity of the forming NPL4 aggregates in the first place? This issue is speculative at present, and it remains to be seen whether some structural features of ATR, possibly shared by additional proteins, such as unstructured regions or high dependency on chaperones, could be involved. Alternatively, the recruitment to aggregates might share the mechanism of the reported ATR recruitment into areas of high topological stress within the nuclear envelope [41]. ATR might be sequestrated by the aggregates also through direct interaction with NPL4 or due to the global proteotoxic stress-related changes in the cell. The latter scenario would partially resemble the so-called β-sheets-containing protein aggregates that sequester and mislocalize several proteins involved in RNA metabolism and nucleocytoplasmic transport [42]. Alternatively, liquid–liquid phase separation might also be involved in this process. A recent study [43] revealed that acute hyperosmotic stress induces phase separation of the proteasomes and formation of discrete puncta in the nucleus. Interestingly, these structures also contained K48-ubiquitinated proteins or p97 segregase, the proteins also found in NPL4 clusters, raising the question of whether phase separation plays a role in the case of NPL4 aggregation or attraction of other proteins. These questions need to be addressed by dedicated future studies, to help us better understand the effects of

NPL4 aggregates on cellular physiology, providing clues about why so many seemingly unrelated phenotypes have so far been described after DSF treatment.

Last but not least, our present results are also highly relevant from the clinical point of view, not least because protein aggregation represents an unorthodox and so far largely unexplored mechanism of action for anticancer drugs. This rather unique mechanism may also contribute to the observed synergistic effects of DSF/copper with either ionizing radiation [44] or the DNA damage-inducing drug temozolomide [45] a combination currently tested in several clinical trials focusing on glioblastoma patients [46–48], as well as a combination of DSF with cisplatin [49]. We hope that the data we report here will inspire further research in this rapidly evolving area of biomedicine, and yield additional effective therapies based on combining DSF/copper (CuET) with other currently used DNA damage-related therapeutic modalities.

or exacerbates

Overall, based on our present results we suggest that CuET (DSF/copper) evokes and/ replication stress in tumor cells while concomitantly precluding the ATR-mediated pro-survival response to such stress, thereby collectively creating a toxic scenario (understandably more severe in BRCA1/2-defective cells) reminiscent of 'killing two birds with one stone.'

Author Contributions: D.M., Z.S., M.M., and J.B. conceived the study, D.M. and Z.S. designed and performed most experiments, K.C. contributed the laser microirradiation data. J.M.M.-M. performed alkaline comet assay. D.M., Z.S., M.M., and J.B. interpreted the results and wrote the manuscript, which was approved by all authors. All authors have read and agreed to the published version of the manuscript.

Acknowledgments: We thank M. Tarsounas (Oxford, UK) for the human H1299 cell lines with the regulatable expression of shBRCA1 and shBRCA2 and Mgr. Tatana Stosova for help with FIGE (Palacky University, Olomouc, Czech Republic).

References

1. Collins, F.S. Mining for therapeutic gold. *Nat. Rev. Drug Discov.* **2011**, *10*, 397. [CrossRef] [PubMed]
2. McMahon, A.; Chen, W.; Li, F. Old wine in new bottles: Advanced drug delivery systems for disulfiram-based cancer therapy. *J. Control. Release* **2020**, *319*, 352–359. [CrossRef] [PubMed]
3. Skrott, Z.; Mistrik, M.; Andersen, K.K.; Friis, S.; Majera, D.; Gursky, J.; Ozdian, T.; Bartkova, J.; Turi, Z.; Moudry, P.; et al. Alcohol-abuse drug disulfiram targets cancer via p97 segregase adaptor NPL4. *Nature* **2017**, *552*, 194–199. [CrossRef] [PubMed]
4. Skrott, Z.; Majera, D.; Gursky, J.; Buchtova, T.; Hajduch, M.; Mistrik, M.; Bartek, J. Disulfiram's anti-cancer activity reflects targeting NPL4, not inhibition of aldehyde dehydrogenase. *Oncogene* **2019**, *38*, 6711–6722. [CrossRef]
5. Tacconi, E.M.; Lai, X.; Folio, C.; Porru, M.; Zonderland, G.; Badie, S.; Michl, J.; Sechi, I.; Rogier, M.; Matía García, V.; et al. BRCA1 and BRCA2 tumor suppressors protect against endogenous acetaldehyde toxicity. *EMBO Mol. Med.* **2017**, *9*, 1398–1414. [CrossRef]
6. Lorenti Garcia, C.; Mechilli, M.; Proietti De Santis, L.; Schinoppi, A.; Katarzyna, K.; Palitti, F. Relationship between DNA lesions, DNA repair and chromosomal damage induced by acetaldehyde. *Mutat. Res. Mol. Mech. Mutagen.* **2009**, *662*, 3–9. [CrossRef]
7. Bartkova, J.; Hořejší, Z.; Koed, K.; Krämer, A.; Tort, F.; Zieger, K.; Guldberg, P.; Sehested, M.; Nesland, J.M.; Lukas, C.; et al. DNA damage response as a candidate anti-cancer barrier in early human tumorigenesis. *Nature* **2005**, *434*, 864–870. [CrossRef]
8. Bartkova, J.; Rezaei, N.; Liontos, M.; Karakaidos, P.; Kletsas, D.; Issaeva, N.; Vassiliou, L.-V.F.; Kolettas, E.; Niforou, K.; Zoumpourlis, V.C.; et al. Oncogene-induced senescence is part of the tumorigenesis barrier imposed by DNA damage checkpoints. *Nature* **2006**, *444*, 633–637. [CrossRef]

9. Gorgoulis, V.G.; Vassiliou, L.-V.F.; Karakaidos, P.; Zacharatos, P.; Kotsinas, A.; Liloglou, T.; Venere, M.; DiTullio, R.A.; Kastrinakis, N.G.; Levy, B.; et al. Activation of the DNA damage checkpoint and genomic instability in human precancerous lesions. *Nature* **2005**, *434*, 907–913. [CrossRef]
10. Halazonetis, T.D.; Gorgoulis, V.G.; Bartek, J. An Oncogene-Induced DNA Damage Model for Cancer Development. *Science* **2008**, *319*, 1352–1355. [CrossRef]
11. Bartek, J.; Bartkova, J.; Lukas, J. DNA damage signalling guards against activated oncogenes and tumour progression. *Oncogene* **2007**, *26*, 7773–7779. [CrossRef] [PubMed]
12. Jackson, S.P.; Bartek, J. The DNA-damage response in human biology and disease. *Nature* **2009**, *461*, 1071–1078. [CrossRef] [PubMed]
13. Gaillard, H.; García-Muse, T.; Aguilera, A. Replication stress and cancer. *Nat. Rev. Cancer* **2015**, *15*, 276–289. [CrossRef]
14. Bartek, J.; Mistrik, M.; Bartkova, J. Thresholds of replication stress signaling in cancer development and treatment. *Nat. Struct. Mol. Biol.* **2012**, *19*, 5–7. [CrossRef]
15. Zeman, M.K.; Cimprich, K.A. Causes and consequences of replication stress. *Nat. Cell Biol.* **2014**, *16*, 2–9. [CrossRef] [PubMed]
16. Berti, M.; Vindigni, A. Replication stress: Getting back on track. *Nat. Struct. Mol. Biol.* **2016**, *23*, 103–109. [CrossRef]
17. Eykelenboom, J.K.; Harte, E.C.; Canavan, L.; Pastor-Peidro, A.; Calvo-Asensio, I.; Llorens-Agost, M.; Lowndes, N.F. ATR Activates the S-M Checkpoint during Unperturbed Growth to Ensure Sufficient Replication Prior to Mitotic Onset. *Cell Rep.* **2013**, *5*, 1095–1107. [CrossRef]
18. Toledo, L.I.; Altmeyer, M.; Rask, M.-B.; Lukas, C.; Larsen, D.H.; Povlsen, L.K.; Bekker-Jensen, S.; Mailand, N.; Bartek, J.; Lukas, J. ATR Prohibits Replication Catastrophe by Preventing Global Exhaustion of RPA. *Cell* **2014**, *156*, 374. [CrossRef]
19. Bekker-Jensen, S.; Lukas, C.; Kitagawa, R.; Melander, F.; Kastan, M.B.; Bartek, J.; Lukas, J. Spatial organization of the mammalian genome surveillance machinery in response to DNA strand breaks. *J. Cell Biol.* **2006**, *173*, 195–206. [CrossRef]
20. Jackson, D.A.; Pombo, A. Replicon Clusters Are Stable Units of Chromosome Structure: Evidence That Nuclear Organization Contributes to the Efficient Activation and Propagation of S Phase in Human Cells. *J. Cell Biol.* **1998**, *140*, 1285–1295. [CrossRef]
21. Mistrik, M.; Vesela, E.; Furst, T.; Hanzlikova, H.; Frydrych, I.; Gursky, J.; Majera, D.; Bartek, J. Cells and Stripes: A novel quantitative photo-manipulation technique. *Sci. Rep.* **2016**, *6*, 19567. [CrossRef] [PubMed]
22. Maya-Mendoza, A.; Moudry, P.; Merchut-Maya, J.M.; Lee, M.; Strauss, R.; Bartek, J. High speed of fork progression induces DNA replication stress and genomic instability. *Nature* **2018**, *559*, 279–284. [CrossRef] [PubMed]
23. Budzowska, M.; Kanaar, R. Mechanisms of Dealing with DNA Damage-Induced Replication Problems. *Cell Biochem. Biophys.* **2009**, *53*, 17–31. [CrossRef] [PubMed]
24. Bianco, J.N.; Poli, J.; Saksouk, J.; Bacal, J.; Silva, M.J.; Yoshida, K.; Lin, Y.-L.; Tourrière, H.; Lengronne, A.; Pasero, P. Analysis of DNA replication profiles in budding yeast and mammalian cells using DNA combing. *Methods* **2012**, *57*, 149–157. [CrossRef]
25. Quinet, A.; Carvajal-Maldonado, D.; Lemacon, D.; Vindigni, A. DNA Fiber Analysis: Mind the Gap! *Methods Enzymology* **2017**, *591*, 55–82.
26. Couch, F.B.; Bansbach, C.E.; Driscoll, R.; Luzwick, J.W.; Glick, G.G.; Betous, R.; Carroll, C.M.; Jung, S.Y.; Qin, J.; Cimprich, K.A.; et al. ATR phosphorylates SMARCAL1 to prevent replication fork collapse. *Genes Dev.* **2013**, *27*, 1610–1623. [CrossRef]
27. Sogo, J.M. Fork Reversal and ssDNA Accumulation at Stalled Replication Forks Owing to Checkpoint Defects. *Science* **2002**, *297*, 599–602. [CrossRef]

28. Byun, T.S.; Pacek, M.; Yee, M.C.; Walter, J.C.; Cimprich, K.A. Functional uncoupling of MCM helicase and DNA polymerase activities activates the ATR-dependent checkpoint. *Genes Dev.* **2005**, *19*, 1040–1052. [CrossRef]
29. Lee, Z.; Elledge, S.J. Sensing DNA Damage Through ATRIP Recognition of RPA-ssDNA Complexes. *Science* **2003**, *300*, 1542–1548. [CrossRef]
30. Liao, H.; Ji, F.; Helleday, T.; Ying, S. Mechanisms for stalled replication fork stabilization: New targets for synthetic lethality strategies in cancer treatments. *EMBO Rep.* **2018**, *19*. [CrossRef]
31. Petermann, E.; Orta, M.L.; Issaeva, N.; Schultz, N.; Helleday, T. Hydroxyurea-Stalled Replication Forks Become Progressively Inactivated and Require Two Different RAD51-Mediated Pathways for Restart and Repair. *Mol. Cell* **2010**, *37*, 492–502. [CrossRef] [PubMed]
32. Whelan, D.R.; Lee, W.T.C.; Yin, Y.; Ofri, D.M.; Bermudez-Hernandez, K.; Keegan, S.; Fenyo, D.; Rothenberg, E. Spatiotemporal dynamics of homologous recombination repair at single collapsed replication forks. *Nat. Commun.* **2018**, *9*, 3882. [CrossRef] [PubMed]
33. Davies, A.A.; Masson, J.Y.; McIlwraith, M.J.; Stasiak, A.Z.; Stasiak, A.; Venkitaraman, A.R.; West, S.C. Role of BRCA2 in control of the RAD51 recombination and DNA repair protein. *Mol. Cell* **2001**, *7*, 273–282. [CrossRef]
34. Majera, D.; Skrott, Z.; Bouchal, J.; Bartkova, J.; Simkova, D.; Gachechiladze, M.; Steigerova, J.; Kurfurstova, D.; Gursky, J.; Korinkova, G.; et al. Targeting genotoxic and proteotoxic stress-response pathways in human prostate cancer by clinically available PARP inhibitors, vorinostat and disulfiram. *Prostate* **2019**, *79*, 352–362. [CrossRef]
35. Ramadan, K. p97/VCP- and Lys48-linked polyubiquitination form a new signaling pathway in DNA damage response. *Cell Cycle* **2012**, *11*, 1062–1069. [CrossRef] [PubMed]
36. Ramadan, K.; Halder, S.; Wiseman, K.; Vaz, B. Strategic role of the ubiquitin-dependent segregase p97 (VCP or Cdc48) in DNA replication. *Chromosoma* **2017**, *126*, 17–32. [CrossRef]
37. Meerang, M.; Ritz, D.; Paliwal, S.; Garajova, Z.; Bosshard, M.; Mailand, N.; Janscak, P.; Hübscher, U.; Meyer, H.; Ramadan, K. The ubiquitin-selective segregase VCP/p97 orchestrates the response to DNA double-strand breaks. *Nat. Cell Biol.* **2011**, *13*, 1376. [CrossRef]
38. Bergink, S.; Ammon, T.; Kern, M.; Schermelleh, L.; Leonhardt, H.; Jentsch, S. Role of Cdc48/p97 as a SUMO-targeted segregase curbing Rad51–Rad52 interaction. *Nat. Cell Biol.* **2013**, *15*, 526–532. [CrossRef]
39. Singh, A.N.; Oehler, J.; Torrecilla, I.; Kilgas, S.; Li, S.; Vaz, B.; Guérillon, C.; Fielden, J.; Hernandez-Carralero, E.; Cabrera, E.; et al. The p97-Ataxin 3 complex regulates homeostasis of the DNA damage response E3 ubiquitin ligase RNF8. *EMBO J.* **2019**, *38*, e102361. [CrossRef]
40. Davis, E.J.; Lachaud, C.; Appleton, P.; Macartney, T.J.; Näthke, I.; Rouse, J. DVC1 (C1orf124) recruits the p97 protein segregase to sites of DNA damage. *Nat. Struct. Mol. Biol.* **2012**, *19*, 1093–1100. [CrossRef]
41. Kumar, A.; Mazzanti, M.; Mistrik, M.; Kosar, M.; Beznoussenko, G.V.; Mironov, A.A.; Garrè, M.; Parazzoli, D.; Shivashankar, G.V.; Scita, G.; et al. ATR Mediates a Checkpoint at the Nuclear Envelope in Response to Mechanical Stress. *Cell* **2014**, *158*, 633–646. [CrossRef] [PubMed]
42. Woerner, A.C.; Frottin, F.; Hornburg, D.; Feng, L.R.; Meissner, F.; Patra, M.; Tatzelt, J.; Mann, M.; Winklhofer, K.F.; Hartl, F.U.; et al. Cytoplasmic protein aggregates interfere with nucleocytoplasmic transport of protein and RNA. *Science* **2016**, *351*, 173–176. [CrossRef] [PubMed]
43. Yasuda, S.; Tsuchiya, H.; Kaiho, A.; Guo, Q.; Ikeuchi, K.; Endo, A.; Arai, N.; Ohtake, F.; Murata, S.; Inada, T.; et al. Stress- and ubiquitylation-dependent phase separation of the proteasome. *Nature* **2020**, *578*, 296–300. [CrossRef] [PubMed]
44. Wang, Y.; Li, W.; Patel, S.S.; Cong, J.; Zhang, N.; Sabbatino, F.; Liu, X.; Qi, Y.; Huang, P.; Lee, H.; et al. Blocking the formation of radiation induced breast cancer stem cells. *Oncotarget* **2014**, *5*, 3743–3755. [CrossRef]
45. Lun, X.; Wells, J.C.; Grinshtein, N.; King, J.C.; Hao, X.; Dang, N.-H.; Wang, X.; Aman, A.; Uehling, D.; Datti, A.; et al. Disulfiram when Combined with Copper Enhances the Therapeutic Effects of Temozolomide for the Treatment of Glioblastoma. *Clin. Cancer Res.* **2016**, *22*, 3860–3875. [CrossRef]
46. Huang, J.; Campian, J.L.; Gujar, A.D.; Tsien, C.; Ansstas, G.; Tran, D.D.; DeWees, T.A.; Lockhart, A.C.; Kim, A.H. Final results of a phase I dose-escalation, dose-expansion study of adding disulfiram with or without copper to adjuvant temozolomide for newly diagnosed glioblastoma. *J. Neurooncol.* **2018**, *138*, 105–111. [CrossRef]

47. Huang, J.; Campian, J.L.; Gujar, A.D.; Tran, D.D.; Lockhart, A.C.; DeWees, T.A.; Tsien, C.I.; Kim, A.H. A phase I study to repurpose disulfiram in combination with temozolomide to treat newly diagnosed glioblastoma after chemoradiotherapy. *J. Neurooncol.* **2016**, *128*, 259–266. [CrossRef]
48. Jakola, A.S.; Werlenius, K.; Mudaisi, M.; Hylin, S.; Kinhult, S.; Bartek, J.J.; Salvesen, O.; Carlsen, S.M.; Strandeus, M.; Lindskog, M.; et al. Disulfiram repurposing combined with nutritional copper supplement as add-on to chemotherapy in recurrent glioblastoma (DIRECT): Study protocol for a randomized controlled trial. *F1000Research* **2018**, *7*, 1797. [CrossRef]
49. Nechushtan, H.; Hamamreh, Y.; Nidal, S.; Gotfried, M.; Baron, A.; Shalev, Y.I.; Nisman, B.; Peretz, T.; Peylan-Ramu, N. A Phase IIb Trial Assessing the Addition of Disulfiram to Chemotherapy for the Treatment of Metastatic Non-Small Cell Lung Cancer. *Oncologist* **2015**, *20*, 366–367. [CrossRef]

12

Ferlin Overview: From Membrane to Cancer Biology

Olivier Peulen [1,*], Gilles Rademaker [1], Sandy Anania [1], Andrei Turtoi [2,3,4], Akeila Bellahcène [1] and Vincent Castronovo [1]

1 Metastasis Research Laboratory, Giga Cancer, University of Liège, B4000 Liège, Belgium
2 Tumor Microenvironment Laboratory, Institut de Recherche en Cancérologie de Montpellier, INSERM U1194, 34000 Montpellier, France
3 Institut du Cancer de Montpeiller, 34000 Montpellier, France
4 Université de Montpellier, 34000 Montpellier, France
* Correspondence: olivier.peulen@uliege.be

Abstract: In mammal myocytes, endothelial cells and inner ear cells, ferlins are proteins involved in membrane processes such as fusion, recycling, endo- and exocytosis. They harbour several C2 domains allowing their interaction with phospholipids. The expression of several Ferlin genes was described as altered in several tumoural tissues. Intriguingly, beyond a simple alteration, myoferlin, otoferlin and Fer1L4 expressions were negatively correlated with patient survival in some cancer types. Therefore, it can be assumed that membrane biology is of extreme importance for cell survival and signalling, making Ferlin proteins core machinery indispensable for cancer cell adaptation to hostile environments. The evidences suggest that myoferlin, when overexpressed, enhances cancer cell proliferation, migration and metabolism by affecting various aspects of membrane biology. Targeting myoferlin using pharmacological compounds, gene transfer technology, or interfering RNA is now considered as an emerging therapeutic strategy.

Keywords: ferlin; myoferlin; dysferlin; otoferlin; C2 domain; plasma membrane

---

1. Introduction

Ferlin is a family of proteins involved in vesicle fusions. To date, more than 760 articles in Pubmed refer to one of its members. Most of these publications are related to muscle biology, while less than 50 are directly related to cancer. However, the emerging idea of targeting plasma membranes [1] and the discovery of a significant correlation between Ferlin gene expression and cancer patient survival, brings attention to cancer. This review focused attention on the roles of these proteins, first in a healthy context, then in cancer.

During the maturation of spermatids to motile spermatozoa in *Caenorhabditis elegans* worm, large vesicles called membranous organelles fuse with the spermatid plasma membrane. This step requires a functional FER-1 protein encoded by the fer-1 gene (*fertilization defective-1*) [2]. When FER-1 was identified and sequenced, no other known proteins had strong resemblance to it. Subsequently, homologs were found by sequence similarity in mammals, forming a family of similar proteins now called ferlins. In humans, a first *C. elegans* fer-1 homolog gene was discovered and the protein encoded by this gene was named dysferlin [3]. Shortly after, a second human FER-1-Like gene was identified. The product of the gene was named otoferlin [4]. The human EST database mining revealed a dysferlin paralog called myoferlin [5,6]. Three new members joined the ferlin gene family: FER1L4, a pseudogene; FER1L5; and FER1L6. The main features of ferlins are summarized in Table 1.

Table 1. Short description of *C. elegans* and human ferlin genes and proteins.

Protein Name (Uniprot Number)	Gene Name	Chromosome Mapping	Main Protein Size
Sperm vesicle fusion protein FER-1 (Q17388)	fer-1		2034 AA (235 KDa)
Dysferlin (O75923)	Fer1-Like 1 Fer1L1	2p13.2	2080 AA (237 KDa)
Otoferlin (Q9HC10)	Fer1-Like Fer1L2	2p23.3	1997 AA (227 KDa)
Myoferlin (Q9NZM1)	Fer1-Like 3 Fer1L3	10q23.33	2061 AA (230 KDa)
FER1L4 (A9Z1Z3)	Fer1-Like 4 Fer1L4	20q11.22	pseudogene
FER1L5 (A0AVI2)	Fer1-Like 5 Fer1L5	2q11.2	2057 AA (238 KDa)
FER1L6 (Q2WGJ9)	Fer1-Like 6 Fer1L6	8q24.13	1857 AA (209 KDa)

The dysferlin mutations were involved in Limb-Girdle muscular dystrophy 2B (LGMD2B), a autosomal recessive degenerative myopathy, and in Miyoshi muscular dystrophy 1 (MMD1), a late-onset muscular dystrophy [3,7]. The otoferlin mutations were described in the non-syndromic prelingual deafness (DFNB9) and in the auditory neuropathy autosomal recessive 1 (AUNB1) [4,8,9]. Nowadays, myoferlin and the 3 last members of the ferlin family are still not linked to human genetic diseases. However, myoferlin was proposed as a modifier protein for muscular dystrophy phenotype [5] and studies of myoferlin-null mice demonstrated impaired myoblast fusion and myofiber formation during muscle development and regeneration [10]. More recently, a truncated variant of myoferlin was associated with Limb-Girdle type muscular dystrophy and cardiomyopathy [11]. Here under, this review discusses that ferlins, mainly myoferlin, are involved in neoplastic diseases and are potential therapeutic targets.

2. Genomic Organization of Ferlin Gene Family

Ferlin genomic organization has not been extensively investigated. Nonetheless, valuable information was obtained from sequencing and subsequent gene annotation (www.ensembl.org In *C. elegans*, fer-1 gene is approximately 8.6 kb in length and composed of 21 exons [2]. In humans, dysferlin gene (DYSF) is composed of 55 exons [12], and encodes 19 splice variant transcripts. Otoferlin gene (OTOF) contains 47 exons and encodes 7 splice variants. One of them is retaining an intronic sequence from other locus and is not coding for protein. An alternate splicing results in a neuronal-specific domain for otoferlin, regulated by the inclusion of exon 47 [8]. Myoferlin gene (MYOF), is composed of 54 exons and encodes for 9 splice variants. Four of them are not translated to protein and the shortest retains an intronic sequence. Myoferlin promoter includes several consensus-binding sites, such as for Myc, MEF2, CEBP, Sp1, AP1, and NFAT. The latter is able to bind endogenous NFATc1 and NFATc3 [13]. FER1L5 encodes 7 splice variants obtained by the arrangement of 53 exons. Five transcripts are known to encode proteins when the 2 shortest are retaining intronic sequences and do not encode protein. FER1L6 gene is composed of 41 exons and encodes a unique transcript. The main features of ferlin genes are summarized in Table 2.

Table 2. Short description of *C. elegans* and human ferlin genes and transcripts.

Gene Name	Gene Length	Number of Exons	Transcript Size	Number of Variants
Fer-1	8.6 kb	21	6.2 kb	3
Fer1-Like 1 Fer1L1 (DYSF)	233 kb	55	0.5–6.7 kb	19
Fer1-Like 2 Fer1L2 (OTOF)	121 kb	47	0.5–7.2 kb	7
Fer1-Like 3 Fer1L3 (MYOF)	180 kb	54	0.4–6.7 kb	9
Fer1-Like 4 Fer1L4	48 kb	43	0.2–5.9 kb	13
Fer1-Like 5 Fer1L5	64 kb	53	3.5–6.5 kb	7
Fer1-Like 6 Fer1L6	278 kb	41	6 kb	1

3. Ferlin's Structure and Localization

Caenorrhabditis elegans FER-1 is a large protein rich in charged residues. Charged amino acids are distributed throughout the whole protein length such that no particularly acidic or basic domains are observed. The hydrophobicity plot described a 35 amino acid long hydrophobic region at the C-terminal end [2]. To the authors' knowledge, it has never been experimentally demonstrated. Similarity studies suggest that this region might be a transmembrane domain. FER-1 sequence analysis with Pfam protein families database [14] revealed the existence of 4 C2 domains and several other domains.

Ferlins are proteins harboring multi-C2 domains. These structural domains are ~130 amino acid long independently folded modules found in several eukaryotic proteins. They were identified in classical Protein Kinase C (PKC) as the second conserved domain out of four. The typical C2 domain is composed of a beta-sandwich made of 8 beta-strands coordinating calcium ions, participating to their ability to bind phospholipids (for review [15]). However, some C2 domains have lost their capacity to bind calcium but still bind membranes [16]. A large variety of proteins containing C2 domains have been identified, and most of them are involved in membrane biology, such as vesicular transport (synaptotagmin), GTPase regulation (Ras GTPase activating protein) or lipid modification (phospholipase C) (for review [17]).

Human ferlin proteins harbour 5 to 7 C2 domains as described in the Pfam database (Figure 1A). According to this database, in humans, 342 proteins harbour C2 domains. However, the occurrence of multiple tandem C2 domains is uncommon. Only three vertebrate protein families contain more than two C2 domains: The multiple C2 domain and transmembrane region proteins (MCTP) [18], the E-Syt (extended synaptotagmins) [19], and the ferlins. The typical feature of a C2 domain is its ability to interact with two or three calcium ions. The prototype of this domain is the C2A contained in PKC that binds phospholipids in a calcium-dependent manner. Several other distinct C2 domain subtypes, e.g. those found in PI3K and in PTEN, do not have calcium binding abilities and instead specialize in protein-protein interactions [16,17]. In classical Ca^{2+}-binding C2 domains, 5 aspartate residues are involved in the ion binding [20]. Clustal omega alignment of ferlin C2 domains with PKC and synaptotagmin I C2 domains revealed that the 5 Ca^{2+}-binding aspartic acids were conserved or substituted by a glutamic acid in the C2E and C2F domains of all human paralogs (Figure 1B). The aspartic acid to glutamic acid substitution is considered as highly conservative and observed in some non-ferlin Ca^{2+}-binding C2 domains [21]. Some ferlins showed more C2 domains with Ca^{2+}-binding potential, e.g. dysferlin and myoferlin C2C and C2D, otoferlin C2D and fer1L6 C2D [22]. The phylogenic tree created by neighbour-joining of a Clustal omega alignment of C2 domain sequences shows that a C2 domain is more similar to others at a similar position in ortholog proteins than it is to the other C2 domains within the same protein [23]. A Clustal omega alignment reveals an evolutionary distribution of the ferlin proteins into two main subgroups (Figure 1C): The type 1 ferlins containing a DysF domain and the type-2 ferlins without the DysF domain [22]. This domain is present in yeast peroxisomal proteins where its established function is to regulate the peroxisome size and number [24]. In mammals, despite the fact that its solution structure was resolved [25] and that many pathogenic point mutations occur in this region [26,27], the function of this domain remains unknown.

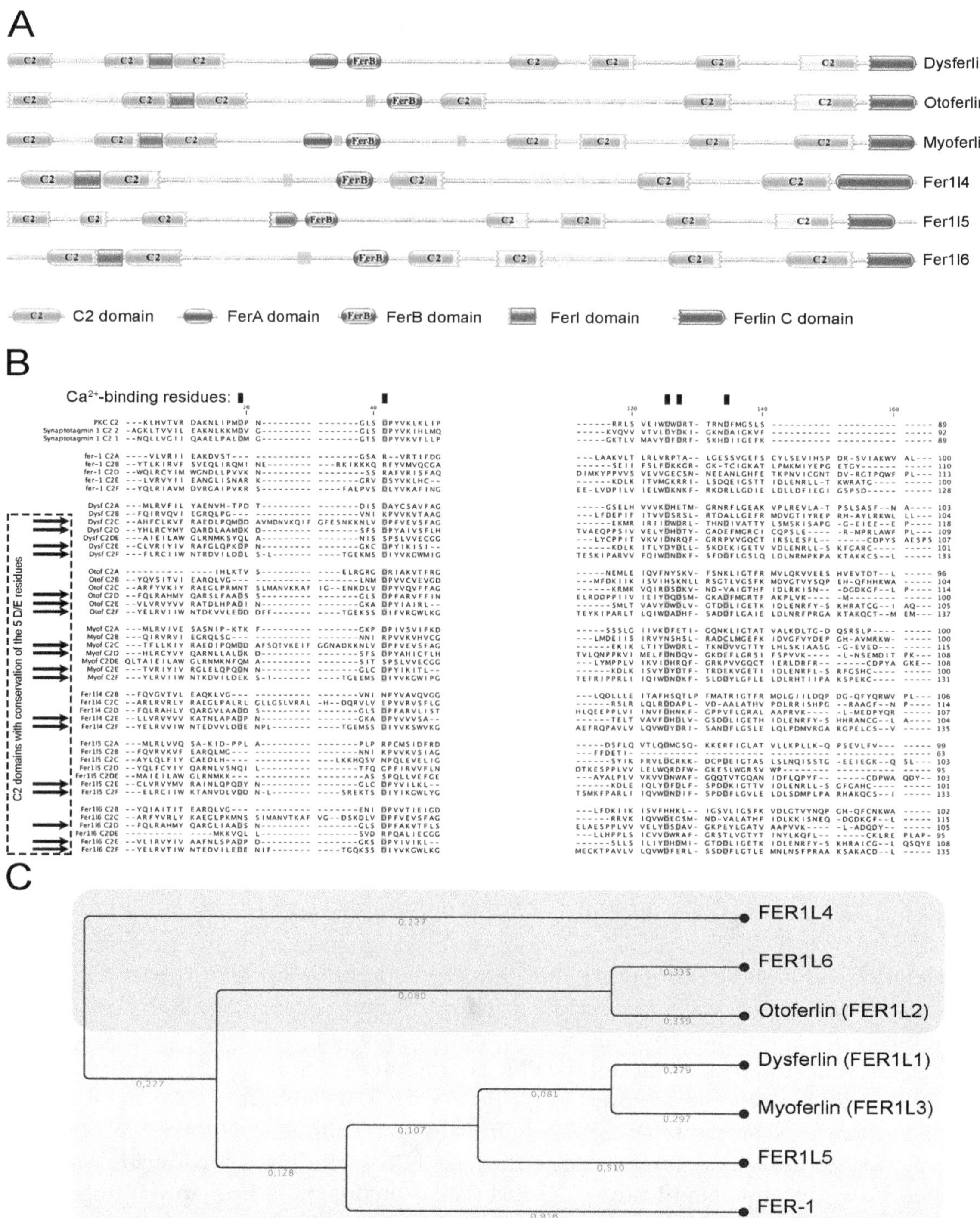

Figure 1. Structure and phylogenic relation of ferlin proteins. (**A**) Schematic structure of FER-1 human homologs as produced by Pfam protein families' database. (**B**) Clustal omega multiple alignment of ferlin C2 domains. Conserved Ca^{2+}-binding site are highlighted in red (aspartic acid—D) or yellow (glutamic acid—E). (**C**) Cladogram of clustal omega alignment indicating type 1 ferlins in blue and type 2 ferlins in yellow. The branch length is indicated in grey.

Immunodetection of a myoferlin-haemagglutinin fusion protein in non-permeabilised COS-7 cells confirmed the presence of the C-terminal domain of the protein in the extracellular compartment [28], supporting the functionality of the putative trans-membrane region. The sublocalisation of ferlins was further studied, indicating robust membrane localisation for dysferlin, myoferlin and Fer1L6 while only low levels of otoferlin were at the plasma membrane and Fer1L5 was intracellular. Dysferlin and myoferlin were localised within the endo-lysosomal pathway accumulating in late endosomes and in recycling compartment. GFP-myoferlin fusion protein revealed that myoferlin was colocalized with lysosomal markers in NIH3T3 cells [29]. Otoferlin has been shown to move from the trans-Golgi network to the plasma membrane and inversely. Fer1L5 was cytosolic while Fer1L6 was detected in a specific sub-compartment of the trans-Golgi network compartment [30].

4. Ferlin's Interactions with Phospholipids

Ferlins are regarded as intrinsic membrane proteins through their putative transmembrane region. However, they can also interact with membranes by other domains. Experimentally, myoferlin C2A was the single C2 domain able to bind to phospholipid vesicles. A significant presence of the negatively charged phosphatidylserine (PS) was required for this interaction. Myoferlin C2A binding to PS-containing vesicles did not occur with calcium concentration similar to the one observed in the basal physiological condition (0.1 μM). Indeed, the half-maximal binding was observed at 1 μM [31], suggesting that the C2A domain is involved in specific processes inside the cell requiring Ca^{2+} release from intracellular stock, like in Ca^{2+}-regulated exocytosis. When cells are stimulated by various means, including depolarization and ligand binding, the cytosolic Ca^{2+} concentration increases to the concentration up to 1 μM or more [32], similar to the one required by myoferlin C2A domain to bind lipids. It appears that dysferlin C2A domain has the same binding properties as myoferlin C2A domain. However, its half-maximal lipid binding was higher (4.5 μM) [31]. A recent publication confirmed that myoferlin and dysferlin C2A domains exhibit different Ca^{2+} affinities. However, they describe myoferlin C2A domain with a lower Ca^{2+} affinity than the dysferlin homolog C2 domain, and a marginal binding of myoferlin C2A domain to phospholipid mixture containing PS [33]. The binding of dysferlin C2A to PS was confirmed and extended to several phosphoinositide monophosphates in a Ca^{2+}-dependent fashion. Therrien et al. observed that all remaining dysferlin C2 domains were able to bind to PS but independently of Ca^{2+} [34]. The laurdan fluorescence emission experiments suggest that dysferlin and myoferlin contribute to increase the lipid order in lipid vesicles. The magnitude of this observation was calcium-enhanced and C2 domains within both N- and C-termini of ferlins influenced lipid packing. The experiments conducted with individual recombinant ferlin's C2A-C domains demonstrated that all of them are able to increase lipid order [35].

The authors described in the first part of this review the conservation of the 5 Ca^{2+}-binding aspartate residues in the C2D-F domains of otoferlin making them putative Ca^{2+}-binding sites. In addition to its C2D-F domains, otoferlin is also able to bind Ca^{2+} via its C2B and C2C domains [36]. Despite the fact that C2A domain from otoferlin does not possess all five aspartate residues, its ability to bind Ca^{2+} is still under debate. Therrien and colleagues showed that otoferlin C2A domain can bind PS in a Ca^{2+}-dependent fashion, suggesting an interaction with this ion [34]. This interaction was confirmed by a direct measure of otoferlin-binding to liposomes in the presence of Ca^{2+} (1 mM). Moreover, C2A-C domains seem to bind lipids also under calcium free conditions [36]. At the opposite, a spectroscopy analysis indicates that otoferlin C2A domain is unable to coordinate Ca^{2+} ion [37].

Floatation assays were unable to confirm the interaction between otoferlin C2A and lipids. This may be due to the presence of a shorter membrane-interacting loop at the top of the domain [37]. As for dysferlin and myoferlin, otoferlin increases lipid order in vesicles. However, its C2A does not participate to the phenomenon [35].

Ferlin proteins contain also a FerA domain recently described as a four-helix bundle fold with its own Ca^{2+}-dependent phospholipid-binding activity [38].

5. Ferlin's Main Functions in Non-Neoplastic Cells and Tissues

5.1. *In Mammal Muscle Cells*

Dysferlin and myoferlin have a specific temporal pattern of expression in an in vitro model of muscle development. Myoferlin was highly expressed in myoblasts that have elongated prior to fusion to syncytial myotubes. After fusion, myoferlin expression was decreased. The dysferlin expression increased concomitantly with the fusion and maturation of myotubes [31]. A proteomic analysis revealed the interacting partners of dysferlin during muscle differentiation [39]. It appeared that the number of partners decreases during the differentiation process, while the core-set of partners is large (115 proteins). Surprisingly, the dysferlin homolog myoferlin was consistently co-immunoprecipitated with dysferlin. The gene ontology analysis of the core-set proteins indicates that the highest ranked clusters are related to vesicle trafficking. In the C2C12 myoblast model, immunoprecipitation experiments showed that myoferlin interacts with the Eps15 Homology Domain 2 (EHD2) apparently through a NPF (asparagine-proline-phenylalanine) motif in its C2B domain [40]. EHD2 has been implicated in endocytic recycling. It was inferred that the interaction between EHD2 and myoferlin might indirectly regulate disassembly or reorganization of the cytoskeleton that accompanies myoblast fusion.

Dysferlin-null mice develop a slowly progressive muscular dystrophy with a loss of plasma membrane integrity. The presence of a stable and functional dystrophin–glycoprotein complex (DGC), involved in muscle injury-susceptibility when altered, suggests that dysferlin has a role in sarcolemma repair process. This was confirmed in dysferlin-null mice by a markedly delayed membrane resealing, even in the presence of Ca^{2+} [41]. Pharmacological experiments conducted in skeletal muscles demonstrated that dysferlin modulates smooth reticulum Ca^{2+} release and that in its absence injuries cause an increased ryanodine receptor (RyR1)-mediated Ca^{2+} leak from the smooth reticulum into the cytoplasm [42]. In the SJL/J mice model of dysferlinopathy, annexin-1 and -2 co-precipitate with muscle dysferlin and co-localise at sarcolemma in an injury-dependent manner [43]. An immunofluorescence analysis of mitochondrial respiratory chain complexes in the muscles from the patients with dysferlinopathy revealed complex I- and complex IV-deficient myofibers [44]. This report is particularly interesting in light of the dysferlin_v1 alternate transcript discovered in skeletal muscle [45] and harboring a mitochondrial importation signal [39].

Intriguingly, at the site of membrane injury, only the C-terminal extremity of dysferlin was immunodetected. It was reported than dysferlin was cleaved by calpain [46], one of its interacting proteins [39]. The cleavage generate a C-terminal fragment called mini-dysferlin$_{C72}$ bearing two cytoplasmic C2 domains anchored by a transmembrane domain [46]. Myoferlin expression is also up regulated in damaged myofibers and in surrounding mononuclear muscle and inflammatory cells [13]. As it was observed for dysferlin, myoferlin can be cleaved by calpain to produce a mini-myoferlin module composed of the C2E and C2F domains [47].

Membrane repair requires the accumulation and fusion of vesicles with each other and with plasma membrane at the disruption point. A role for dysferlin and myoferlin in these processes is consistent with the presence of several C2 domains and with their homology with FER-1 having a role in vesicle fusion. Moreover, mini-dysferlin and mini-myoferlin bear structural resemblance to synaptotagmin, a well-known actor in synaptic vesicle fusion with the presynaptic membrane [48].

In mouse skeletal muscle, myoferlin was found at the nuclear and plasma membrane [5]. It is highly expressed in myoblasts before their fusion to myotubes [10,31] and found to be highly concentrated at the site of apposed myoblast and myotube membranes, and at site of contact between two myotubes [10]. Myoblast fusion requires a Ca^{2+} concentration increase to 1.4 μM [49], similar to the one reported for myoferlin C2A binding to phospholipids [31]. Myoferlin-null mice myoblasts show impaired fusion in vitro, producing mice with smaller muscles and smaller myofibers in vivo [10]. All together, these observations support a role for myoferlin in the maturation of myotubes and the formation of large myotubes that arise from the fusion of myoblasts to multinucleated myotubes.

Interestingly, myoferlin-null mice are unresponsive to IGF-1 for the myoblast fusion to the pre-existing myofibers. Mechanistic experiments indicate a defect in IGF-1 internalization and a redirection of the IGF1R to the lysosomal degradation pathway instead of recycling. As expected, myoferlin-null myoblasts lacked the IGF1-induced increase in AKT and MAPK activity downstream to IGFR [50].

The defects in myoblast fusion and muscle repair observed in myoferlin-null mice are reminiscent of what was reported in muscle lacking nuclear factor of activated T-cells (NFAT). Demonbreun and colleagues suggested that in injured myofibers, the membrane damages induce an intracellular increase of Ca^{2+} concentration producing a calcineurin-dependent NFAT activation and subsequent translocation to the nucleus. The activated NFAT can therefore bind to its response element on the myoferlin promoter [13].

Using HeLa and HEK293T cell lines overexpressing ADAM-12, it was discovered that myoferlin was one of the ten most abundant interacting partners of ADAM-12 [51]. Though this was discovered in an artificial overexpressing model using cancer cells, it can be considered as pertinent in the context of muscle cell repair. Indeed, ADAM-12 is a marker of skeletal muscle regeneration interacting with the actin-binding protein α-actinin-2 in the context of myoblast fusion [52].

The differentiating myoblast C2C12 expressed Fer1L5 at the protein level with an expression pattern similar to dysferlin throughout myoblast differentiation. Fer1L5 shares with myoferlin a NPF motif in its C2B domain. As in myoferlin, this motif was described as interacting with EHD2, but also with EHD1 [53].

5.2. *In mammal Inner Ear Cells*

In adult mouse cochlea, otoferlin gene expression is limited to inner hair cells (IHC) [4]. In these cells, the strongest immunostaining of otoferlin was associated with the basolateral region, where the afferent synaptic contacts are located, suggesting that otoferlin is a component of the IHC presynaptic machinery. Ultrastructural observations confirmed the association of otoferlin with the synaptic vesicles. It appears that otoferlin is not necessary for the synapse formation [54], but rather regulates the Ca^{2+}-induced synaptic vesicle exocytosis [36].

At molecular level, otoferlin interacts with plasma membrane t-SNARE (*soluble N-ethylmaleimide-sensitive-factor attachment protein receptor)* proteins (syntaxin 1 and SNAP-25) in a Ca^{2+}-dependent manner [54]. Supporting this discovery, both t-SNARE proteins are known to interact with synaptotagmin I, a C2 domain harbouring protein, in the context of the classical synaptic vesicles docking [55,56]. It was reported that otoferlin relies on C2F domain for its Ca^{2+}-dependent interaction with t-SNARE [57–59]. However, others suggest a Ca^{2+}-dependent interaction through the C2C, C2D, C2E and C2F domains and a Ca^{2+}-independent interaction via the C2A and C2B domains. The SNARE-mediated membrane fusion was reconstituted with proteoliposomes. This assay indicates that in presence of Ca^{2+}, otoferlin accelerates the fusion process [36], suggesting that otoferlin operates as a calcium-sensor for SNARE-mediated membrane fusion.

5.3. *In Mammal Endothelial Cells*

Bernatchez and colleagues reported that dysferlin and myoferlin are abundant in caveolae-enriched membrane microdomains/lipid rafts (CEM/LR) isolated from human endothelial cells and are highly expressed in mouse blood vessels [28,60]. As observed for dysferlin in muscle cells, myoferlin regulates the endothelial cell membrane resealing after physical damage. In endothelial cells, myoferlin silencing reduced or abolished the ERK-1/2, JNK or PLCγ phosphorylation by VEGF, resulting from a loss of VEGFR-2 stabilization at the membrane. Indeed, myoferlin silencing caused an increase in VEGFR2 polyubiquitination, which leads to its degradation [28]. In contrast to what was observed in myoferlin-silenced endothelial cells, dysferlin gene silencing decrease neither VEGFR2 expression nor its downstream signalling. However, dysferlin-siRNA treated endothelial cells showed a near-complete inhibition of proliferation when they were sub-confluent. The proliferation decrease seems to be due to an impaired attachment rather than to cell death, as supported by adhesion assays and PECAM-1 poly-ubiquitination that leads to its degradation. Co-immunoprecipitation and co-localisation experiments support the formation of a molecular complex between dysferlin and PECAM-1. This PECAM-1 degradation leads, in dysferlin-null mice, to a blunted VEGF-induced angiogenesis [60]. Another angiogenic tyrosine kinase receptor Tie-2 (tyrosine kinase with Ig and epidermal growth factor homology domains-2) is significantly less expressed at the plasma membrane when myoferlin is silenced in endothelial cells [61]. In this case, it appears that proteasomal degradation plays a minor role in the down regulation of the receptor. Strikingly, G-protein coupled receptors (GCPR) were unaffected by the decrease of myoferlin expression, suggesting a selective effect on receptor tyrosine kinases (RTK).

It was also reported that in endothelial cells, myoferlin is required for an efficient clathrin and caveolae/raft-dependent endocytosis, is co-localized with Dynamin-2 protein [62] and that the FASL-induced lysosome fusion to plasma membrane is mediated by dysferlin C2A domain [63].

5.4. Other Mammal's Cells

Dysferlin and myoferlin are expressed in both basal and ciliated airway epithelial cells from healthy human lungs [64]. In the airway epithelial cell line (16HBE), dysferlin and myoferlin were immuno-detected at the plasma membrane, Golgi membrane and in cytoplasm but not in the nuclei. The silencing of myoferlin in these cells induces the loss of zonula occludens (ZO)-1, inducing apoptosis [64].

Myoferlin was also detected in exosomes from human eye trabecular meshwork cells [65] and in phagocytes where it participates to the fusion between lysosomes and the plasma membrane, thus promoting the release of lysosomal contents [29].

The Fer1L5 gene expression was largely restricted to the pancreas, where it was alternatively spliced by removing exon 51 [30].

6. Ferlins in Cancer, Potential Targets to Kill Cancer

It is clear from the data above that ferlins are consistently involved in membrane processes requiring membrane fusion, including endocytosis, exocytosis, membrane repair, recycling and remodelling. Membrane processes are of extreme importance for cell survival and signalling, making them core machinery for cancer cell adaptation to hostile environments.

Considering that ferlins have been only scarcely investigated in cancer, the authors next sought to mine publicly available databases and gain information regarding ferlin's expression or mutation in tumors. Using the FireBrowse gene expression viewer (firebrowse.org), The Cancer Genome Atlas (TCGA) RNAseq data of all ferlin's genes in neoplastic tissues were investigated in order to obtain a differential expression in comparison to their normal counterparts. It appears that all ferlin genes are modulated in several cancer types. Myoferlin and fer1l4 genes are more frequently up regulated than down regulated, while dysferlin, fer1l5, and fer1l6 are more frequently down regulated (Figure 2).

Experimentally, a myoferlin gene was discovered as highly expressed in several tumour tissues including the pancreas [66,67], breast [68], kidneys [68], and head and neck squamous cell carcinoma (HNSCC) [69]. This expression was confirmed at a protein level in tumour tissue and/or cell lines, from the pancreas [70–73], breast [74,75], lungs [75], melanoma [75], hepatocellular carcinoma [76], HNSCC [77], clear cell renal carcinoma [78,79], and endometroid carcinoma [80]. Myoferlin was also detected at a protein level in microvesicles/exosomes derived from several cancer cells including the bladder [81], colon [82–85], ovary [86], prostate [87], breast and pancreas, where it plays a role in vesicle fusion with the recipient endothelial cells [88].

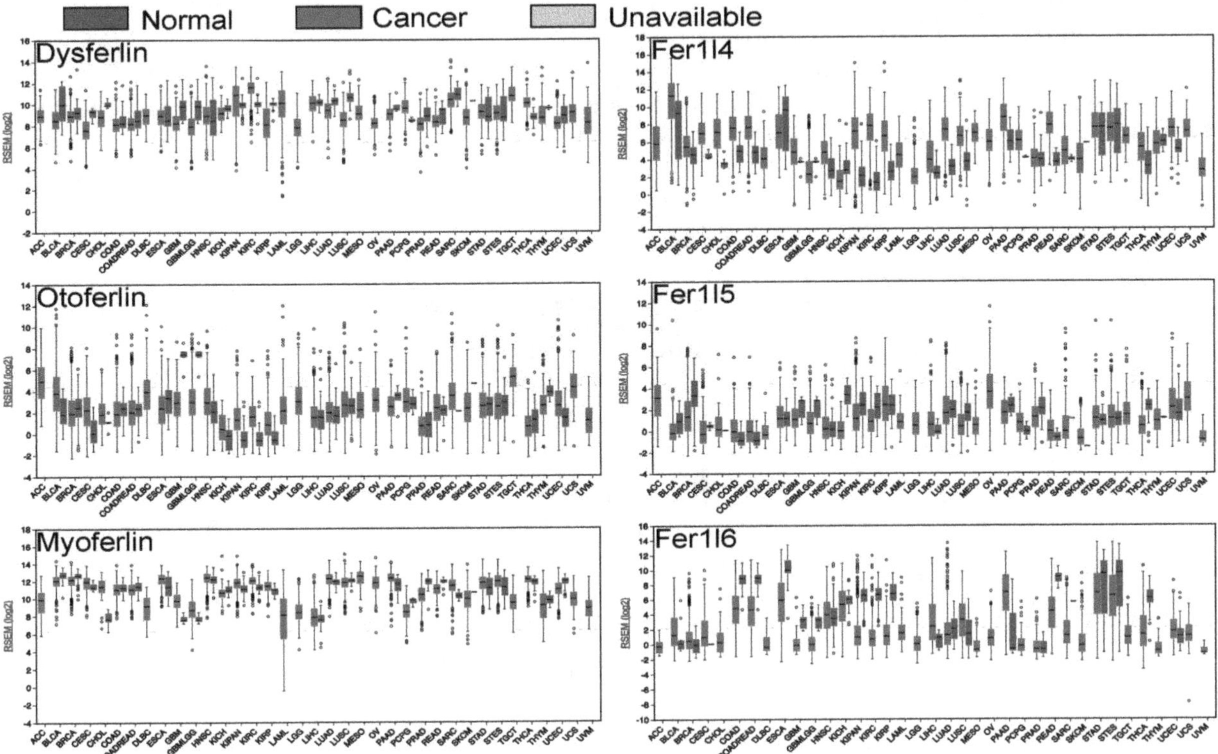

Figure 2. Ferlin gene expression in several cancers (red) and their normal counterparts (blue). Cancer tissues from adrenocortical carcinoma (ACC), bladder urothelial carcinoma (BLCA), breast invasive carcinoma (BRCA), cervical squamous cell carcinoma and endocervical adenocarcinoma (CESC), cholangiocarcinoma (CHOL), colon adenocarcinoma (COAD), colorectal adenocarcinoma (COADREAD), lymphoid neoplasm diffuse large B-cell lymphoma (DLBC), esophageal carcinoma (ESCA), glioblastoma multiforme (GBM), glioma (GBMLGG), head and neck squamous cell carcinoma (HNSC), kidney chromophobe (KICH), pan-kidney cohort (KIPAN), kidney renal clear cell carcinoma (KIRC), kidney renal papillary cell carcinoma (KIRP), acute myeloid leukemia (LAML), brain lower grade glioma (LGG), liver hepatocellular carcinoma (LIHC), lung adenocarcinoma (LUAD), lung squamous cell carcinoma (LUBC), mesothelioma (MESO), ovarian serous cystadenocarcinoma (OV), pancreatic adenocarcinoma (PAAD), pheochromocytoma and paraganglioma (PCPG), prostate adenocarcinoma (PRAD), rectum adenocarcinoma (READ), sarcoma (SARC), skin cutaneous melanoma (SKCM), stomach adenocarcinoma (STAD), stomach and esophageal carcinoma (STES), testicular germ cell tumours (TGCT), thyroid carcinoma (THCA), thymoma (THYM), uterine corpus endometrial carcinoma (UCEC), uterine carcinosarcoma (UCS), uveal melanoma (UVM).

This review then explored the mutations occurring in ferlin genes in tumours using Tumorportal (http://www.tumorportal.org) [89]. Several mutations were reported in ferlin genes in a few cancer types. However, none of them were considered as significant. Survival was also analysed (Table 3) using a pan-cancer method available online (OncoLnc–http://www.oncolnc.org) and combining mRNAs, miRNAs, and lncRNAs expression [90]. Noticeably, otoferlin expression was strongly significantly correlated with survival in renal clear cell carcinoma (KIRC–$p < 10^{-5}$); myoferlin expression was strongly significantly correlated with survival in brain lower grade glioma (LGG–$p < 10^{-4}$) and pancreatic adenocarcinoma (PAAD–$p < 10^{-4}$), and Fer1l4 expression was strongly significantly correlated with survival in bladder urothelial carcinoma (BLCA–$p < 10^{-5}$) and kidney renal clear cell carcinoma (KIRC–$p < 10^{-5}$). The 5 more significant correlations between ferlin's expression and the overall survival were represented as Kaplan-Meier curves with their associated log-rank p-value (Figure 3).

Table 3. Survival analysis by a Cox regression.

Positive Association			Negative Association		
Cohort	**Cox Coefficient**	**p-Value**	**Cohort**	**Cox Coefficient**	**p-Value**
		DYSF EXPRESSION			
CESC	0.266	$4.20e^{-02}$	SARC	−0.277	$1.00e^{-02}$
STAD	0.171	$4.80e^{-02}$	KIRC	−0.220	$1.00e^{-02}$
		OTOF EXPRESSION			
KIRC	**0.377**	$\mathbf{1.50e^{-06}}$	BLCA	−0.275	$4.50e^{-04}$
KIRP	0.413	$4.90e^{-03}$	SKCM	−0.169	$1.40e^{-02}$
		MYOF EXPRESSION			
LGG	**0.441**	$\mathbf{1.40e^{-05}}$	SKCM	−0.163	$1.90e^{-02}$
PAAD	**0.561**	$\mathbf{1.70e^{-05}}$			
LAML	0.215	$4.70e^{-02}$			
		FER1L4 EXPRESSION			
KIRC	**0.356**	$\mathbf{5.20e^{-06}}$	**BLCA**	**−0.383**	$\mathbf{2.90e^{-06}}$
KIRP	0.492	$1.10e^{-03}$	SKCM	−0.225	$1.10e^{-03}$
LGG	0.244	$4.00e^{-03}$			
		FER1L5 EXPRESSION			
LUAD	−0.199	$1.30e^{-02}$			
		FER1L6 EXPRESSION			
KIRC	−0.160	$4.80e^{-02}$			
READ	−0.401	$4.90e^{-02}$			

Ferlin gene expression from cohorts with cancer was submitted to a survival analysis with a Cox regression. The red rows indicate a negative Cox coefficient, the green rows indicate positive Cox coefficient. The bold p-values were considered as highly significant ($p < 10^{-4}$). Bladder urothelial carcinoma (BLCA), cervical squamous cell carcinoma and endocervical adenocarcinoma (CESC), kidney renal clear cell carcinoma (KIRC), kidney renal papillary cell carcinoma (KIRP), acute myeloid leukemia (LAML), brain lower grade glioma (LGG), lung adenocarcinoma (LUAD), pancreatic adenocarcinoma (PAAD), rectum adenocarcinoma (READ), sarcoma (SARC), skin cutaneous melanoma (SKCM), stomach adenocarcinoma (STAD).

Interestingly, a recent publication points out specific single nucleotide polymorphisms in dysferlin genes as significantly associated with pancreas cancer patient survival [91]. Mining the TCGA database, a high Fer1L4 expression was reported as a predictor of a poor prognosis in glioma [92,93] and as an oncogenic driver in several human cancers [94]. However, several other publications pointed it out as a predictor of good prognosis in osteosarcoma [95], gastric cancer [96], endometrial carcinoma [97].

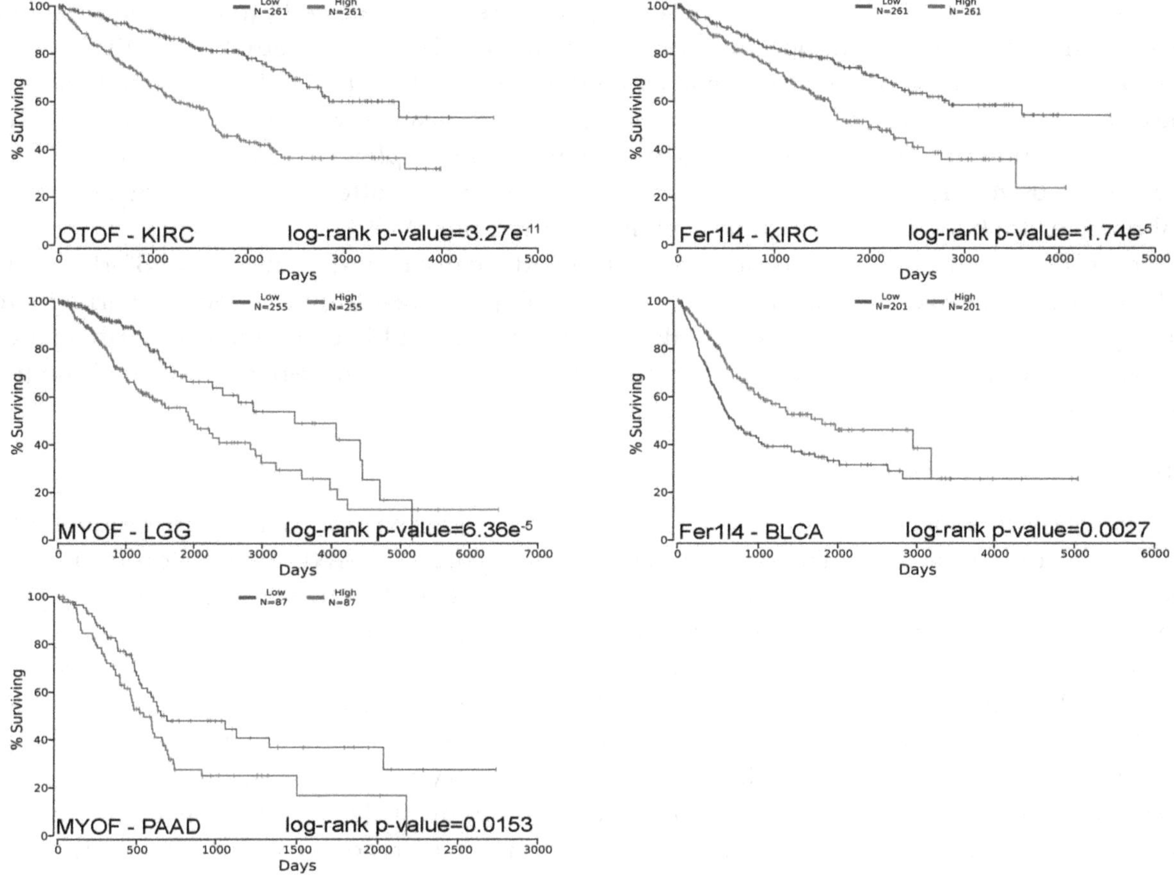

Figure 3. Kaplan-Meier survival curves of patient cohorts with different cancer types. Ferlin gene expression was segregated in low (blue) and high (red) expression according to median in kidney renal clear cell carcinoma (KIRC), brain lower grade glioma (LGG), bladder urothelial carcinoma (BLCA), and pancreatic adenocarcinoma (PAAD).

6.1. Breast Cancer and Melanoma

A mathematical model was proposed to examine the role of myoferlin in cancer cell invasion. This model confirms the experimental observation of decreased invasion of the myoferlin-null breast MDA-MB-231 cell line, and predicts that the pro-invasion effect of myoferlin may be in large partly mediated by MMPs [98]. The model was further validated in vitro suggesting a mesenchymal to epithelial transition (MET) when myoferlin was knockdown [99,100]. Using the same cell model, Blackstone and colleagues showed that myoferlin depletion increased cell adhesion to PET substrate by enhancing focal adhesion kinase (FAK) and its associated protein paxillin (PAX) phosphorylation [101]. Interestingly, myoferlin was reported as regulating the cell migration through a TGF-β1 autocrine loop [102]. Recently, related results were reported in melanoma [103]. Myoferlin expression was first correlated with vasculogenic mimicry (VM) in patients, then its in vitro depletion in A375 cell line impaired VM, migration, and invasion by decreasing MMP-2 production.

Several evidences, obtained from normal endothelial cells, indicate that myoferlin is involved in RTKs recycling (see above). Our group showed that MDA-MB-231 and -468 cells depleted for myoferlin were unable to migrate and to undergo EMT upon EGF stimulation. The authors discovered that myoferlin depletion altered the EGFR fate after ligand binding, most probably by inhibiting the non-clathrin mediated endocytosis [104]. Unexpectedly, myoferlin seemed to be physically associated with lysosomal fraction in MCF-7 cells [105], supporting its involvement in the membrane receptor recycling.

The co-localisation of myoferlin with caveolin-1 [104], the main component of caveolae considered as a metabolic hub [106] prompted our group to investigate the implication of myoferlin in energy metabolism.

In this context, the authors showed in triple-negative breast cancer cells that myoferlin-silencing produces an accumulation of monounsaturated fatty acids (C16:1). Its depletion further decreased oxygen consumption switching the cell metabolism toward glycolysis [107]. This was the first report of the role of myoferlin in mitochondrial function and cell metabolism. A recent report describing the link between dysferlin mutations and mitochondrial respiratory complexes in muscular dysferlinopathy emerged (see above) [44]. It is also intriguing that dysferlin_v1 alternate transcript discovered in skeletal muscle [45] harbours a mitochondrial importation signal [39].

Several breast cancer cell lines and tissues showed a calpain-independent myoferlin cleavage, regardless of cell injuries and subsequent Ca^{2+} influx [108]. The resulting cleaved myoferlin increases ERK phosphorylation in an overexpressing HEK293 system. It would be of interest to further study the link between mini-myoferlin and KRAS mutated cancers as ERK is a mid-pathway signalling protein in this context.

6.2. Pancreas and Colon Cancers

In pancreas adenocarcinoma (PAAD), myoferlin is overexpressed in high grade PAAD in comparison to low grade [73]. The patients with high myoferlin PAAD had a significantly worse prognosis than those with low myoferlin PAAD, with myoferlin appearing as an independent prognosis factor. The experiments undertaken with pancreatic cell lines and siRNA-mediated silencing demonstrated that myoferlin requested to maintain a high proliferation rate. The authors reported that myoferlin is a key element in VEGF exocytosis by PAAD cell lines, correlating with microvessel density in PAAD tissue [109]. Recently, it was demonstrated that myoferlin is critical to maintain mitochondrial structure and oxidative phosphorylation [110]. This discovery was extended to colon cancer where myoferlin seemed also to protect cells from p53-driven apoptosis [111]. The concept claiming that metastatic dissemination relies on oxidative phosphorylation is broadly accepted [112,113]. Based on these reports, the authors discovered that myoferlin was overexpressed in PAAD cells with a high metastatic potential, where it controls mitochondrial respiration [114].

Recently, FER1L4 methylated DNA marker in pancreatic juice has been strongly associated with pancreatic ductal adenocarcinoma suggesting its use as a biomarker for early detection [115].

6.3. Lung Cancer

In mice bearing solid LLC lung tumours, the intratumoral injection of myoferlin siRNA mixed with a lipidic vector reduced the tumour volume by 73%. The observed reduction was neither the consequence of a difference in blood vessel density nor of VEGF secretion. However, a significant reduction of the proportion of the Ki67-positive cells indicated a decrease in cell proliferation [75]. Myoferlin was reported as expressed in human non-small cell lung cancer tissues where it was correlated with VEGFR2, thyroid transcription factor (TTF)-1 and transformation-related protein (p63), especially in the low stage tumours [116].

Recently, it was suggested that long non-coding RNA Fer1L4 negatively controlled proliferation and migration of lung cancer cells, probably through the PI3K/AKT pathway [117]. The same observation was made in osteosarcoma cells [118], esophageal squamous cell carcinoma [119], and hepatocellular carcinoma [120].

6.4. Liver Cancer

In the hepatocellular carcinoma (HCC) cell line, the silencing of the transcriptional coactivator of the serum response factor (SRF), Megakaryoblastic Leukemia 1/2 (MKL1/2), induced a reduction of myoferlin gene expression. It was shown by chromatin immunoprecipitation that MKL1/2 binds effectively to the myoferlin promoter [76]. As in other cancer types, HCC required myoferlin to proliferate and perform invasion or anchorage-independent cell growth. Its depletion enhanced EGFR phosphorylation, in agreement with the concept of myoferlin being a regulator of RTK recycling.

6.5. *Head and Neck Cancer*

A myoferlin expression pattern was investigated in oropharyngeal squamous carcinoma (OPSCC). It was reported that myoferlin was overexpressed in 50% of the cases and significantly associated with worse survival. Moreover, HPV-negative patients had significantly higher expressions of myoferlin. A subgroup survival analysis indicates the interaction between these two parameters as HPV-negative has the worst prognosis when myoferlin is highly expressed. Nuclear myoferlin expression appeared to be highly predictive of the clinical outcome and associated with IL-6 and nanog overexpression [77]. Upon HNSCC cell line stimulation with IL-6, myoferlin dissociates from EHD2 and binds activated STAT3 to drive it in the nucleus. The observation was extended to breast cancer cell lines [69].

6.6. *Gastric Cancer*

Recently, a profiling study reported that FER1L4 was a long non-coding RNA (lncRNA) strongly downregulated in gastric cancer tissue [96], in plasma from gastric cancer patients [121] and in human gastric cancer cell lines [122]. In gastric cancer tissues, FER1L4 lncRNA was associated with the tumour diameter, differentiation state, tumour classification, invasion, metastasis, TNM stage and serum CA72-4. Interestingly, the abundance of this lncRNA decreases in plasma shortly after surgery [121]. The same team reported that the FER1L4 lncRNA is a target of miR-106a-5p [122,123]. The cell depletion in FER1L4 lncRNA resulted in an increase in miR-106a-5p and in a decrease of its endogenous target PTEN, suggesting a competing endogenous RNA (ceRNA) [124] role for FER1L4 lncRNA [122]. The control of miR-106a-5p by FER1L4 lncRNA was extended to colon cancer [125] and HCC [126], while it was described over miR-18a-5p in osteosarcoma [127].

6.7. *Gynecological Cancers*

Lnc Fer1L4 was briefly investigated in ovarian cancer where it was described as downregulated in cancer cells in comparison to normal ovarian epithelial cells [128]. Interestingly, the Fer1L4 expression correlates negatively with the paclitaxel resistance and its re-expression restore the paclitaxel sensitivity through the inhibition of a MAPK signalling pathway.

7. Conclusions

This review clearly shows that all ferlin proteins are membrane-based molecular actors sharing structural similarities. Far beyond their well-described involvement in physiological membrane fusion, several correlations apparently link ferlins, and most particularly myoferlin, to cancer prognosis. However, further investigations are still needed to discover the direct link between myoferlin and cancer biology. Encouragingly, there are many indications that myoferlin depletion interferes with growth factor exocytosis, surface receptor fate determination, exosome composition, and metabolism, indicating the future research axes.

Self-sufficiency in growth factor signalling is a hallmark of cancer cells. Cancer cells overproduce the growth factor to stimulate unregulated proliferation in an autocrine, juxtacrine or paracrine fashions. In this context, myoferlin could be considered as a cancer growth promoter as it helps the exocytosis of the growth factors, at least VEGF. In normal cells, myoferlin was described as involved in receptor tyrosine kinase (EGFR and VEGFR) recycling or expression, allowing as such, the cell response to the growth factors. Knowing that some cancer cells exhibit mutations in tyrosine kinase receptors, which lead to a constitutive receptor activation triggering the downstream pathways, it can be speculated that myoferlin depletion could impede cell proliferation in these cases. This role was indeed described in breast cancer cells [104].

Exosomes are small extracellular vesicles released on exocytosis of multivesicular bodies filled with intraluminal vesicles. They represent an important role in intercellular communication, serving as carrier for the transfer of miRNA and proteins between cells. The exosomes are increasingly described as cancer biomarkers [129] and involved in the preparation of the tumour microenvironment [130].

Interestingly, myoferlin was demonstrated to be present in exosomes isolated from several cancer cell types. However, the biological significance of this localization has still to be investigated.

Metabolism recently integrated the hallmarks of cancer [131], and mitochondria were recognised as key players in cancer metabolism [132]. The indications that myoferlin is necessary for optimal mitochondrial function is a promising avenue in the search for an innovative therapy.

Myoferlin, being overexpressed in several cancer types, offers very promising advantages for cancer diagnosis and targeting. Targeting myoferlin at the expression or functional levels remains, however, the next challenge. Interestingly, recent studies identified new small compounds interacting with the myoferlin C2D domain and demonstrating promising anti-tumoral/metastasis properties in breast and pancreas cancer [133,134].

Gene transfer strategies have undergone profound development in recent years and this is particularly applicable for recessive disorders. The adeno-associated virus (AAV) is a non-pathogenic vector used in a treatment strategy aiming at delivering full-length dysferlin or shorter variants to skeletal muscle in dysferlin-null mice. Several well documented reports demonstrate an improvement in the outcome measures after dysferlin gene therapy [135–138]. Similar AAV vectors were used as a gene delivery system in cancer [139,140], allowing the dream of myoferlin negative-dominant delivery to cancer cells. Moreover, the sleeping beauty transposon system [141] may overcome some of the limitations associated with viral gene transfer vectors and transient non-viral gene delivery approaches that are being used in the majority of ongoing clinical trials.

8. Statistical Methods

The multivariate Cox regressions (Table 3) were performed with the coxph function from the R survival library. For each cancer and data type, OncoLnc attempted to construct a model with gene expression, sex, age, and grade or histology as multivariates [90]. The clinical information was obtained from TCGA and only patients who contained all the necessary clinical information were included in the analysis. The patients were split into low and high expressing according to the median gene expression.

Acknowledgments: The results published here are in whole or part based upon data generated by the TCGA Research Network: http://cancergenome.nih.gov/. AB is a Research Director at the National Fund for Scientific Research (FNRS), Belgium. SA is supported by a FNRS FRIA grant. AT acknowledges LabEx MAbImprove for financial support.

References

1. Bernardes, N.; Fialho, A.M. Perturbing the Dynamics and Organization of Cell Membrane Components: A New Paradigm for Cancer-Targeted Therapies. *Int. J. Mol. Sci.* **2018**, *19*, 3871. [CrossRef] [PubMed]
2. Achanzar, W.E.; Ward, S. A nematode gene required for sperm vesicle fusion. *J. Cell Sci.* **1997**, *110*, 1073–1081. [PubMed]
3. Bashir, R.; Britton, S.; Strachan, T.; Keers, S.; Vafiadaki, E.; Lako, M.; Richard, I.; Marchand, S.; Bourg, N.; Argov, Z.; et al. A gene related to caenorhabditis elegans spermatogenesis factor fer-1 is mutated in limb-girdle muscular dystrophy type 2B. *Nat. Genet.* **1998**, *20*, 37–42. [CrossRef] [PubMed]
4. Yasunaga, S.; Grati, M.; Cohen-Salmon, M.; El-Amraoui, A.; Mustapha, M.; Salem, N.; El-Zir, E.; Loiselet, J.; Petit, C. A mutation in OTOF, encoding otoferlin, a FER-1-like protein, causes DFNB9, a nonsyndromic form of deafness. *Nat. Genet.* **1999**, *21*, 363–369. [CrossRef] [PubMed]
5. Davis, D.B.; Delmonte, A.J.; Ly, C.T.; McNally, E.M. Myoferlin, a candidate gene and potential modifier of muscular dystrophy. *Hum. Mol. Genet.* **2000**, *9*, 217–226. [CrossRef] [PubMed]
6. Britton, S.; Freeman, T.; Vafiadaki, E.; Keers, S.; Harrison, R.; Bushby, K.; Bashir, R. The third human FER-1-like protein is highly similar to dysferlin. *Genomics* **2000**, *68*, 313–321. [CrossRef]

7. Liu, J.; Aoki, M.; Illa, I.; Wu, C.; Fardeau, M.; Angelini, C.; Serrano, C.; Urtizberea, J.A.; Hentati, F.; Hamida, M.B.; et al. Dysferlin, a novel skeletal muscle gene, is mutated in Miyoshi myopathy and limb girdle muscular dystrophy. *Nat. Genet.* **1998**, *20*, 31–36. [CrossRef] [PubMed]
8. Choi, B.Y.; Ahmed, Z.M.; Riazuddin, S.; Bhinder, M.A.; Shahzad, M.; Husnain, T.; Griffith, A.J.; Friedman, T.B. Identities and frequencies of mutations of the otoferlin gene (OTOF) causing DFNB9 deafness in Pakistan. *Clin. Genet.* **2009**, *75*, 237–243. [CrossRef]
9. Tekin, M.; Akcayoz, D.; Incesulu, A. A novel missense mutation in a C2 domain of OTOF results in autosomal recessive auditory neuropathy. *Am. J. Med. Genet. A* **2005**, *138*, 6–10. [CrossRef]
10. Doherty, K.R.; Cave, A.; Davis, D.B.; Delmonte, A.J.; Posey, A.; Earley, J.U.; Hadhazy, M.; McNally, E.M. Normal myoblast fusion requires myoferlin. *Development* **2005**, *132*, 5565–5575. [CrossRef]
11. Kiselev, A.; Vaz, R.; Knyazeva, A.; Sergushichev, A.; Dmitrieva, R.; Khudiakov, A.; Jorholt, J.; Smolina, N.; Sukhareva, K.; Fomicheva, Y.; et al. Truncating variant in myof gene is associated with limb-girdle type muscular dystrophy and cardiomyopathy. *Front. Genet.* **2019**, *10*, 608. [CrossRef] [PubMed]
12. Aoki, M.; Liu, J.; Richard, I.; Bashir, R.; Britton, S.; Keers, S.M.; Oeltjen, J.; Brown, H.E.; Marchand, S.; Bourg, N.; et al. Genomic organization of the dysferlin gene and novel mutations in Miyoshi myopathy. *Neurology* **2001**, *57*, 271–278. [CrossRef] [PubMed]
13. Demonbreun, A.R.; Lapidos, K.A.; Heretis, K.; Levin, S.; Dale, R.; Pytel, P.; Svensson, E.C.; McNally, E.M. Myoferlin regulation by NFAT in muscle injury, regeneration and repair. *J. Cell Sci.* **2010**, *123*, 2413–2422. [CrossRef] [PubMed]
14. Finn, R.D.; Coggill, P.; Eberhardt, R.Y.; Eddy, S.R.; Mistry, J.; Mitchell, A.L.; Potter, S.C.; Punta, M.; Qureshi, M.; Sangrador-Vegas, A.; et al. The Pfam protein families database: Towards a more sustainable future. *Nucleic Acids Res.* **2016**, *44*, D279–D285. [CrossRef] [PubMed]
15. Corbalan-Garcia, S.; Gómez-Fernández, J.C. Signaling through C2 domains: More than one lipid target. *Biochim. Biophys. Acta* **2014**, *1838*, 1536–1547. [CrossRef] [PubMed]
16. Zhang, D.; Aravind, L. Identification of novel families and classification of the C2 domain superfamily elucidate the origin and evolution of membrane targeting activities in eukaryotes. *Gene* **2010**, *469*, 18–30. [CrossRef]
17. Nalefski, E.A.; Falke, J.J. The C2 domain calcium-binding motif: Structural and functional diversity. *Protein Sci.* **1996**, *5*, 2375–2390. [CrossRef]
18. Shin, O.-H.; Han, W.; Wang, Y.; Südhof, T.C. Evolutionarily conserved multiple C2 domain proteins with two transmembrane regions (MCTPs) and unusual Ca^{2+} binding properties. *J. Biol. Chem.* **2005**, *280*, 1641–1651. [CrossRef]
19. Min, S.-W.; Chang, W.-P.; Südhof, T.C. E-Syts, a family of membranous Ca^{2+}-sensor proteins with multiple C2 domains. *Proc. Natl. Acad. Sci. USA* **2007**, *104*, 3823–3828. [CrossRef]
20. Rizo, J.; Sudhof, T.C. C2-domains, structure and function of a universal Ca^{2+}-binding domain. *J. Biol. Chem.* **1998**, *273*, 15879–15882. [CrossRef]
21. Von Poser, C.; Ichtchenko, K.; Shao, X.; Rizo, J.; Sudhof, T.C. The evolutionary pressure to inactivate. A subclass of synaptotagmins with an amino acid substitution that abolishes Ca^{2+} binding. *J. Biol. Chem.* **1997**, *272*, 14314–14319. [CrossRef] [PubMed]
22. Lek, A.; Lek, M.; North, K.N.; Cooper, S.T. Phylogenetic analysis of ferlin genes reveals ancient eukaryotic origins. *BMC Evol. Biol.* **2010**, *10*, 231. [CrossRef] [PubMed]
23. Washington, N.L.; Ward, S. FER-1 regulates Ca^{2+}-mediated membrane fusion during C. elegans spermatogenesis. *J. Cell Sci.* **2006**, *119*, 2552–2562. [CrossRef] [PubMed]
24. Yan, M.; Rachubinski, D.A.; Joshi, S.; Rachubinski, R.A.; Subramani, S. Dysferlin domain-containing proteins, Pex30p and Pex31p, localized to two compartments, control the number and size of oleate-induced peroxisomes in Pichia pastoris. *Mol. Biol. Cell.* **2008**, *19*, 885–898. [CrossRef] [PubMed]
25. Patel, P.; Harris, R.; Geddes, S.M.; Strehle, E.-M.; Watson, J.D.; Bashir, R.; Bushby, K.; Driscoll, P.C.; Keep, N.H. Solution Structure of the Inner DysF Domain of Myoferlin and Implications for Limb Girdle Muscular Dystrophy Type 2B. *J. Mol. Biol.* **2008**, *379*, 981–990. [CrossRef] [PubMed]
26. Fuson, K.; Rice, A.; Mahling, R.; Snow, A.; Nayak, K.; Shanbhogue, P.; Meyer, A.G.; Redpath, G.M.I.; Hinderliter, A.; Cooper, S.T.; et al. Alternate splicing of dysferlin C2A confers Ca^{2+}-dependent and Ca^{2+}-independent binding for membrane repair. *Structure* **2014**, *22*, 104–115. [CrossRef] [PubMed]

27. Aartsma-Rus, A.; Van Deutekom, J.C.T.; Fokkema, I.F.; Van Ommen, G.-J.B.; Den Dunnen, J.T. Entries in the Leiden Duchenne muscular dystrophy mutation database: An overview of mutation types and paradoxical cases that confirm the reading-frame rule. *Muscle Nerve* **2006**, *34*, 135–144. [CrossRef] [PubMed]
28. Bernatchez, P.N.; Acevedo, L.; Fernandez-Hernando, C.; Murata, T.; Chalouni, C.; Kim, J.; Erdjument-Bromage, H.; Shah, V.; Gratton, J.-P.; McNally, E.M.; et al. Myoferlin regulates vascular endothelial growth factor receptor-2 stability and function. *J. Biol. Chem.* **2007**, *282*, 30745–30753. [CrossRef]
29. Miyatake, Y.; Yamano, T.; Hanayama, R. Myoferlin-Mediated Lysosomal Exocytosis Regulates Cytotoxicity by Phagocytes. *J. Immunol.* **2018**, *201*, 3051–3057. [CrossRef]
30. Redpath, G.M.I.; Sophocleous, R.A.; Turnbull, L.; Whitchurch, C.B.; Cooper, S.T. Ferlins Show Tissue-Specific Expression and Segregate as Plasma Membrane/Late Endosomal or Trans-Golgi/Recycling Ferlins. *Traffic* **2016**, *17*, 245–266. [CrossRef]
31. Davis, D.B.; Doherty, K.R.; Delmonte, A.J.; McNally, E.M. Calcium-sensitive phospholipid binding properties of normal and mutant ferlin C2 domains. *J. Biol. Chem.* **2002**, *277*, 22883–22888. [CrossRef] [PubMed]
32. Bootman, M.D.; Rietdorf, K.; Hardy, H.; Dautova, Y.; Corps, E.; Pierro, C.; Stapleton, E.; Kang, E.; Proudfoot, D. Calcium Signalling and Regulation of Cell Function. In *eLS*; John Wiley & Sons, Ltd.: Chichester, UK, 2012; pp. 1–14.
33. Harsini, F.M.; Bui, A.A.; Rice, A.M.; Chebrolu, S.; Fuson, K.L.; Turtoi, A.; Bradberry, M.; Chapman, E.R.; Sutton, R.B. Structural Basis for the Distinct Membrane Binding Activity of the Homologous C2A Domains of Myoferlin and Dysferlin. *J. Mol. Biol.* **2019**, *431*, 2112–2126. [CrossRef] [PubMed]
34. Therrien, C.; Fulvio, S.D.; Pickles, S.; Sinnreich, M. Characterization of lipid binding specificities of dysferlin C2 domains reveals novel interactions with phosphoinositides. *Biochemistry* **2009**, *48*, 2377–2384. [CrossRef] [PubMed]
35. Marty, N.J.; Holman, C.L.; Abdullah, N.; Johnson, C.P. The C2 domains of otoferlin, dysferlin, and myoferlin alter the packing of lipid bilayers. *Biochemistry* **2013**, *52*, 5585–5592. [CrossRef] [PubMed]
36. Johnson, C.P.; Chapman, E.R. Otoferlin is a calcium sensor that directly regulates SNARE-mediated membrane fusion. *J. Cell Biol.* **2010**, *191*, 187–197. [CrossRef] [PubMed]
37. Helfmann, S.; Neumann, P.; Tittmann, K.; Moser, T.; Ficner, R.; Reisinger, E. The Crystal Structure of the C2A Domain of Otoferlin Reveals an Unconventional Top Loop Region. *J. Mol. Biol.* **2011**, *406*, 479–490. [CrossRef]
38. Harsini, F.M.; Chebrolu, S.; Fuson, K.L.; White, M.A.; Rice, A.M.; Sutton, R.B. FerA is a Membrane-Associating Four-Helix Bundle Domain in the Ferlin Family of Membrane-Fusion Proteins. *Sci. Rep.* **2018**, *8*, 10949. [CrossRef]
39. De Morrée, A.; Hensbergen, P.J.; van Haagen, H.H.; Dragan, I.; Deelder, A.M.; AC't Hoen, P.; Frants, R.R.; van der Maarel, S.M. Proteomic analysis of the dysferlin protein complex unveils its importance for sarcolemmal maintenance and integrity. *PLoS ONE* **2010**, *5*, e13854. [CrossRef]
40. Doherty, K.R.; Demonbreun, A.R.; Wallace, G.Q.; Cave, A.; Posey, A.D.; Heretis, K.; Pytel, P.; McNally, E.M. The endocytic recycling protein EHD2 interacts with myoferlin to regulate myoblast fusion. *J. Biol. Chem.* **2008**, *283*, 20252–20260. [CrossRef]
41. Bansal, D.; Miyake, K.; Vogel, S.S.; Groh, S.; Chen, C.-C.; Williamson, R.; McNeil, P.L.; Campbell, K.P. Defective membrane repair in dysferlin-deficient muscular dystrophy. *Nature* **2003**, *423*, 168–172. [CrossRef]
42. Lukyanenko, V.; Muriel, J.M.; Bloch, R.J. Coupling of excitation to Ca^{2+} release is modulated by dysferlin. *J. Physiol.* **2017**, *595*, 5191–5207. [CrossRef] [PubMed]
43. Lennon, N.J.; Kho, A.; Bacskai, B.J.; Perlmutter, S.L.; Hyman, B.T.; Brown, R.H. Dysferlin Interacts with Annexins A1 and A2 and Mediates Sarcolemmal Wound-healing. *J. Biol. Chem.* **2003**, *278*, 50466–50473. [CrossRef] [PubMed]
44. Vincent, A.E.; Rosa, H.S.; Alston, C.L.; Grady, J.P.; Rygiel, K.A.; Rocha, M.C.; Barresi, R.; Taylor, R.W.; Turnbull, D.M. Dysferlin mutations and mitochondrial dysfunction. *Neuromuscul. Disord.* **2016**, *26*, 782–788. [CrossRef]
45. Pramono, Z.A.D.; Lai, P.S.; Tan, C.L.; Takeda, S.; Yee, W.C. Identification and characterization of a novel human dysferlin transcript: Dysferlin_v1. *Hum. Genet.* **2006**, *120*, 410–419. [CrossRef] [PubMed]
46. Lek, A.; Evesson, F.J.; Lemckert, F.A.; Redpath, G.M.I.; Lueders, A.-K.; Turnbull, L.; Whitchurch, C.B.; North, K.N.; Cooper, S.T. Calpains, cleaved mini-dysferlinC72, and L-type channels underpin calcium-dependent muscle membrane repair. *J. Neurosci.* **2013**, *33*, 5085–5094. [CrossRef]

47. Redpath, G.M.I.; Woolger, N.; Piper, A.K.; Lemckert, F.A.; Lek, A.; Greer, P.A.; North, K.N.; Cooper, S.T. Calpain cleavage within dysferlin exon 40a releases a synaptotagmin-like module for membrane repair. *Mol. Biol. Cell.* **2014**, *25*, 3037–3048. [CrossRef] [PubMed]
48. O'Connor, V.; Lee, A.G. Synaptic vesicle fusion and synaptotagmin: 2B or not 2B? *Nat. Neurosci.* **2002**, *5*, 823–824. [CrossRef]
49. Przybylski, R.J.; Szigeti, V.; Davidheiser, S.; Kirby, A.C. Calcium regulation of skeletal myogenesis. II. Extracellular and cell surface effects. *Cell Calcium* **1994**, *15*, 132–142. [CrossRef]
50. Demonbreun, A.R.; Posey, A.D.; Heretis, K.; Swaggart, K.A.; Earley, J.U.; Pytel, P.; McNally, E.M. Myoferlin is required for insulin-like growth factor response and muscle growth. *FASEB J.* **2010**, *24*, 1284–1295. [CrossRef]
51. Zhou, Y.; Xiong, L.; Zhang, Y.; Yu, R.; Jiang, X.; Xu, G. Quantitative proteomics identifies myoferlin as a novel regulator of A Disintegrin and Metalloproteinase 12 in HeLa cells. *J. Proteom.* **2016**, *148*, 94–104. [CrossRef]
52. Galliano, M.F.; Huet, C.; Frygelius, J.; Polgren, A.; Wewer, U.M.; Engvall, E. Binding of ADAM12, a marker of skeletal muscle regeneration, to the muscle-specific actin-binding protein, α-actinin-2, is required for myoblast fusion. *J. Biol. Chem.* **2000**, *275*, 13933–13939. [CrossRef] [PubMed]
53. Posey, A.D.; Pytel, P.; Gardikiotes, K.; Demonbreun, A.R.; Rainey, M.; George, M.; Band, H.; McNally, E.M. Endocytic recycling proteins EHD1 and EHD2 interact with fer-1-like-5 (Fer1L5) and mediate myoblast fusion. *J. Biol. Chem.* **2011**, *286*, 7379–7388. [CrossRef] [PubMed]
54. Roux, I.; Safieddine, S.; Nouvian, R.; Grati, M.; Simmler, M.-C.; Bahloul, A.; Perfettini, I.; Le Gall, M.; Rostaing, P.; Hamard, G.; et al. Otoferlin, defective in a human deafness form, is essential for exocytosis at the auditory ribbon synapse. *Cell* **2006**, *127*, 277–289. [CrossRef] [PubMed]
55. Chapman, E.R.; Hanson, P.I.; An, S.; Jahn, R. Ca^{2+} regulates the interaction between synaptotagmin and syntaxin 1. *J. Biol. Chem.* **1995**, *270*, 23667–23671. [CrossRef] [PubMed]
56. Mohrmann, R.; de Wit, H.; Connell, E.; Pinheiro, P.S.; Leese, C.; Bruns, D.; Davletov, B.; Verhage, M.; Sørensen, J.B. Synaptotagmin interaction with SNAP-25 governs vesicle docking, priming, and fusion triggering. *J. Neurosci.* **2013**, *33*, 14417–14430. [CrossRef] [PubMed]
57. Ramakrishnan, N.A.; Drescher, M.J.; Drescher, D.G. Direct interaction of otoferlin with syntaxin 1A, SNAP-25, and the L-type voltage-gated calcium channel Cav1.3. *J. Biol. Chem.* **2009**, *284*, 1364–1372. [CrossRef] [PubMed]
58. Ramakrishnan, N.A.; Drescher, M.J.; Morley, B.J.; Kelley, P.M.; Drescher, D.G. Calcium regulates molecular interactions of otoferlin with soluble NSF attachment protein receptor (SNARE) proteins required for hair cell exocytosis. *J. Biol. Chem.* **2014**, *289*, 8750–8766. [CrossRef]
59. Hams, N.; Padmanarayana, M.; Qiu, W.; Johnson, C.P. Otoferlin is a multivalent calcium-sensitive scaffold linking SNAREs and calcium channels. *Proc. Natl. Acad. Sci. USA* **2017**, *114*, 8023–8028. [CrossRef] [PubMed]
60. Sharma, A.; Yu, C.; Leung, C.; Trane, A.; Lau, M.; Utokaparch, S.; Shaheen, F.; Sheibani, N.; Bernatchez, P. A new role for the muscle repair protein dysferlin in endothelial cell adhesion and angiogenesis. *Arterioscler. Thromb. Vasc. Biol.* **2010**, *30*, 2196–2204. [CrossRef]
61. Yu, C.; Sharma, A.; Trane, A.; Utokaparch, S.; Leung, C.; Bernatchez, P. Myoferlin gene silencing decreases Tie-2 expression in vitro and angiogenesis in vivo. *Vascul. Pharmacol.* **2011**, *55*, 26–33. [CrossRef]
62. Bernatchez, P.N.; Sharma, A.; Kodaman, P.; Sessa, W.C. Myoferlin is critical for endocytosis in endothelial cells. *Am. J. Physiol. Cell. Physiol.* **2009**, *297*, C484–C492. [CrossRef] [PubMed]
63. Han, W.Q.; Xia, M.; Xu, M.; Boini, K.M.; Ritter, J.K.; Li, N.J.; Li, P.L. Lysosome fusion to the cell membrane is mediated by the dysferlin C2A domain in coronary arterial endothelial cells. *J. Cell Sci.* **2012**, *125*, 1225–1234. [CrossRef] [PubMed]
64. Leung, C.; Shaheen, F.; Bernatchez, P.; Hackett, T.-L. Expression of myoferlin in human airway epithelium and its role in cell adhesion and zonula occludens-1 expression. *PLoS ONE* **2012**, *7*, e40478. [CrossRef] [PubMed]
65. Stamer, W.D.; Hoffman, E.A.; Luther, J.M.; Hachey, D.L.; Schey, K.L. Protein profile of exosomes from trabecular meshwork cells. *J. Proteom.* **2011**, *74*, 796–804. [CrossRef] [PubMed]
66. Iacobuzio-Donahue, C.A.; Maitra, A.; Shen-Ong, G.L.; van Heek, T.; Ashfaq, R.; Meyer, R.; Walter, K.; Berg, K.; Hollingsworth, M.A.; Cameron, J.L.; et al. Discovery of Novel Tumor Markers of Pancreatic Cancer using Global Gene Expression Technology. *Am. J. Pathol.* **2002**, *160*, 1239–1249. [CrossRef]
67. Han, H.; Bearss, D.J.; Browne, L.W.; Calaluce, R.; Nagle, R.B.; Von Hoff, D.D. Identification of differentially expressed genes in pancreatic cancer cells using cDNA microarray. *Cancer Res.* **2002**, *62*, 2890–2896. [PubMed]

68. Amatschek, S.; Koenig, U.; Auer, H.; Steinlein, P.; Pacher, M.; Gruenfelder, A.; Dekan, G.; Vogl, S.; Kubista, E.; Heider, K.-H.; et al. Tissue-wide expression profiling using cDNA subtraction and microarrays to identify tumor-specific genes. *Cancer Res.* **2004**, *64*, 844–856. [CrossRef]
69. Yadav, A.; Kumar, B.; Lang, J.C.; Teknos, T.N.; Kumar, P. A muscle-specific protein "myoferlin" modulates IL-6/STAT3 signaling by chaperoning activated STAT3 to nucleus. *Oncogene* **2017**, *36*, 6374–6382. [CrossRef]
70. McKinney, K.Q.; Lee, Y.Y.; Choi, H.S.; Groseclose, G.; Iannitti, D.A.; Martinie, J.B.; Russo, M.W.; Lundgren, D.H.; Han, D.K.; Bonkovsky, H.L.; et al. Discovery of putative pancreatic cancer biomarkers using subcellular proteomics. *J. Proteom.* **2011**, *74*, 79–88. [CrossRef]
71. Turtoi, A.; Musmeci, D.; Wang, Y.; Dumont, B.; Somja, J.; Bevilacqua, G.; De Pauw, E.; Delvenne, P.; Castronovo, V. Identification of novel accessible proteins bearing diagnostic and therapeutic potential in human pancreatic ductal adenocarcinoma. *J. Proteome Res.* **2011**, *10*, 4302–4313. [CrossRef]
72. McKinney, K.Q.; Lee, J.-G.; Sindram, D.; Russo, M.W.; Han, D.K.; Bonkovsky, H.L.; Hwang, S.-I. Identification of differentially expressed proteins from primary versus metastatic pancreatic cancer cells using subcellular proteomics. *Cancer Genom. Proteom.* **2012**, *9*, 257–263.
73. Wang, W.S.; Liu, X.H.; Liu, L.X.; Lou, W.H.; Jin, D.Y.; Yang, P.Y.; Wang, X.L. ITRAQ-based quantitative proteomics reveals myoferlin as a novel prognostic predictor in pancreatic adenocarcinoma. *J. Proteom.* **2013**, *91*, 453–465. [CrossRef] [PubMed]
74. Adam, P.J.; Boyd, R.; Tyson, K.L.; Fletcher, G.C.; Stamps, A.; Hudson, L.; Poyser, H.R.; Redpath, N.; Griffiths, M.; Steers, G.; et al. Comprehensive proteomic analysis of breast cancer cell membranes reveals unique proteins with potential roles in clinical cancer. *J. Biol. Chem.* **2003**, *278*, 6482–6489. [CrossRef] [PubMed]
75. Leung, C.; Yu, C.; Lin, M.I.; Tognon, C.; Bernatchez, P. Expression of myoferlin in human and murine carcinoma tumors: Role in membrane repair, cell proliferation, and tumorigenesis. *Am. J. Pathol.* **2013**, *182*, 1900–1909. [CrossRef] [PubMed]
76. Hermanns, C.; Hampl, V.; Holzer, K.; Aigner, A.; Penkava, J.; Frank, N.; Martin, D.E.; Maier, K.C.; Waldburger, N.; Roessler, S.; et al. The novel MKL target gene myoferlin modulates expansion and senescence of hepatocellular carcinoma. *Oncogene* **2017**, *36*, 3464–3476. [CrossRef] [PubMed]
77. Kumar, B.; Brown, N.V.; Swanson, B.J.; Schmitt, A.C.; Old, M.; Ozer, E.; Agrawal, A.; Schuller, D.E.; Teknos, T.N.; Kumar, P. High expression of myoferlin is associated with poor outcome in oropharyngeal squamous cell carcinoma patients and is inversely associated with HPV-status. *Oncotarget* **2016**, *7*, 18665–18677. [CrossRef] [PubMed]
78. Song, D.H.; Ko, G.H.; Lee, J.H.; Lee, J.S.; Yang, J.W.; Kim, M.H.; An, H.J.; Kang, M.H.; Jeon, K.N.; Kim, D.C. Prognostic role of myoferlin expression in patients with clear cell renal cell carcinoma. *Oncotarget* **2017**, *8*, 89033–89039. [CrossRef]
79. Koh, H.M.; An, H.J.; Ko, G.H.; Lee, J.H.; Lee, J.S.; Kim, D.C.; Seo, D.H.; Song, D.H. Identification of Myoferlin Expression for Prediction of Subsequent Primary Malignancy in Patients With Clear Cell Renal Cell Carcinoma. *In Vivo* **2019**, *33*, 1103–1108. [CrossRef]
80. Kim, M.H.; Song, D.H.; Ko, G.H.; Lee, J.H.; Kim, D.C.; Yang, J.W.; Lee, H.I.; An, H.J.; Lee, J.S. Myoferlin expression and its correlation with FIGO histologic grading in early-stage endometrioid carcinoma. *J. Pathol. Transl. Med.* **2018**, *52*, 93–97. [CrossRef]
81. Welton, J.L.; Khanna, S.; Giles, P.J.; Brennan, P.; Brewis, I.A.; Staffurth, J.; Mason, M.D.; Clayton, A. Proteomics analysis of bladder cancer exosomes. *Mol. Cell. Proteom.* **2010**, *9*, 1324–1338. [CrossRef]
82. Mathivanan, S.; Lim, J.W.E.; Tauro, B.J.; Ji, H.; Moritz, R.L.; Simpson, R.J. Proteomics analysis of A33 immunoaffinity-purified exosomes released from the human colon tumor cell line LIM1215 reveals a tissue-specific protein signature. *Mol. Cell. Proteom.* **2010**, *9*, 197–208. [CrossRef] [PubMed]
83. Beckler, M.D.; Higginbotham, J.N.; Franklin, J.L.; Ham, A.-J.; Halvey, P.J.; Imasuen, I.E.; Whitwell, C.; Li, M.; Liebler, D.C.; Coffey, R.J. Proteomic analysis of exosomes from mutant KRAS colon cancer cells identifies intercellular transfer of mutant KRAS. *Mol. Cell. Proteom.* **2013**, *12*, 343–355. [CrossRef] [PubMed]
84. Ji, H.; Greening, D.W.; Barnes, T.W.; Lim, J.W.; Tauro, B.J.; Rai, A.; Xu, R.; Adda, C.; Mathivanan, S.; Zhao, W.; et al. Proteome profiling of exosomes derived from human primary and metastatic colorectal cancer cells reveal differential expression of key metastatic factors and signal transduction components. *Proteomics* **2013**, *13*, 1672–1686. [CrossRef] [PubMed]

85. Choi, D.-S.; Choi, D.-Y.; Hong, B.S.; Jang, S.C.; Kim, D.-K.; Lee, J.; Kim, Y.-K.; Kim, K.P.; Gho, Y.S. Quantitative proteomics of extracellular vesicles derived from human primary and metastatic colorectal cancer cells. *J. Extracell. Vesicles* **2012**, *1*, 18704. [CrossRef] [PubMed]
86. Liang, B.; Peng, P.; Chen, S.; Li, L.; Zhang, M.; Cao, D.; Yang, J.; Li, H.; Gui, T.; Li, X.; et al. Characterization and proteomic analysis of ovarian cancer-derived exosomes. *J. Proteom.* **2013**, *80*, 171–182. [CrossRef] [PubMed]
87. Sandvig, K.; Llorente, A. Proteomic analysis of microvesicles released by the human prostate cancer cell line PC-3. *Mol. Cell. Proteom.* **2012**, *11*, M111-012914. [CrossRef]
88. Blomme, A.; Fahmy, K.; Peulen, O.J.; Costanza, B.; Fontaine, M.; Struman, I.; Baiwir, D.; De Pauw, E.; Thiry, M.; Bellahcène, A.; et al. Myoferlin is a novel exosomal protein and functional regulator of cancer-derived exosomes. *Oncotarget* **2016**, *7*, 83669–83683. [CrossRef]
89. Lawrence, M.S.; Stojanov, P.; Mermel, C.H.; Robinson, J.T.; Garraway, L.A.; Golub, T.R.; Meyerson, M.; Gabriel, S.B.; Lander, E.S.; Getz, G. Discovery and saturation analysis of cancer genes across 21 tumour types. *Nature* **2014**, *505*, 495–501. [CrossRef]
90. Anaya, J. OncoLnc: Linking TCGA survival data to mRNAs, miRNAs, and lncRNAs. *PeerJ Comp. Sci.* **2016**, *2*, e67. [CrossRef]
91. Tang, H.; Wei, P.; Chang, P.; Li, Y.; Yan, D.; Liu, C.; Hassan, M.; Li, D. Genetic polymorphisms associated with pancreatic cancer survival: A genome-wide association study. *Int. J. Cancer* **2017**, *141*, 678–686. [CrossRef]
92. Ding, F.; Tang, H.; Nie, D.; Xia, L. Long non-coding RNA Fer-1-like family member 4 is overexpressed in human glioblastoma and regulates the tumorigenicity of glioma cells. *Oncol. Lett.* **2017**, *14*, 2379–2384. [CrossRef] [PubMed]
93. Xia, L.; Nie, D.; Wang, G.; Sun, C.; Chen, G. FER1L4/miR-372/E2F1 works as a ceRNA system to regulate the proliferation and cell cycle of glioma cells. *J. Cell. Mol. Med.* **2019**, *23*, 3224–3233. [CrossRef] [PubMed]
94. You, Z.; Ge, A.; Pang, D.; Zhao, Y.; Xu, S. Long noncoding RNA FER1L4 acts as an oncogenic driver in human pan-cancer. *J. Cell. Physiol.* **2019**, *1859*, 46. [CrossRef] [PubMed]
95. Chen, Z.-X.; Chen, C.-P.; Zhang, N.; Wang, T.-X. Low-expression of lncRNA FER1L4 might be a prognostic marker in osteosarcoma. *Eur. Rev. Med. Pharmacol. Sci.* **2018**, 22, 2310–2314.
96. Song, H.; Sun, W.; Ye, G.; Ding, X.; Liu, Z.; Zhang, S.; Xia, T.; Xiao, B.; Xi, Y.; Guo, J. Long non-coding RNA expression profile in human gastric cancer and its clinical significances. *J. Transl. Med.* **2013**, *11*, 225. [CrossRef] [PubMed]
97. Kong, Y.; Ren, Z. Overexpression of LncRNA FER1L4 in endometrial carcinoma is associated with favorable survival outcome. *Eur. Rev. Med. Pharmacol. Sci.* **2018**, *22*, 8113–8118.
98. Eisenberg, M.C.; Kim, Y.; Li, R.; Ackerman, W.E.; Kniss, D.A.; Friedman, A. Mechanistic modeling of the effects of myoferlin on tumor cell invasion. *Proc. Natl. Acad. Sci. USA* **2011**, *108*, 20078–20083. [CrossRef]
99. Li, R.; Ackerman, W.E.; Mihai, C.; Volakis, L.I.; Ghadiali, S.; Kniss, D.A. Myoferlin depletion in breast cancer cells promotes mesenchymal to epithelial shape change and stalls invasion. *PLoS ONE* **2012**, *7*, e39766. [CrossRef]
100. Volakis, L.I.; Li, R.; Ackerman, W.E.; Mihai, C.; Bechel, M.; Summerfield, T.L.; Ahn, C.S.; Powell, H.M.; Zielinski, R.; Rosol, T.J.; et al. Loss of myoferlin redirects breast cancer cell motility towards collective migration. *PLoS ONE* **2014**, *9*, e86110. [CrossRef]
101. Blackstone, B.N.; Li, R.; Ackerman, W.E.; Ghadiali, S.N.; Powell, H.M.; Kniss, D.A. Myoferlin depletion elevates focal adhesion kinase and paxillin phosphorylation and enhances cell-matrix adhesion in breast cancer cells. *Am. J. Physiol. Cell. Physiol.* **2015**, *308*, C642–C649. [CrossRef]
102. Barnhouse, V.R.; Weist, J.L.; Shukla, V.C.; Ghadiali, S.N.; Kniss, D.A.; Leight, J.L. Myoferlin regulates epithelial cancer cell plasticity and migration through autocrine TGF-β1 signaling. *Oncotarget* **2018**, *9*, 19209–19222. [CrossRef] [PubMed]
103. Zhang, W.; Zhou, P.; Meng, A.; Zhang, R.; Zhou, Y. Down-regulating Myoferlin inhibits the vasculogenic mimicry of melanoma via decreasing MMP-2 and inducing mesenchymal-to-epithelial transition. *J. Cell. Mol. Med.* **2017**, *155*, 739. [CrossRef] [PubMed]
104. Turtoi, A.; Blomme, A.; Bellahcène, A.; Gilles, C.; Hennequière, V.; Peixoto, P.; Bianchi, E.; Noël, A.; De Pauw, E.; Lifrange, E.; et al. Myoferlin is a key regulator of EGFR activity in breast cancer. *Cancer Res.* **2013**, *73*, 5438–5448. [CrossRef] [PubMed]
105. Nylandsted, J.; Becker, A.C.; Bunkenborg, J.; Andersen, J.S.; Dengjel, J.; Jäättelä, M. ErbB2-associated changes in the lysosomal proteome. *Proteomics* **2011**, *11*, 2830–2838. [CrossRef] [PubMed]

106. Örtegren, U.; Aboulaich, N.; Öst, A.; Strålfors, P. A new role for caveolae as metabolic platforms. *Trends Endocrinol. Metab.* **2007**, *18*, 344–349. [CrossRef] [PubMed]
107. Blomme, A.; Costanza, B.; de Tullio, P.; Thiry, M.; Van Simaeys, G.; Boutry, S.; Doumont, G.; Di Valentin, E.; Hirano, T.; Yokobori, T.; et al. Myoferlin regulates cellular lipid metabolism and promotes metastases in triple-negative breast cancer. *Oncogene* **2017**, *36*, 2116–2130. [CrossRef] [PubMed]
108. Piper, A.-K.; Ross, S.E.; Redpath, G.M.; Lemckert, F.A.; Woolger, N.; Bournazos, A.; Greer, P.A.; Sutton, R.B.; Cooper, S.T. Enzymatic cleavage of myoferlin releases a dual C2-domain module linked to ERK signalling. *Cell. Signal.* **2017**, *33*, 30–40. [CrossRef]
109. Fahmy, K.; Gonzalez, A.; Arafa, M.; Peixoto, P.; Bellahcène, A.; Turtoi, A.; Delvenne, P.; Thiry, M.; Castronovo, V.; Peulen, O.J. Myoferlin plays a key role in VEGFA secretion and impacts tumor-associated angiogenesis in human pancreas cancer. *Int. J. Cancer* **2016**, *138*, 652–663. [CrossRef]
110. Rademaker, G.; Hennequière, V.; Brohée, L.; Nokin, M.-J.; Lovinfosse, P.; Durieux, F.; Gofflot, S.; Bellier, J.; Costanza, B.; Herfs, M.; et al. Myoferlin controls mitochondrial structure and activity in pancreatic ductal adenocarcinoma, and affects tumor aggressiveness. *Oncogene* **2018**, *66*, 1–15. [CrossRef]
111. Rademaker, G.; Costanza, B.; Bellier, J.; Herfs, M.; Peiffer, R.; Agirman, F.; Maloujahmoum, N.; Habraken, Y.; Delvenne, P.; Bellahcène, A.; et al. Human colon cancer cells highly express myoferlin to maintain a fit mitochondrial network and escape p53-driven apoptosis. *Oncogenesis* **2019**, *8*, 21. [CrossRef]
112. LeBleu, V.S.; O'Connell, J.T.; Gonzalez Herrera, K.N.; Wikman, H.; Pantel, K.; Haigis, M.C.; de Carvalho, F.M.; Damascena, A.; Domingos Chinen, L.T.; Rocha, R.M.; et al. PGC-1α mediates mitochondrial biogenesis and oxidative phosphorylation in cancer cells to promote metastasis. *Nat. Cell Biol.* **2014**, *16*, 992–1003. [CrossRef] [PubMed]
113. Porporato, P.E.; Payen, V.L.; Pérez-Escuredo, J.; De Saedeleer, C.J.; Danhier, P.; Copetti, T.; Dhup, S.; Tardy, M.; Vazeille, T.; Bouzin, C.; et al. A mitochondrial switch promotes tumor metastasis. *Cell Rep.* **2014**, *8*, 754–766. [CrossRef] [PubMed]
114. Rademaker, G.; Costanza, B.; Anania, S.; Agirman, F.; Maloujahmoum, N.; Di Valentin, E.; Goval, J.J.; Bellahcène, A.; Castronovo, V.; Peulen, O.J. Myoferlin Contributes to the Metastatic Phenotype of Pancreatic Cancer Cells by Enhancing Their Migratory Capacity through the Control of Oxidative Phosphorylation. *Cancers* **2019**, *11*, 853. [CrossRef] [PubMed]
115. Majumder, S.; Raimondo, M.; Taylor, W.R.; Yab, T.C.; Berger, C.K.; Dukek, B.A.; Cao, X.; Foote, P.H.; Wu, C.W.; Devens, M.E.; et al. Methylated DNA in Pancreatic Juice Distinguishes Patients with Pancreatic Cancer from Controls. *Clin. Gastroenterol. Hepatol.* **2019**. [CrossRef] [PubMed]
116. Song, D.H.; Ko, G.H.; Lee, J.H.; Lee, J.S.; Lee, G.-W.; Kim, H.C.; Yang, J.W.; Heo, R.W.; Roh, G.S.; Han, S.-Y.; et al. Myoferlin expression in non-small cell lung cancer: Prognostic role and correlation with VEGFR-2 expression. *Oncol. Lett.* **2016**, *11*, 998–1006. [CrossRef] [PubMed]
117. Gao, X.; Wang, N.; Wu, S.; Cui, H.; An, X.; Yang, Y. Long non-coding RNA FER1L4 inhibits cell proliferation and metastasis through regulation of the PI3K/AKT signaling pathway in lung cancer cells. *Mol. Med. Rep.* **2019**, *20*, 182–190. [CrossRef] [PubMed]
118. Ma, L.; Zhang, L.; Guo, A.; Liu, L.C.; Yu, F.; Diao, N.; Xu, C.; Wang, D. Overexpression of FER1L4 promotes the apoptosis and suppresses epithelial-mesenchymal transition and stemness markers via activating PI3K/AKT signaling pathway in osteosarcoma cells. *Pathol. Res. Pract.* **2019**, *215*, 152412. [CrossRef] [PubMed]
119. Ma, W.; Zhang, C.-Q.; Li, H.-L.; Gu, J.; Miao, G.-Y.; Cai, H.-Y.; Wang, J.-K.; Zhang, L.-J.; Song, Y.-M.; Tian, Y.-H.; et al. LncRNA FER1L4 suppressed cancer cell growth and invasion in esophageal squamous cell carcinoma. *Eur. Rev. Med. Pharmacol. Sci.* **2018**, *22*, 2638–2645. [PubMed]
120. Wang, X.; Dong, K.; Jin, Q.; Ma, Y.; Yin, S.; Wang, S. Upregulation of lncRNA FER1L4 suppresses the proliferation and migration of the hepatocellular carcinoma via regulating PI3K/AKT signal pathway. *J. Cell. Biochem.* **2019**, *120*, 6781–6788. [CrossRef]
121. Liu, Z.; Shao, Y.; Tan, L.; Shi, H.; Chen, S.; Guo, J. Clinical significance of the low expression of FER1L4 in gastric cancer patients. *Tumour Biol.* **2014**, *35*, 9613–9617. [CrossRef] [PubMed]
122. Xia, T.; Chen, S.; Jiang, Z.; Shao, Y.; Jiang, X.; Li, P.; Xiao, B.; Guo, J. Long noncoding RNA FER1L4 suppresses cancer cell growth by acting as a competing endogenous RNA and regulating PTEN expression. *Sci. Rep.* **2015**, *5*, 13445. [CrossRef] [PubMed]
123. Xia, T.; Liao, Q.; Jiang, X.; Shao, Y.; Xiao, B.; Xi, Y.; Guo, J. Long noncoding RNA associated-competing endogenous RNAs in gastric cancer. *Sci. Rep.* **2014**, *4*, 6088. [CrossRef] [PubMed]

124. Salmena, L.; Poliseno, L.; Tay, Y.; Kats, L.; Pandolfi, P.P. A ceRNA hypothesis: The rosetta stone of a hidden RNA language? *Cell* **2011**, *146*, 353–358. [CrossRef] [PubMed]
125. Yue, B.; Sun, B.; Liu, C.; Zhao, S.; Zhang, D.; Yu, F.; Yan, D. Long non-coding RNA Fer-1-like protein 4 suppresses oncogenesis and exhibits prognostic value by associating with miR-106a-5p in colon cancer. *Cancer Sci.* **2015**, *106*, 1323–1332. [CrossRef] [PubMed]
126. Wu, J.; Huang, J.; Wang, W.; Xu, J.; Yin, M.; Cheng, N.; Yin, J. Long non-coding RNA Fer-1-like protein 4 acts as a tumor suppressor via miR-106a-5p and predicts good prognosis in hepatocellular carcinoma. *Cancer Biomark.* **2017**, *20*, 55–65. [CrossRef]
127. Fei, D.; Zhang, X.; Liu, J.; Tan, L.; Xing, J.; Zhao, D.; Zhang, Y. Long Noncoding RNA FER1L4 Suppresses Tumorigenesis by Regulating the Expression of PTEN Targeting miR-18a-5p in Osteosarcoma. *Cell. Physiol. Biochem.* **2018**, *51*, 1364–1375. [CrossRef] [PubMed]
128. Liu, S.; Zou, B.; Tian, T.; Luo, X.; Mao, B.; Zhang, X.; Lei, H. Overexpression of the lncRNA FER1L4 inhibits paclitaxel tolerance of ovarian cancer cells via the regulation of the MAPK signaling pathway. *J. Cell. Biochem.* **2018**, *120*, 7581–7589. [CrossRef]
129. Théry, C. Cancer: Diagnosis by extracellular vesicles. *Nature* **2015**, *523*, 161–162. [CrossRef]
130. Ciardiello, C.; Cavallini, L.; Spinelli, C.; Yang, J.; Reis-Sobreiro, M.; de Candia, P.; Minciacchi, V.R.; Di Vizio, D. Focus on Extracellular Vesicles: New Frontiers of Cell-to-Cell Communication in Cancer. *Int. J. Mol. Sci.* **2016**, *17*, 175. [CrossRef]
131. Hanahan, D.; Weinberg, R.A. Hallmarks of cancer: The next generation. *Cell* **2011**, *144*, 646–674. [CrossRef]
132. Anderson, R.G.; Ghiraldeli, L.P.; Pardee, T.S. Mitochondria in cancer metabolism, an organelle whose time has come? *Biochim. Biophys. Acta Rev. Cancer* **2018**, *1870*, 96–102. [CrossRef] [PubMed]
133. Zhang, T.; Jingjie, L.; He, Y.; Yang, F.; Hao, Y.; Jin, W.; Wu, J.; Sun, Z.; Li, Y.; Chen, Y.; et al. A small molecule targeting myoferlin exerts promising anti-tumor effects on breast cancer. *Nat. Commun.* **2018**, *9*, 3726. [CrossRef] [PubMed]
134. Li, Y.; He, Y.; Shao, T.; Pei, H.; Guo, W.; Mi, D.; Krimm, I.; Zhang, Y.; Wang, P.; Wang, X.; et al. Modification and Biological Evaluation of a Series of 1,5-Diaryl-1,2,4-triazole Compounds as Novel Agents against Pancreatic Cancer Metastasis through Targeting Myoferlin. *J. Med. Chem.* **2019**, *62*, 4949–4966. [CrossRef] [PubMed]
135. Sondergaard, P.C.; Griffin, D.A.; Pozsgai, E.R.; Johnson, R.W.; Grose, W.E.; Heller, K.N.; Shontz, K.M.; Montgomery, C.L.; Liu, J.; Clark, K.R.; et al. AAV.Dysferlin Overlap Vectors Restore Function in Dysferlinopathy Animal Models. *Ann. Clin. Transl. Neurol.* **2015**, *2*, 256–270. [CrossRef] [PubMed]
136. Escobar, H.; Schöwel, V.; Spuler, S.; Marg, A.; Izsvák, Z. Full-length Dysferlin Transfer by the Hyperactive Sleeping Beauty Transposase Restores Dysferlin-deficient Muscle. *Mol. Ther. Nucleic Acids* **2016**, *5*, e277. [CrossRef] [PubMed]
137. Potter, R.A.; Griffin, D.A.; Sondergaard, P.C.; Johnson, R.W.; Pozsgai, E.R.; Heller, K.N.; Peterson, E.L.; Lehtimäki, K.K.; Windish, H.P.; Mittal, P.J.; et al. Systemic Delivery of Dysferlin Overlap Vectors Provides Long-Term Gene Expression and Functional Improvement for Dysferlinopathy. *Hum. Gene Ther.* **2017**. hum.2017.062. [CrossRef]
138. Llanga, T.; Nagy, N.; Conatser, L.; Dial, C.; Sutton, R.B.; Hirsch, M.L. Structure-Based Designed Nano-Dysferlin Significantly Improves Dysferlinopathy in BLA/J Mice. *Mol. Ther.* **2017**, *25*, 2150–2162. [CrossRef]
139. Lee, J.H.; Kim, Y.; Yoon, Y.-E.; Kim, Y.-J.; Oh, S.-G.; Jang, J.-H.; Kim, E. Development of efficient adeno-associated virus (AAV)-mediated gene delivery system with a phytoactive material for targeting human melanoma cells. *New Biotechnol.* **2017**, *37*, 194–199. [CrossRef]
140. Chow, R.D.; Guzman, C.D.; Wang, G.; Schmidt, F.; Youngblood, M.W.; Ye, L.; Errami, Y.; Dong, M.B.; Martinez, M.A.; Zhang, S.; et al. AAV-mediated direct in vivo CRISPR screen identifies functional suppressors in glioblastoma. *Nat. Neurosci.* **2017**, *20*, 1329–1341. [CrossRef]
141. Hodge, R.; Narayanavari, S.A.; Izsvák, Z.; Ivics, Z. Wide Awake and Ready to Move: 20 Years of Non-Viral Therapeutic Genome Engineering with the Sleeping Beauty Transposon System. *Hum. Gene Ther.* **2017**, *28*, 842–855. [CrossRef]

13

Dexamethasone Inhibits Spheroid Formation of Thyroid Cancer Cells Exposed to Simulated Microgravity

Daniela Melnik [1], Jayashree Sahana [2], Thomas J. Corydon [2,3], Sascha Kopp [1,4], Mohamed Zakaria Nassef [1], Markus Wehland [1,4], Manfred Infanger [1,4], Daniela Grimm [2,4,5] and Marcus Krüger [1,4,*]

[1] Clinic for Plastic, Aesthetic and Hand Surgery, Otto von Guericke University, Leipziger Str. 44, 39120 Magdeburg, Germany; daniela.melnik@med.ovgu.de (D.M.); sascha.kopp@med.ovgu.de (S.K.); mohamed.nassef@med.ovgu.de (M.Z.N.); markus.wehland@med.ovgu.de (M.W.); manfred.infanger@med.ovgu.de (M.I.)

[2] Department of Biomedicine, Aarhus University, Hoegh-Guldbergsgade 10, 8000 Aarhus C, Denmark; jaysaha@biomed.au.dk (J.S.); corydon@biomed.au.dk (T.J.C.); dgg@biomed.au.dk (D.G.)

[3] Department of Ophthalmology, Aarhus University Hospital, Palle Juul-Jensens Boulevard 99, 8200 Aarhus N, Denmark

[4] Research Group "Magdeburger Arbeitsgemeinschaft für Forschung unter Raumfahrt- und Schwerelosigkeitsbedingungen" (MARS), Otto von Guericke University, Universitätsplatz 2, 39106 Magdeburg, Germany

[5] Department of Microgravity and Translational Regenerative Medicine, Otto von Guericke University, Pfälzer Platz, 39106 Magdeburg, Germany

* Correspondence: marcus.krueger@med.ovgu.de

Abstract: Detachment and the formation of spheroids under microgravity conditions can be observed with various types of intrinsically adherent human cells. In particular, for cancer cells this process mimics metastasis and may provide insights into cancer biology and progression that can be used to identify new drug/target combinations for future therapies. By using the synthetic glucocorticoid dexamethasone (DEX), we were able to suppress spheroid formation in a culture of follicular thyroid cancer (FTC)-133 cells that were exposed to altered gravity conditions on a random positioning machine. DEX inhibited the growth of three-dimensional cell aggregates in a dose-dependent manner. In the first approach, we analyzed the expression of several factors that are known to be involved in key processes of cancer progression such as autocrine signaling, proliferation, epithelial–mesenchymal transition, and anoikis. Wnt/β-catenin signaling and expression patterns of important genes in cancer cell growth and survival, which were further suggested to play a role in three-dimensional aggregation, such as *NFKB2*, *VEGFA*, *CTGF*, *CAV1*, *BCL2*(*L1*), or *SNAI1*, were clearly affected by DEX. Our data suggest the presence of a more complex regulation network of tumor spheroid formation involving additional signal pathways or individual key players that are also influenced by DEX.

Keywords: glucocorticoids; 3D growth; nuclear factor kappa-light-chain-enhancer of activated B-cells (NF-κB); epithelial–mesenchymal transition; anoikis; proliferation

---

1. Introduction

Glucocorticoids (GCs) are a class of steroid hormones involved in many physiological processes such as metabolism, proliferation, differentiation, and survival of cells [1]. GCs induce their pharmacodynamic effects through binding to glucocorticoid receptors (GRs) [2], which interact downstream with signaling molecules in the cytoplasm or are able to translocate into the nucleus, where they repress the activity of other transcription factors (such as nuclear factor kappa-light-chain-enhancer of activated B-cells, NF-κB, or activator protein 1, AP-1) or initiate transcription of genes associated with anti-inflammatory and immunosuppressive effects (via binding to specific glucocorticoid response elements, GREs) (Figure 1A) [3,4]. Due to these properties, GCs are utilized in the treatment of a variety of immunological disorder treatments to reduce pain and electrolyte imbalance, but also to enhance the anti-tumor effect of chemotherapeutics and prevent adverse effects caused by cytotoxic agents [5–7]. The synthetic GC dexamethasone (DEX; Figure 1B) is commonly administered as a supportive care co-medication to reduce cancer-related fatigue in patients with advanced disease [8]. DEX was further reported to inhibit proliferation of different cancer cells in vitro and in vivo [9–13]. Effective inhibition of tumor growth was suggested to be associated with downregulation of JAK3/STAT3, hypoxia inducible factor 1α, vascular endothelial growth factor (VEGF), and interleukin-6 [12,14,15]. Nevertheless, the exact mechanism by which DEX suppresses cancer cell growth is still unclear.

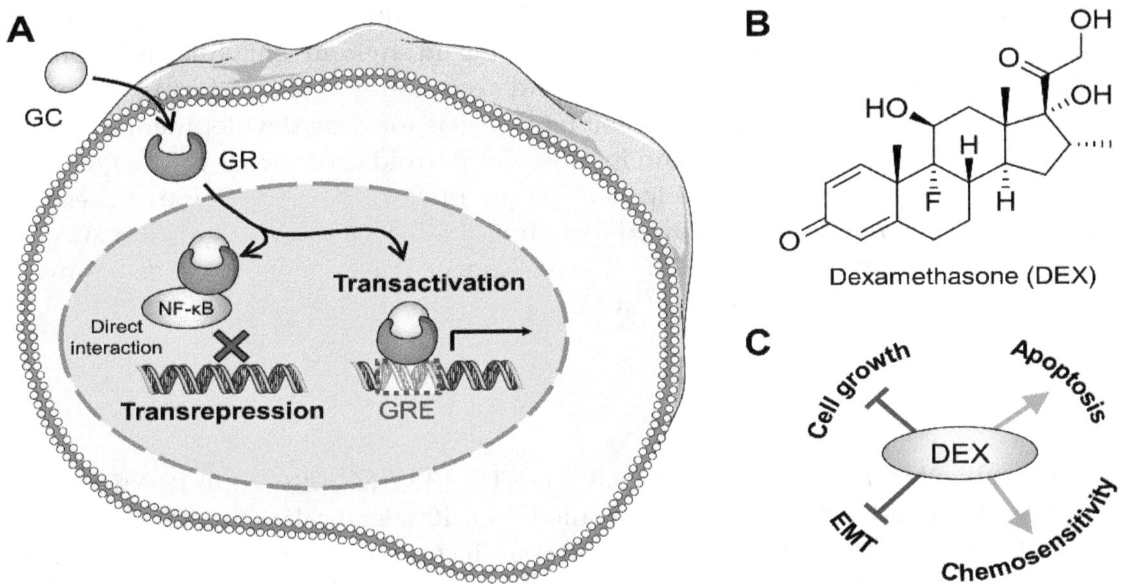

Figure 1. (**A**) Sketch showing the genomic actions of glucocorticoids (GCs) such as dexamethasone (DEX). When bound to DEX, the glucocorticoid receptor (GR) complex translocates into the nucleus and modifies the synthesis of several metabolic proteins. This is done either through directly binding to glucocorticoid response elements (GREs) on the DNA or through influencing the activity of transcription factors (i.e., nuclear factor kappa-light-chain-enhancer of activated B-cells, NF-κB); (**B**) Chemical structure of DEX; (**C**) Described effects of DEX on cancer cells. Parts of the figure are drawn using pictures from Servier Medical Art .

Over the last 50 years, the incidence of thyroid cancer has increased worldwide and the incidence rate is still on the rise. The result of improved diagnostic procedures, an elevated prevalence of individual risk factors (e.g., obesity), and increased exposure to environmental risk factors (e.g., iodine levels), thyroid cancer is the most common form of endocrine malignancy today [16] and is expected to become the fourth leading type of cancer across the globe [17]. Especially poorly differentiated thyroid tumors are aggressive and tend to metastasize. The prognosis for differentiated thyroid cancer is related to the capability of tumor cells to accumulate radioiodine. Due to de-differentiation, some tumor cells may lose their iodine uptake capability, leaving only extremely limited treatment options, despite intensive searches for new drugs and targets. Therefore, novel approaches to control thyroid cancer progression are required.

Metastasis is the most limiting factor in cancer therapy and responsible for 90% of cancer-related deaths [18]. During the development of metastatic competence, carcinoma cells change their adhesive properties, secrete proteinases, and become motile, which allows them to detach from their primary tumor [19]. Therefore, tumor cells respond to mechanical signals, sensed by integrins or other adhesion receptors [20,21], and chemical signals, sensed by chemokines or growth factor receptors [22] causing changes in their transcriptional profile. The process which enables tumor cells to achieve migration and invasion is called epithelial–mesenchymal transition (EMT) and represents a driving force in tumorigenesis [23]. In the course of EMT, essential proteins for epithelial cell–cell adhesion, such as E-cadherin, are downregulated, thus weakening epithelial tissue integrity and polarization of epithelial cell layers [24]. Under normal circumstances, detached epithelial cells undergo apoptosis, a phenomenon termed anoikis. Cancer cells acquire resistance to anoikis to survive after they have left the primary tumor. In this way, they are able to travel via the circulatory and lymphatic systems disseminating throughout the body. EMT and anoikis resistance are critical steps of the metastatic cascade and potential targets to impact a natural molecular prerequisite for the aggressive metastatic spread of cancer [25,26].

Microgravity (μg) has become a powerful tool in cancer research by enabling metastasis-like cell detachment and formation of three-dimensional (3D) multicellular spheroids (MCS) [27–30]. Experiments in μg contribute to drug discovery by providing an environment which is helpful to detect changes in gene expression and protein synthesis and secretion that occur during the progression from 2D to 3D growth and which might represent new targets for drug development against thyroid cancer. A couple of these proteins were found in follicular thyroid cancer cells by analyzing multiple pilot studies, performed in μg, with the help of semantic methods [31,32]. Some of these potential drugs, including DEX, were recently reviewed [33]. In this study, we investigate the effects of DEX supplementation on the growth of follicular thyroid cancer (FTC) cells exposed to simulated μg produced by a random positioning machine (RPM).

2. Materials and Methods

2.1. Cell Culture

The human follicular thyroid carcinoma cell line FTC-133 was cultured in RPMI-1640 medium (Life Technologies, Carlsbad, CA, USA), supplemented with 10% fetal calf serum (FCS; Sigma-Aldrich, St. Louis, MO, USA), and 1% penicillin/streptomycin (Life Technologies) at 37 °C and 5% CO_2 until use for the experiment. For RPM experiments FTC-133 cells were seeded at a density of 1×10^6 cells per flask either in T25 cell culture flasks (Sarstedt, Nümbrecht, Germany) for mRNA and protein extraction or in slide flasks (Sarstedt) for immunofluorescence staining. Cells were given at least 24 h to attach to the bottom of the flasks.

2.2. Dexamethasone Treatment

Water-soluble DEX (dexamethasone–cyclodextrin complex) was purchased from Sigma-Aldrich. Then, 24 h after seeding, cells were synchronized in RPMI-1640 medium with 0.25% FCS and 1% penicillin/streptomycin for 4 h. Afterwards, the cells were cultured according to Section 2.1, supplemented with DEX concentrations of 10 nM, 100 nM, or 1000 nM [34].

2.3. Random Positioning Machine

The used desktop-RPM (Dutch Space, Leiden, Netherlands) was located in an incubator with 37 °C/5% CO_2 and operated in real random mode, with a constant angular velocity of 60°/s. Before the run, the flasks were filled up completely and air bubble-free with medium to avoid shear stress. The slide and culture flasks were installed on the prewarmed RPM. After 4 h (short-term experiments) or 3 days (long-term experiments), the cells were photographed and fixed with 4% paraformaldehyde (PFA; Carl Roth, Karlsruhe, Germany) for immunostaining. For RNA and protein extraction adherent cells were harvested by adding ice-cold phosphate-buffered saline (PBS; Life Technologies) and using cell scrapers. The suspensions were centrifuged at 3000× g for 10 min at 4 °C followed by discarding the PBS and storage of cell pellets at −150 °C. MCS were collected by centrifuging supernatant at

3000× g for 10 min at 4 °C and subsequent storage at −150 °C. Corresponding static controls were prepared in parallel under the same conditions and stored next to the device in an incubator.

2.4. Phase Contrast Microscopy

Cells were observed and photographed using an Axiovert 25 Microscope (Carl Zeiss Microscopy, Jena, Germany) equipped with a Canon EOS 550D camera (Canon, Tokio, Japan).

2.5. Immunofluorescence Microscopy

Immunofluorescence staining was performed to visualize possible translocal alteration of NF-κB proteins and β-catenin by dexamethasone in cells. The PFA-fixed cells were permeabilized with 0.1% Triton™ X-100 for 15 min and blocked with 3% bovine serum albumin (BSA) for 45 min at ambient temperature. Afterwards, the cells were labeled with primary NF-κB p65 rabbit polyclonal antibody #PA1-186 (Invitrogen, Carlsbad, CA, USA) at 1 μg/mL or β-catenin mouse monoclonal antibody #MA1-300 (Invitrogen) at a dilution of 1:200 in 0.1% BSA and incubated overnight at 4 °C in a moist chamber. The next day, cells were washed three times with PBS before incubation with the secondary Alexa Fluor 488 (AF488)-conjugated anti-rabbit (Cell Signaling Technology, Danvers, MA, USA) or anti-mouse antibody (Invitrogen) at a dilution of 1:1000 for 1 h at ambient temperature. Cells were washed again three times with PBS and mounted with Fluoroshield™ with DAPI (4′,6-diamidino-2-phenylindole) (Sigma-Aldrich). The slides were subsequently investigated with a Zeiss LSM 710 confocal laser scanning microscope (Carl Zeiss) [35].

2.6. mRNA Isolation and Quantitative Real-Time PCR

RNA isolation and quantitative real-time PCR were performed according to routine protocols [36–38]. Briefly, RNA was isolated by using the RNeasy Mini Kit (Qiagen, Venlo, Netherlands) according to the manufacturer's protocol and quantified with a spectrophotometer. Afterwards, cDNA was produced with the High Capacity cDNA Reverse Transcription Kit (Applied Biosystems, Foster City, CA, USA) following manufacturer's instructions. To determine the expression level of the target genes shown in Table S1, quantitative real-time PCR was performed applying the Fast SYBR™ Green Master Mix (Applied Biosystems) and the 7500 Fast Real-Time PCR System (Applied Biosystems). Primers were designed to have a $T_m \approx 60$ °C and to span exon/exon boundaries using Primer-BLAST [39] (Supplementary Materials). Primer were synthesized by TIB Molbio (Berlin, Germany). All samples were measured in triplicates and analyzed by the comparative threshold cycle ($\Delta\Delta C_T$) method with 18S rRNA as reference.

2.7. Western Blot Analysis

Western blot analysis was performed with routine protocols as described previously [36]. The control and DEX-treated samples were collected after 4 h and 3 days, solubilized in lysis buffer and compared to the control samples without DEX. Each condition included three batches with a total number of 24 samples (4 h) and 33 samples (3 days), respectively. Following lysis and centrifugation, aliquots of 40 μg total protein were subjected to SDS-PAGE and Western blotting. The samples were loaded onto Criterion XT 4–12% precast gels (Bio-Rad, Hercules, CA, USA), run for 1 h at 150 V and transferred to a polyvinylidene difluoride membrane using TurboBlot (Bio-Rad) (100 V, 30 min). Cyclophilin B was used as a loading control. Membranes were blocked with TBS-T containing 0.3% I-Block (Applied Biosystems) for 2 h at ambient temperature. For detection of the proteins shown in Table S2, the membranes were incubated overnight at 4 °C in TBS-T containing 0.3% I-Block solutions of the antibodies. The next day, membranes were washed three times with TBS-T for 5 min and incubated for 2 h at ambient temperature with a horseradish peroxidase (HRP)-linked antibody (Cell Signaling Technology) diluted 1:1000 in TBS-T with 0.3% I-Block. The respective protein bands were visualized using Clarity ECL Western Blot Substrate (Bio-Rad). Images were captured with Image Quant LAS 4000 mini (GE Healthcare, Chicago, IL, USA) and analyzed using ImageJ software (imagej.net) for densitometric quantification.

2.8. *Terminal Deoxynucleotidyl Transferase dUTP Nick-End Labeling (TUNEL) Assay*

The Click-iT™ Plus TUNEL assay (Invitrogen) was used for apoptosis detection. FTC-133 cells were cultured in slide flasks (Sarstedt) under static culture conditions or exposed to the RPM, supplemented without or with 1000 nM DEX. After 4 h or 3 days cells were fixed with 4% PFA and prepared for the evaluation of apoptosis. The staining procedure was performed according to the manufacturer's recommendation. A positive control sample was treated with DNase I (Epicentre, Madison, WI, USA) to induce DNA fragmentation. The stained cells were examined using a Zeiss LSM 800 confocal laser scanning microscope (Carl Zeiss) equipped with an external light source and an objective with a calibrated 630× magnification.

2.9. *Ki-67 Proliferation Assay*

Cells were cultured and prepared as described in Section 2.5. Cells were labeled with an AF488 recombinant anti-Ki-67 antibody #ab197234 (Abcam, Cambridge, UK) at a dilution of 1:100 in 0.1% BSA and incubated overnight at 4 °C. The next day, cells were washed three times with PBS and mounted with Fluoroshield™ with DAPI (Sigma-Aldrich). The cell proliferation was evaluated by a Zeiss LSM 800 confocal laser scanning microscope (Carl Zeiss) and an objective with a calibrated 230× magnification. Five microscopic images for each condition were analyzed using ImageJ (imagej.net). The percentage of Ki-67 positive cells was counted for each condition and normalized to the control.

2.10. *Spheroid Formation Assay*

Approximately 1×10^6 cells per flasks were seeded into T25 cell culture flasks (Sarstedt). After 24 h the culture flasks were filled up completely (air bubble-free) with media and were installed on the prewarmed RPM (37 °C, 5% CO_2). To investigate the ability of MCS formation, two RPM running time points were considered: media was completely removed from culture flasks after 24 h and after 48 h exposure to the RPM. Flasks were re-filled with fresh media for a further 24 h run on the RPM. After each run, cells were examined and photographed.

2.11. *Statistics*

Statistical evaluation was performed using GraphPad Prism 7.01 (GraphPad Software, San Diego, CA, USA). The nonparametric Mann–Whitney U test was used to compare DEX-free with DEX-treated samples as well as static and µg conditions. All data are presented as mean ± standard deviation (SD) with a significance level of $p < 0.05$.

3. Results

Based on the knowledge that NF-κB seems to play a crucial role in spheroid formation of MCF-7 breast cancer cells [34] and that NF-κB subunit p65 (RelA) accumulates in thyroid cancer cells on the RPM [40], we decided to target RelA in µg-grown thyroid cancer cells using DEX. Therefore, we cultured the human follicular thyroid cancer cell line FTC-133 on an RPM in the presence of three different DEX concentrations (10, 100, 1000 nM). After three days on the RPM, the cells showed a DEX dose-dependent inhibition of spheroid formation in µg (Figure 2).

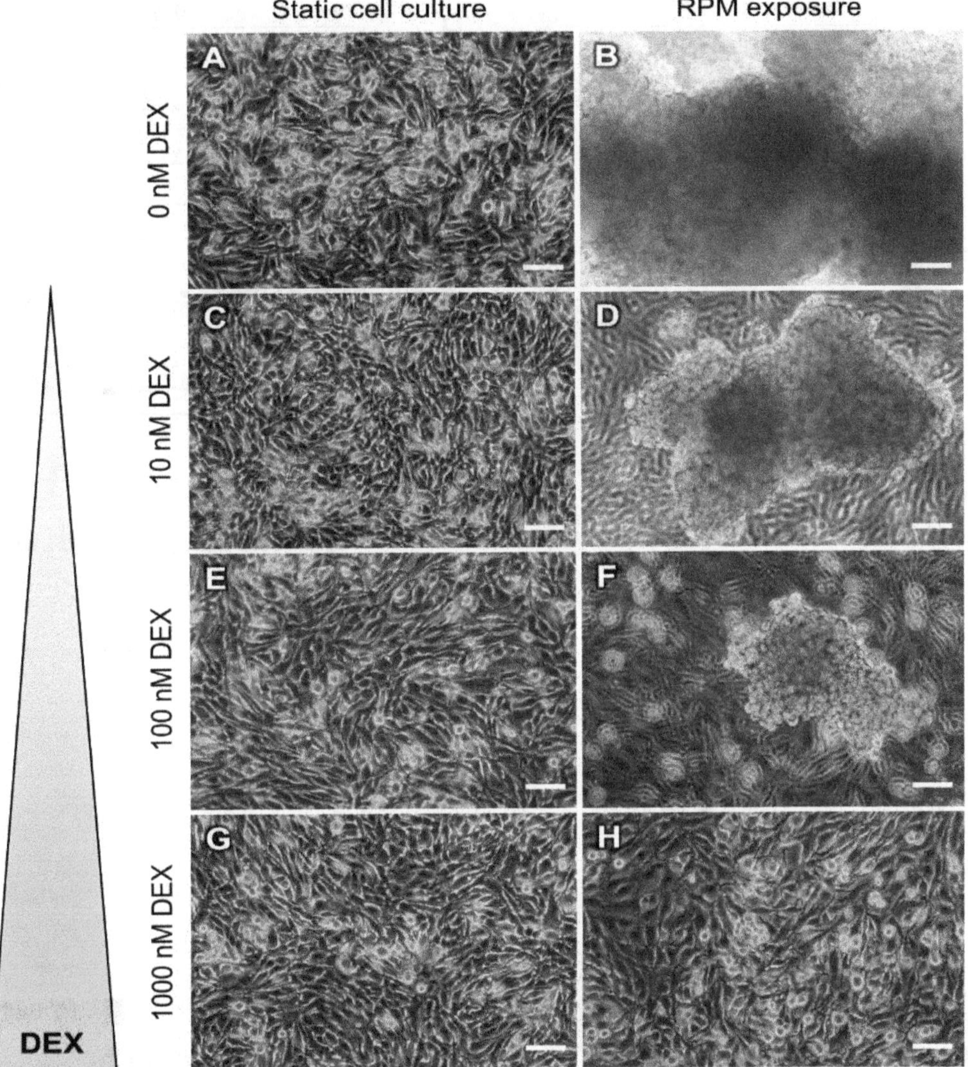

Figure 2. Impact of DEX on the spheroid formation ability of follicular thyroid cancer (FTC)-133 cells exposed to a random positioning machine (RPM). (**A,B**) After three days cells showed a dose-dependent inhibition of spheroid formation when treated with (**C,D**) 10 nM DEX, (**E,F**) 100 nM DEX, or (**G,H**) 1000 nM DEX on the RPM (right column). Scale bars: 100 μm.

3.1. NF-κB Pathway

NF-κB transcription factors play a fundamental role in the tumorigenesis of many cancer types, including thyroid cancer [41,42] and may be a target in the treatment of advanced thyroid cancer [43]. DEX is known to have inhibitory effects on the NF-κB pathway [44].

We investigated the transcription of the NF-κB family members subunit p50 and its precursor p105 (encoded by *NFKB1*) as well as subunit p52 and its precursor p100 (encoded by *NFKB2*). The mRNA levels of both genes were reduced in MCS cells grown for three days on the RPM and *NFKB2* was upregulated in adherently growing (AD) cells, harvested from the RPM (Figure 3A,B). In addition, we found a dose-dependent inhibitory effect of DEX on the mRNA synthesis of *NFKB2* (Figure 3B) and a less pronounced effect on the mRNA synthesis of *NFKB1* (Figure 3A). In contrast to DEX-treated MCF-7 cells [34], RelA was not translocated into the nucleus of FTC-133 cells in a significant amount after DEX supplementation (Figure 3E,F). Furthermore, RelA expression was not significantly altered by DEX on the transcriptional level (Figure 3C). RelA protein was increased after three days on the RPM and seemed to be augmented by DEX treatment in μg-exposed cells (Figure 3D).

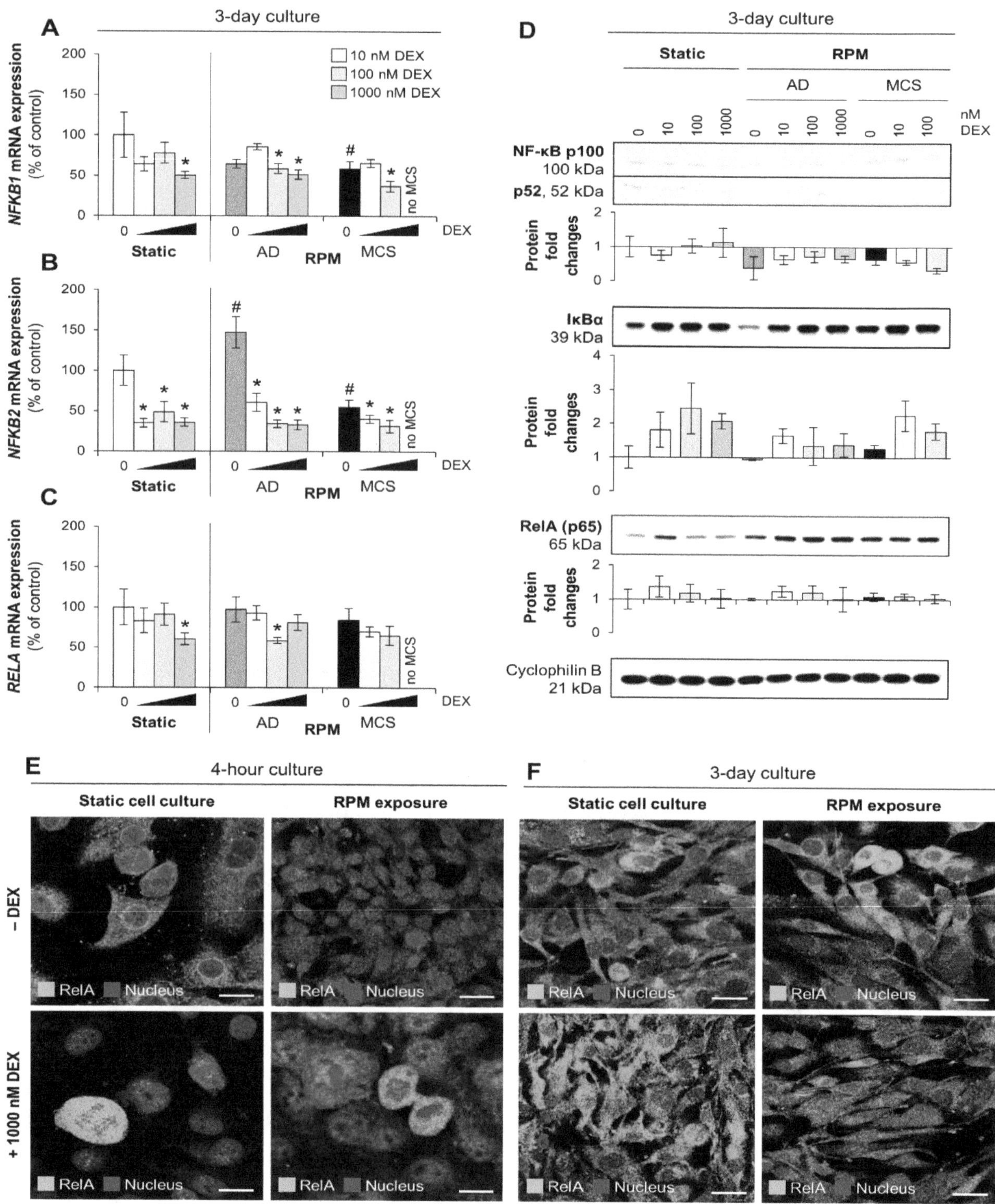

Figure 3. Effect of DEX on NF-κB family members in FTC-133 cells. (**A**) *NFKB1* mRNA expression; (**B**) *NFKB2* mRNA expression; (**C**) *RELA* mRNA expression. Depicted are means of relative mRNA levels ± standard deviations ($n = 5$). *: $p < 0.05$ vs. DEX-free samples. #: $p < 0.05$ vs. static cultures; (**D**) Western blots indicate protein levels of regulated genes after three days. Representatives of each of the three replicates are shown. Diagrams describe relative fold changes to control. AD: adherently growing cells; MCS: multicellular spheroids. (**E**,**F**) Immunofluorescence shows only minor translocation of RelA (green) into the nucleus (blue; 4′,6-diamidino-2-phenylindole (DAPI)-stained) in FTC-133 cells. Scale bars: 20 μm.

NF-κB dimers can be sequestered in the cytoplasm by the inhibitor of κB (IκB) proteins. Therefore, we analyzed the expression of IκBα (encoded by *NFKBIA*), IκBβ (encoded by *NFKBIB*), and IκBε (encoded by *NFKBIE*). The effect of DEX supplementation on *NFKBIA* expression was limited to RPM-exposed cells (Figure 4A), but it tended to upregulate the IκBα protein level in three-day cultures, independent of gravity (Figure 3D). In addition, DEX lowered *NFKBIB* and *NFKBIE* mRNA in cells cultured under normal conditions. The *NFKBIB* mRNA synthesis seemed to be increased (Figure 4B) whereas *NFKBIE* mRNA synthesis was reduced in adherently growing cells on the RPM (Figure 4C). Overall, the mRNA synthesis of all IκB proteins was reduced by long-term exposure to the RPM.

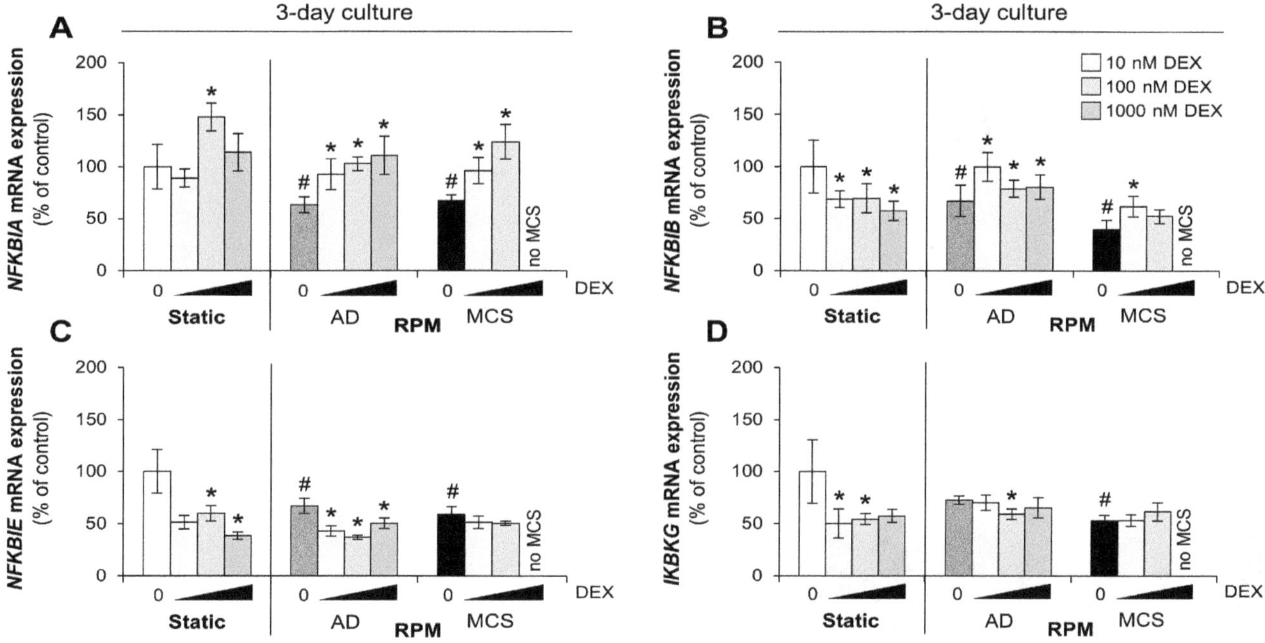

Figure 4. Effect of DEX on NF-κB regulators in FTC-133 cells. (**A**) *NFKBIA* mRNA expression; (**B**) *NFKBIB* mRNA expression; (**C**) *NFKBIE* mRNA expression; (**D**) *IKBKG* mRNA expression. Depicted are means of relative mRNA levels ± standard deviations ($n = 5$). *: $p < 0.05$ vs. DEX-free samples. #: $p < 0.05$ vs. static cultures. AD: adherently growing cells; MCS: multicellular spheroids.

Activation of NF-κB is initiated by the signal-induced degradation of IκB proteins, mainly via activation of IκB kinase (IKK). IKK is composed of the catalytic IKKα/IKKβ heterodimer and the master regulator NEMO (NF-κB essential modulator), also referred as IKKγ (encoded by *IKBKG*). Three-day MCS showed a reduction in *IKBKG* mRNA synthesis. DEX reduced *IKBKG* mRNA synthesis only in static cultured cells after three days. Under all other conditions, transcription was unaffected by DEX supplementation (Figure 4D).

Since NF-κB is obviously not the main target of DEX in suppressing µ*g*-based spheroid formation of FTC-133 cells, we proceeded to illuminate further cancer-related processes which have been reported in connection with DEX (Figure 1C) and that are also involved in the formation of tumor spheroids.

3.2. Growth Factors and Proliferation

Different growth factors are expressed and secreted by cancer cells and contribute to proliferation, survival, and migration. Previous experiments designed to elucidate the growth behavior of cancer cells in µ*g* reveal that especially connective tissue growth factor (CTGF), epidermal growth factor (EGF), transforming growth factor beta (TGF-β), and VEGF were regulated in FTC-133 cells after gravity was omitted [37]. CTGF is a member of the CCN family of secreted, matrix-associated proteins that plays a key role in tumor development, progression, and angiogenesis [45]. CTGF is suggested to regulate cancer cell migration, invasion, angiogenesis, and anoikis [46]. In our experiments, CTGF was upregulated in adherently growing FTC-133 cells after DEX supplementation (Figure 5A). RPM-exposure also enhanced the *CTGF* mRNA level resulting in an additive effect of µg and DEX supplementation. However, the transcription was lower in MCS cells compared to cells in static cultures after three days (Figure 5A).

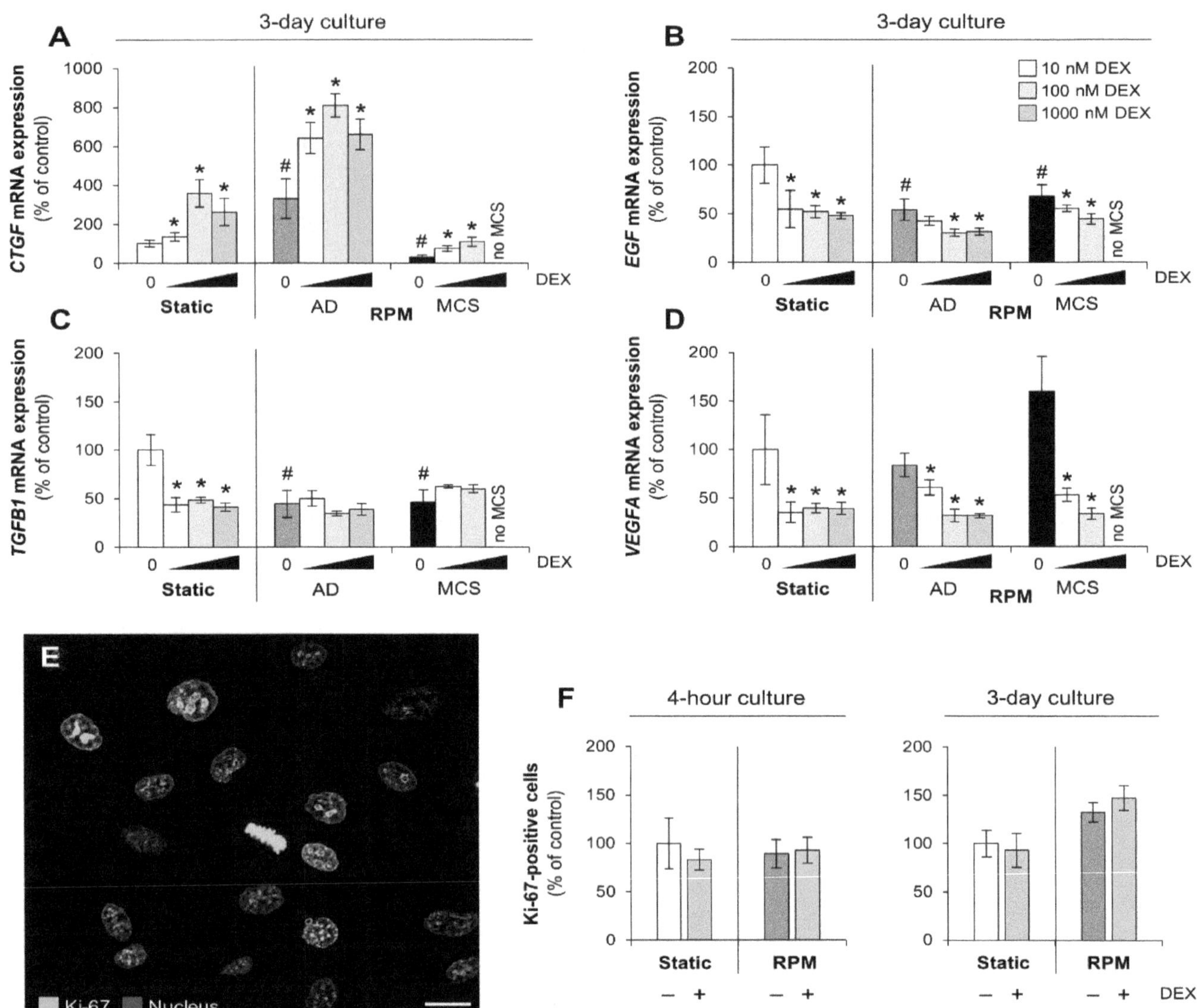

Figure 5. Effect of DEX on autocrine growth factors and proliferation markers in FTC-133 cells. (**A**) *CTGF* mRNA expression; (**B**) *EGF* mRNA expression; (**C**) *TGFB1* mRNA expression; (**D**) *VEGFA* mRNA expression. Depicted are means of relative mRNA levels ± standard deviations ($n = 5$); (**E**) Immunofluorescence. Nuclear expression of Ki-67 indicates proliferating cells; (**F**) Proliferation analysis using Ki-67. *: $p < 0.05$ vs. DEX-free samples. #: $p < 0.05$ vs. static cultures. AD: adherently growing cells; MCS: multicellular spheroids.

TGF-β and EGF represent two physiological regulators of thyroid cell differentiation and proliferation. Whereas EGF is a strong mitogen for follicular thyroid cells [47], TGF-β has a complicated role in cancer. Initially, TGF-β is a tumor suppressor that inhibits the growth of thyrocytes and induces apoptosis [48]. However, at later stages of tumor progression, TGF-β acts as a potent EMT inducer and then it plays a fundamental role in tumor progression and metastasis formation [49–51]. *EGF* mRNA was downregulated both in presence of DEX and in µg (Figure 5B). *TGFB1* mRNA levels were also lower in µg-grown cells, but DEX decreased *TGFB1* mRNA synthesis only in cells from static cultures (Figure 5C). In addition, DEX suppressed VEGF under normal culture conditions and in both cell populations on the

RPM (Figure 5D). In accordance with previous studies that investigated other follicular thyroid cancer cells on the RPM [52], *VEGFA* expression was somewhat increased in MCS cells after three days.

DEX was previously reported to have anti-proliferative effects on human medullary thyroid cancer cells [53]. To prove this effect with follicular thyroid cancer cells and in the context of µ*g*, we searched for cellular markers for proliferation such as the Ki-67 protein (encoded by *MKI67*) [54]. Ki-67 can be detected during all active phases of the cell cycle (G1, S, G2, and M), but not in resting cells (G0). Thus, the nuclear expression of Ki-67 can be evaluated to study tumor proliferation using immunofluorescence microscopy (Figure 5E). In our experiments, neither µ*g* nor DEX had a significant influence on the proliferation of FTC-133 cells (Figure 5F).

3.3. Epithelial and Mesenchymal Characteristics, Wnt/β-catenin Signaling

To find signs for EMT, that is also influenced by µ*g* in cancer cells [55], different epithelial (E-cadherin) and mesenchymal markers (N-cadherin, vimentin, fibronectin, Snail1) were analyzed. In a four-hour culture the E-cadherin mRNA (encoded by *CDH1*) was reduced in cells incubated with DEX (Figure 6A), without significant changes in E-cadherin protein levels (Figure 6H). After three days on the RPM, we found a difference in the *CDH1* gene expression between the two phenotypes: adherently growing cells showed a lower, whereas MCS showed a higher, *CDH1* expression compared to control cells. The elevated *CDH1* expression in spheroids was significantly reduced by DEX supplementation (Figure 6A).

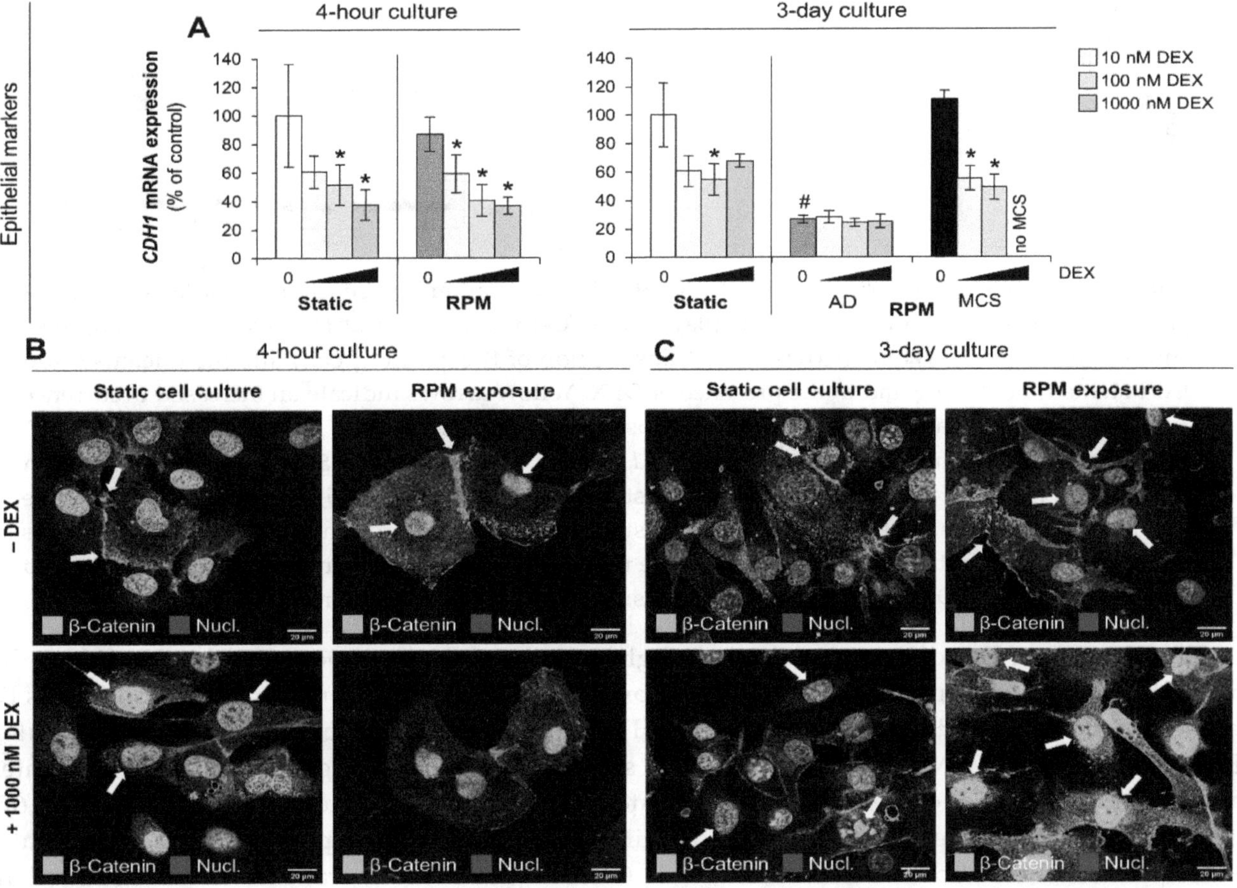

Figure 6. *Cont.*

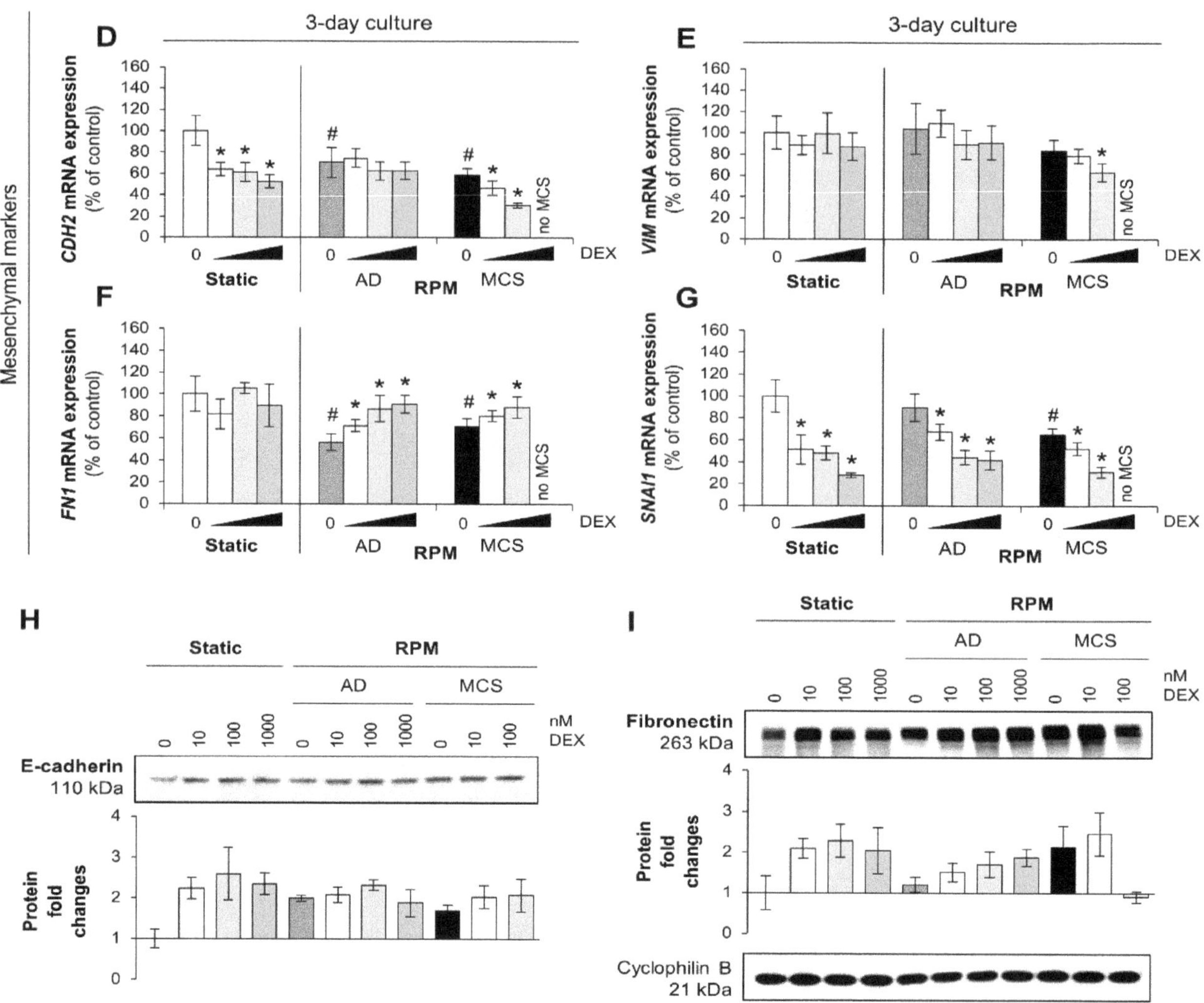

Figure 6. Effect of DEX on the mRNA synthesis of epithelial markers, mesenchymal markers, and other epithelial–mesenchymal transition (EMT) players in FTC-133 cells. (**A**) *CDH1* mRNA expression; (**B**,**C**) Immunofluorescence. White arrows show translocation of β-catenin (green) into the nucleus (blue; DAPI-stained) both in µ*g* and in the presence of DEX. Yellow arrows indicate an increased occurrence of β-catenin on the plasma membrane in the absence of DEX. Scale bars: 20 µm; (**D**) *CDH2* mRNA expression; (**E**) *VIM* mRNA expression; (**F**) *FN1* mRNA expression; (**G**) *SNAI1* mRNA expression. Depicted are means of relative mRNA levels ± standard deviations ($n = 5$). *: $p < 0.05$ vs. DEX-free samples. #: $p < 0.05$ vs. static cultures; (**H**,**I**) Western blots indicate protein levels of regulated genes after 3 days. Representatives of each of the three replicates is shown. Diagrams describe relative fold changes to control. AD: adherently growing cells; MCS: multicellular spheroids.

The amount of E-cadherin protein was slightly higher in cells exposed to the RPM than those from static cell cultures and was not influenced by DEX in µ*g*. Under normal culture conditions DEX seemed to increase E-cadherin levels (Figure 6H). Downstream of the cadherin complex, β-catenin mRNA (encoded by *CTNNB1*) was not influenced significantly by DEX (Figure S3). However, β-catenin was translocated from the plasma membrane into the nucleus in the presence of DEX (Figure 6B,C) suggesting an involvement of the Wnt/β-catenin pathway. This is supported by the fact that the transcription of the E-cadherin repressor Snail1 (encoded by *SNAI1*) was also downregulated after DEX treatment (Figure 6G).

N-cadherin (encoded by *CDH2*) and vimentin (encoded by *VIM*) were identified to promote thyroid tumorigenesis [56,57]. *CDH2* mRNA was upregulated in cells after short-term exposure (Figure S3C) and downregulated after long-term exposure to the RPM (Figure 6D). Similar to *CDH1*, *CDH2* expression in spheroids was reduced by DEX supplementation (Figure 6D). Furthermore, DEX elicited the same reducing effects in control cells of a three-day culture. However, adherently growing cells on the RPM were not influenced by DEX. *VIM* expression was not altered by RPM-exposure, but slightly reduced by high DEX concentrations in MCS cells after three days (Figure 6E). RPM-exposure reduced *FN1* mRNA levels in three-day cultures. This effect could be reversed in the presence of DEX (Figure 6F). Protein levels of fibronectin were also slightly increased after DEX supplementation (Figure 6I).

3.4. Anoikis Factors

There is a further possibility that RPM-based spheroid formation of FTC-133 cells in the presence of DEX is abolished through anoikis of detached cells. Cells undergo apoptosis before aggregates are formed. Unfortunately, live/dead staining of detached cells inside the RPM is technically not possible. Adherent cells showed no signs of apoptosis after DEX treatment and after µ*g*-exposure as visualized by a TUNEL staining (Figure 7A). Caspase-3 cleavage tests were negative, both for adherent and spheroid cells in the presence of DEX (Figure 7B). Additionally, we investigated several factors involved in anoikis on the transcriptional level. The cysteine protease caspase-8 (encoded by *CASP8*) is implicated in apoptosis and involved in the induction of NF-κB nuclear translocation [58]. DEX had only a minor effect on *CASP8* gene expression in our experiments (Figure 7C).

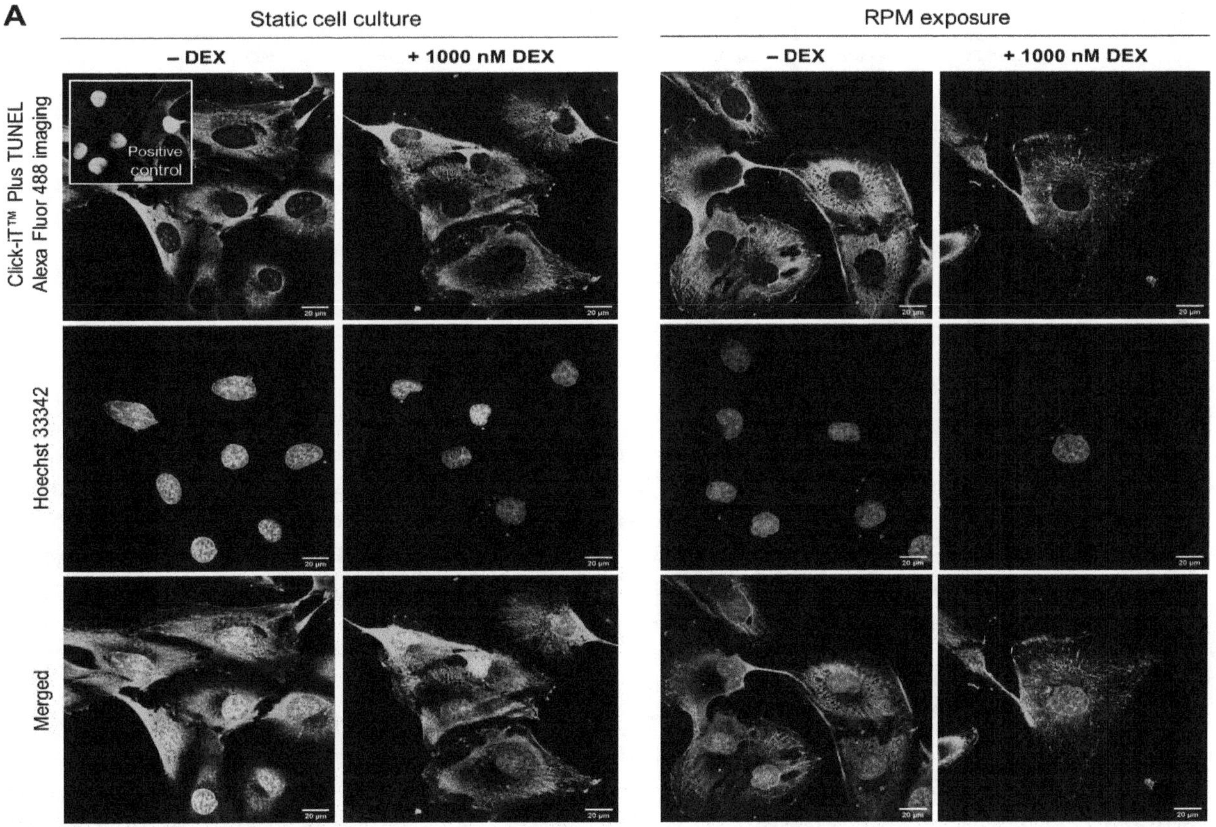

Figure 7. *Cont.*

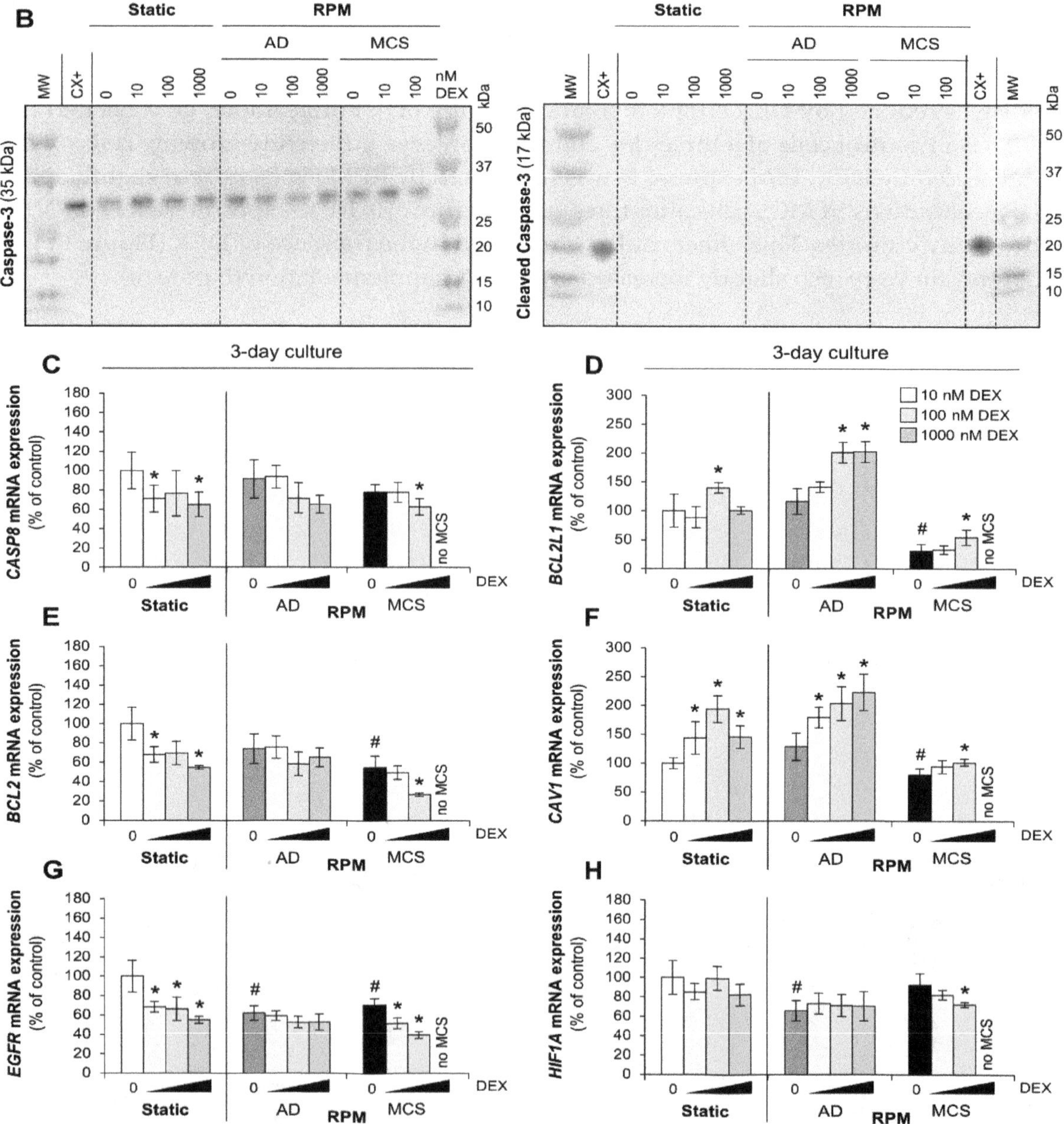

Figure 7. Effect of DEX on apoptosis and anoikis-related proteins in FTC-133 cells. (**A**) No apoptotic cells (green nuclei) were detected by transferase dUTP nick-end labeling (TUNEL) staining after three days. The staining indicates free fluorophores in the cytoplasm in all images except for the positive control. Scale bars: 20 µm; (**B**) Caspase-3 cleavage as an indicator of apoptosis; (**C**) *CASP8* mRNA expression; (**D**) *BCL2L1* mRNA expression; (**E**) *BCL2* mRNA expression; (**F**) *CAV1* mRNA expression; (**G**) *EGFR* mRNA expression; (**H**) *HIF1A* mRNA expression. Depicted are means of relative mRNA levels ± standard deviations ($n = 5$). *: $p < 0.05$ vs. DEX-free samples. #: $p < 0.05$ vs. static cultures. AD: adherently growing cells; MCS: multicellular spheroids.

The anti-apoptotic protein B-cell lymphoma-extra large (Bcl-xL; encoded by *BCL2L1*) has been implicated in the survival of cancer cells by inhibiting the function of the tumor suppressor p53 [59,60]. *BCL2L1* mRNA synthesis was upregulated in FTC-133 cells exposed to the RPM after four hours and reduced by DEX supplementation (Figure S4C). After three days, the *BCL2L1* mRNA synthesis was downregulated in MCS cells, but remained unchanged in adherently growing cells on the RPM. DEX increased *BCL2L1* mRNA after long-term exposure to the RPM (Figure 7D). In contrast, B-cell lymphoma 2 (Bcl-2; encoded by *BCL2*) was further downregulated by DEX in MCS cells (Figure 7E).

A further factor, caveolin-1 (encoded by *CAV1*), was shown to inhibit anchorage-independent growth, anoikis, and invasiveness in human breast cancer cells [61]. Indeed, µ*g* affected the *CAV1* gene expression during spheroid formation: in MCS cells, the *CAV1* mRNA level was reduced. DEX treatment led to an upregulation of caveolin-1 mRNA (Figure 7F).

The loss of coupling between normal integrin and EGF receptor (EGFR) signaling may be further cause for anoikis resistance in tumor cells [62]. We analyzed *EGFR* mRNA synthesis and found a downregulation of EGFR in RPM-grown cells. In addition, DEX decreased *EGFR* transcription in control cells and MCS after three days (Figure 7G).

Hypoxia inducible factor-1 alpha (HIF-1α; encoded by *HIF1A*) is abundantly expressed in most human carcinomas and their metastases. HIF-1α can be induced via EGFR activation and is known to control central metastasis-associated pathways such as angiogenesis, invasion, and resistance to anoikis [63]. Transcription of *HIF1A* was only downregulated in adherently growing cells in three-day RPM cultures and remained unaffected in MCS or by DEX supplementation (Figure 7H).

3.5. Dexamethasone vs. Microgravity—Elucidation of Spheroid Formation Capability

Comparing DEX-induced gene expression data of control cells and transcriptional adaption of FTC-133 cells to µ*g* revealed similar regulation patterns (Figure 8A). We performed an additional two-step RPM culture experiment to check if spheroid formation capability was lost after long-term exposure to µ*g*. Cells that were pre-incubated on the RPM for 48 h showed only marginally reduced spheroid formation during the following 24 h (Figure 8B,C).

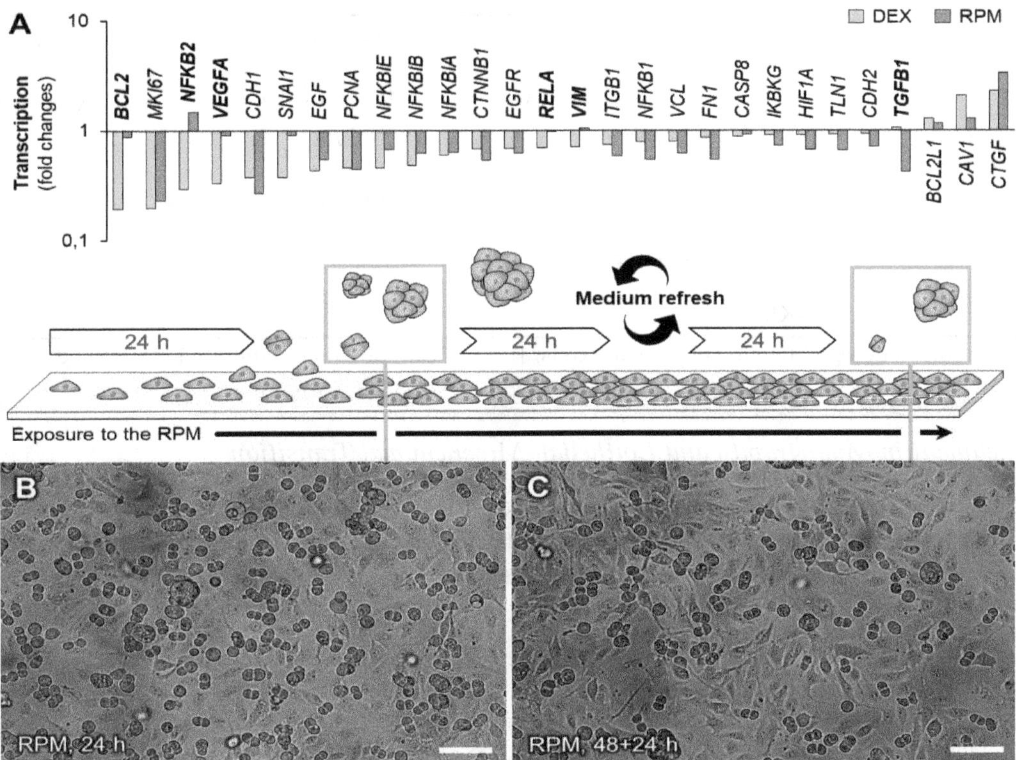

Figure 8. Spheroid formation capability of FTC-133 cells cultured on the RPM. (**A**) Comparison of transcription regulation patterns 4 h after DEX supplementation (yellow bars) and after a three-day RPM-exposure (grey bars). Bold gene symbols indicate fold changes >2.5 or regulation in opposite directions. (**B**) Cells 24 h after the RPM-experiment started; (**C**) Cells 24 h after an initial two-day RPM exposure. Medium was refreshed and spheroids were discarded after the first two days. Although many genes were similarly regulated after DEX supplementation and after a three-day-exposure to the RPM, in contrast to DEX treatment, cells did not lose the ability to form spheroids in µ*g*. Scale bars: 100 µm.

4. Discussion

We investigated the effects of DEX supplementation on the growth of follicular thyroid cancer cells exposed to simulated µ*g*. During a three-day culture on an RPM, cells grew into the form of a large MCS, as it was reported and studied earlier [28,52,64,65]. Previous research revealed that the addition of DEX to spinner flask cultures led to smaller, irregularly shaped spheroids of rat hepatocytes. Higher DEX concentrations inhibited MCS aggregation and promoted MCS disassembly in culture dishes [66]. Kopp et al. [34] described an inhibitory effect of DEX on the MCS formation rate of MCF-7 breast cancer cells cultured on the RPM. However, the authors did not perform any further analyses to elucidate the underlying effects of DEX on MCF-7 cells. After the current study we can confirm similar effects on FTC-133 cells. We found a dose-dependent inhibition of RPM-based spheroid formation by DEX, that was independent from RelA nuclear translocation which was described for DEX-treated breast cancer cells [34]. This finding agrees with the theory of Bauerle et al. [43] that global regulation of thyroid cancer cell growth is not achieved by NF-κB signaling alone and indicates that NF-κB (pathway) may not be the main target of DEX inhibiting the 3D growth of FTC-133 cells in µ*g*. Therefore, we used transcriptional and translational methods to find answers for the changed growth behavior. Interestingly, after DEX supplementation a couple of genes were regulated in the same direction as after a three-day exposure to the RPM. Since the ability of spheroid formation was not suppressed in the RPM-cultures, especially those genes that are of interest, which had a differential expression pattern (Table 1).

Table 1. Significant differences ($p < 0.05$) in mRNA synthesis of adherently growing FTC-133 cells in presence of DEX in static cell culture compared with cells grown without DEX on the RPM.

Process/Pathway	4-Hour Culture	Both Time Points	3-Day Culture
NF-κB pathway	*NFKB1*↑, *NFKBIA*↓, *NFKBIB*↓	*NFKB2*↓, *NFKBIE*↓	*NFKB1*↓, *RELA*↓, *NFKBIA*↑, *IKBKG*↓
Autocrine signaling	*EGF*↓, *TGFB1*↓	*VEGFA*↓	
EMT	*CDH1*↓, *CTNNB1*↓, *VIM*↓,	*CDH2*↓, *SNAI1*↓	*CDH1*↑
Anoikis	*CASP8*↓, *BCL2*↓, *BCL2L1*↓, *EFGR*↓, *HIF1A*↓		*HIF1A*↑
Proliferation	*MKI67*↓, *PCNA*↓		*MKI67*↑

↑: significant upregulation in DEX-treated cells; ↓: significant downregulation in DEX-treated cells.

4.1. Cell Detachment in Microgravity and Epithelial–Mesenchymal Transition

The EMT describes a fundamental process of cancer progression when carcinoma cells lose their epithelial characteristics and acquire a migratory behavior, indicated by mesenchymal markers. This alteration enables them to escape from their epithelial cell community and invade into surrounding tissues, even at distant locations, and contributes to the acquisition and maintenance of stem cell-like properties [49,67]. In previous studies, DEX proved to suppress cell invasion in bladder cancer [68], inhibited hypoxia-induced EMT in colon cancer cells [69], and reduced TGF-β-induced EMT in non-malignant cells [70].

The interaction of DEX-bound GRs with NF-κB affects the expression of several target genes, one of which is TGF-β [71]. TGF-β induces the upregulation mesenchymal markers such as vimentin and downregulation of the epithelial marker E-cadherin, which are considered critical prerequisites for metastasis in numerous human cancers [72]. Therefore, it is not surprising that the expression of E-cadherin and β-catenin in thyroid cancer is associated with better prognosis [73]. Among the set of analyzed genes, *TGFB1* was regulated differently in µ*g* and in the presence of DEX. Hinz [74] suggested that the TGF-β complex functions as an extracellular mechanosensory that can be activated by contractile forces that are transmitted by integrins. Indeed, µ*g* was identified as a possible cause changing TGF-β expression levels [75]. In four-hour cultures stacked on the RPM, the *TGFB1* mRNA was slightly elevated whereas in three-day cultures the mRNA level was attenuated, maybe due to missing forces in µg. DEX supplementation led to a slow downregulation of *TGFB1* expression in static cell cultures or in follicular thyroid cancer cells grown for four hours on the RPM (Figure S2C). This observation could be cell-type specific, as DEX increased *TGFB1* expression in prostate cancer and pancreatic ductal carcinoma cells [76,77]. TGF-β signaling is identified as one of the most altered pathways in ovarian tumor spheroids [78] and cell aggregation proved to be induced by TGF-β in ovarian cancer cells [79]. Therefore, *TGFB1* could be a possible target gene for DEX that may inhibit spheroid formation of FTC-133 cells in an early culture stage at least in part by downregulation of *TGFB1*.

The translocation of β-catenin into the nucleus as well as upregulation of *FN1* mRNAs suggest an activation of the Wnt/β-catenin pathway after DEX supplementation. On the other hand, expression of Snail1 is reduced in the presence of DEX. However, in ovarian adenocarcinoma cells Snail1 is downregulated when TGF-β and Wnt signaling pathways are co-activated [80]. Snail1 acts as an EMT inducer and a potent repressor of E-cadherin [81,82]. The finding that E-cadherin expression correlates with spheroid formation capability suggests that intercellular adhesion plays a key role in 3D growth [83, 84]. Sahana et al. [85] found that the blocking of E-cadherin activity with antibodies promoted µg-driven spheroid formation of MCF-7 cells. Budding of ovarian cancer spheroids from monolayers correlated with the expression of vimentin and lack of cortical E-cadherin [86]. In our experiments the *CDH1* gene was downregulated in adherent cells but remained nearly unchanged in MCS cells of a three-day RPM culture. E-cadherin protein increased after DEX supplementation. This finding is consistent with the observations of Sahana et al. [85] and suggests a quantity-dependent influence of E-cadherin on cancer cell aggregation, that is not directly related to its mRNA synthesis. For renal cell carcinoma, N-cadherin was shown not to be an essential molecule for spheroid formation indicating a somewhat different role from cell–cell adhesion. However, anti-N-cadherin antibodies inhibit spheroid formation in a renal cell carcinoma cell line that expressed N-cadherin alone [87]. Tsai et al. [88] suggested that N-cadherin might play a role in the formation and maintenance of spheroid core structures. Due to a higher affinity of N-cadherin to form homodimers [89], cells with higher N-cadherin expression aggregate first. Indeed, in the spheroid-inducing environment of the RPM, the *CDH2* gene was upregulated after four hours (Figure S3B). DEX reduced *CDH2* expression in these cells as well as in spheroids after three days. This explains the reduced spheroid formation in the presence of DEX, but on the other hand, it suggests a destabilization of formed spheroids.

Fibronectin was downregulated in µg, but upregulated by DEX, in three-day cultures. Thus, it was the only mesenchymal factor showing a significantly altered regulation after DEX supplementation. Abu-Absi et al. [66] previously reported an increase in fibronectin and collagen III mRNA when rat hepatocytes were cultured in spinner flasks in the presence of DEX and suggested that a modification of the extracellular matrix (ECM) contributes to the changes in morphology. It is further known that DEX treatment significantly increases the strength of cell–ECM adhesion in glioblastoma cells and thus decreases their motility [90]. Robinson et al. [91] confirmed in different experiments that fibronectin matrix assembly plays a key role in cell aggregation and spheroid formation. So, it is very likely that DEX alters the ECM composition of FTC-133 cells, including fibronectin, in a way that they are no longer susceptible to 3D aggregation in µg.

Our data indicate that FTC-133 cells were not shifted to a typical mesenchymal phenotype during spheroid formation on the RPM and the phenotype was not strongly influenced by DEX. However, the results confirm the involvement of the Wnt/β-catenin axis and TGF-β-induced signaling in µg-triggered spheroid formation ability. These pathways were affected by DEX and can regulate some individual adhesion and matrix proteins (e.g., E-cadherin and fibronectin) which are important for detachment and 3D aggregation.

4.2. Survival of Detached Cells

At least for adherently growing FTC-133 cells, a cell-based assay showed no apoptotic cells after DEX treatment. For osteoblasts it is known that DEX can cause anoikis, probably due to the decreased integrin β1 expression [92]. In our experiments, indeed we found a downregulation of *ITGB1* transcription in DEX-treated cells as well as lower integrin β1 levels in MCS cells that grew in the presence of DEX (Figure S5).

The induction of anoikis occurs through an interplay of the two apoptotic pathways involving activation of caspase-8 and inhibition of Bcl-2 [26]. Caspase-8 expression was only marginally affected by μg and DEX treatment. We observed a counter-regulation for enhanced *CASP8* mRNA synthesis by DEX in cells after four hours on the RPM (Figure S4A). DEX significantly reduced expression of the anti-apoptotic *BCL2* gene in FTC-133 cells but stimulated the expression of the anti-apoptotic Bcl-xL. An upregulation of Bcl-xL expression by DEX was reported earlier for follicular thyroid cancer cells where it promotes survival [93]. That Bcl-2 plays an important role in the efficacy of DEX was confirmed in a study with myeloma cells where Bcl-2 overexpression was associated with resistance to DEX [94]. Overexpression of Bcl-2 correlates with the progression and metastasis of prostate cancer [95] and was shown to inhibit anoikis at least in intestinal epithelial cells [96]. Looking at apoptosis signaling, there are a some, but not all, indications that anoikis can be induced in FTC-133 cells after DEX treatment.

Apart from the apoptotic pathways, there are other proteins playing important roles in the complex network of survival signaling. It has been reported that inhibition of E-cadherin binding prevented cell–cell aggregation and could induce anoikis in epithelial cells [97,98]. In addition, the overexpression of β-catenin, a downstream regulator of cadherin signaling, resulted in anoikis resistance [99]. Indeed, on the transcriptional level we saw a DEX-mediated downregulation of *CDH1* together with an upregulation of *CTNNB1* in MCS cells.

The integral membrane protein caveolin-1 was identified as an important factor in spheroid formation of thyroid cancer cells in an μg environment [65,100] which further inhibits anchorage-independent growth and anoikis, obviously two independent processes, in MCF-7 breast cancer cells [61]. The *CAV1* gene was downregulated when FTC-133 cells formed MCS on an RPM [100]. We were able to confirm this effect in our experiments. The upregulation of *CAV1* expression in the presence of DEX may suppress caveolin's yet undefined effects on 3D aggregation of thyroid carcinoma cells. Interestingly, caveolin-1 is overexpressed in other metastatic carcinoma cells where it promotes growth [101,102] and resistance to anoikis [61]. Caveolin-1 controls the stability of focal adhesions and contributes to mechanosensing and adaptation in response to mechanical stimuli including cell detachment [103]. Moreno-Vicente et al. [104] demonstrated that caveolin-1 regulates yes-associated protein activity which in turn modulates pathophysiological processes such as ECM remodeling. The authors suggested that this regulation could determine the onset and progression of tumor development. A possible explanation for suppressed spheroid formation would be that a more rigid ECM inhibits the growth into 3D aggregates.

In summary, we found regulatory indications but no clear evidence of anoikis after DEX treatment, as both caspase-3 cleavage and TUNEL staining were negative. Therefore, we suggest that apoptosis does not play a (major) role in inhibition of FTC-133 spheroid formation by DEX.

4.3. Autocrine Signaling

Growth factors have been considered to be involved in spheroid formation of thyroid cancer cells for long time. During the Shenzhou-8 space experiment, extraordinarily large 3D aggregates were formed by FTC-133 cells which showed an altered expression of *EGF* and *CTGF* genes under real μg [105]. A decreased expression of *CTGF* in MCS compared to an increased expression in adherent cells was observed after cultivation of FTC-133 on different μg-devices suggesting an important role for CTGF in spheroid formation [65]. DEX supplementation resulted in an upregulation of *CTGF* mRNA synthesis. In vitro, CTGF was identified to stimulate ECM synthesis, proliferation, or integrin expression and has been implicated in different cancer-related processes, comprising migration, invasion, angiogenesis, and anoikis [46]. Elevated *CTGF* expression levels in primary papillary thyroid carcinoma samples were correlated with metastasis [106]. EGF acts as a strong mitogen for follicular thyroid cells [47] and has been shown to increase the spheroid size in various tumor cell lines [107–109]. Both, DEX and µ*g* reduced *EGF* expression. However, CTGF upregulation and EGF downregulation by DEX cannot explain the inhibition of spheroid formation, especially since adherent cells on the RPM are able to form MCS but show the same gene regulations.

VEGF promotes tumor angiogenesis by stimulating proliferation and survival of endothelial cells and can directly modulate cancer cell behavior [110]. Studies have shown that VEGF expression is upregulated in most human tumors and correlates with the risk for the development of metastasis in papillary thyroid cancer [111,112]. VEGF expression can be upregulated in response to hypoxia and was found in the microenvironment of tumor spheroids formed by HT-29 human colon cancer cells [113]. Furthermore, spheroids formed by FTC-133 cells on an RPM showed an increase in *VEGFA* gene expression [52]. Inhibition of VEGF signaling significantly reduced cell viability of thyroid cancer cells and increased apoptosis in the NPA'87 tumor-derived cell line [114]. DEX was reported to reduce VEGF secretion in some head and neck cancer cells via STAT3 [115]. We can confirm a decreasing effect of DEX on *VEGFA* expression in FTC-133 cells, independently of their exposure to µ*g* or their growth behavior on the RPM. A decrease in VEGF-A by treatment using siRNA or anti-VEGF-A, reduced spheroid formation, proliferation, migration, and invasion of epidermal cancer stem cells [116]. This finding highlights the role of VEGF (signaling) in the formation of solid tumors and could also provide an explanation for the effect of DEX on FTC-133 cells. In T47D breast cancer cells, DEX was shown to affect the PI3K/AKT/mTOR pathway [117] that could also be a possible target in thyroid cancer cells responsible for the suppression of spheroid formation [118].

5. Conclusions

In our study, DEX suppressed spheroid formation of FTC-133 cells cultured on an RPM in a dose-dependent manner. Interestingly, DEX did not influence NF-κB in a way that would explain the inhibition of µ*g*-triggered spheroid formation indicating that NF-κB (pathway) may not be the main target of DEX in FTC-133 cells. However, transcriptional regulation of important individual factors in cancer cell biology, which were previously suggested to play a role in spheroid formation, was clearly affected by DEX. Thereby, our data indicate the presence of a more complex regulation network of spheroid formation also involving other signal pathways, such as Wnt/β-catenin and TGF-β, that regulate adhesion and matrix proteins which are important for cell detachment and 3D growth. According to our results, it will be necessary to carry out a broad transcriptome analysis in order to identify the exact influence of DEX on the growth behavior of follicular thyroid cancer cells. Furthermore, it needs to be clarified whether DEX not only inhibits formation of spheroids but also promotes their disassembly in µ*g*.

Author Contributions: Conceptualization, D.M., M.K., and D.G.; methodology, D.M., J.S., and T.J.C.; software, D.M.; validation, D.M., M.K., and S.K.; formal analysis, D.M.; investigation, D.M., M.K., T.J.C., and M.Z.N.; resources, M.I. and T.J.C.; data curation, D.M., M.K., S.K., and D.G.; writing—original draft preparation, M.K. and D.M.; writing—review and editing, M.K., D.G., S.K., T.J.C., and M.W.; visualization, D.M. and M.K.; supervision, D.G. and M.K.; project administration, D.G.; funding acquisition, D.G. and M.I. All authors have read and agreed to the published version of the manuscript.

Acknowledgments: The authors would like to thank the Institute of Anatomy (Otto von Guericke University), especially Stefan Kahlert and Andrea Kröber, for the technical support. We also acknowledge financial support by the Open Access Publication Fonds of the Otto von Guericke University Magdeburg.

References

1. Kadmiel, M.; Cidlowski, J.A. Glucocorticoid receptor signaling in health and disease. *Trends Pharmacol. Sci.* **2013**, *34*, 518–530. [CrossRef] [PubMed]
2. Mangelsdorf, D.J.; Thummel, C.; Beato, M.; Herrlich, P.; Schütz, G.; Umesono, K.; Blumberg, B.; Kastner, P.; Mark, M.; Chambon, P.; et al. The nuclear receptor superfamily: The second decade. *Cell* **1995**, *83*, 835–839. [CrossRef]
3. Coutinho, A.E.; Chapman, K.E. The anti-inflammatory and immunosuppressive effects of glucocorticoids, recent developments and mechanistic insights. *Mol. Cell. Endocrinol.* **2011**, *335*, 2–13. [CrossRef]
4. Vandevyver, S.; Dejager, L.; Tuckermann, J.; Libert, C. New insights into the anti-inflammatory mechanisms of glucocorticoids: An emerging role for glucocorticoid-receptor-mediated transactivation. *Endocrinology* **2013**, *154*, 993–1007. [CrossRef]
5. Vandewalle, J.; Luypaert, A.; De Bosscher, K.; Libert, C. Therapeutic mechanisms of glucocorticoids. *Trends Endocrinol. Metab.* **2018**, *29*, 42–54. [CrossRef]
6. Herr, I.; Pfitzenmaier, J. Glucocorticoid use in prostate cancer and other solid tumours: Implications for effectiveness of cytotoxic treatment and metastases. *Lancet Oncol.* **2006**, *7*, 425–430. [CrossRef]
7. Wang, H.; Wang, Y.; Rayburn, E.R.; Hill, D.L.; Rinehart, J.J.; Zhang, R. Dexamethasone as a chemosensitizer for breast cancer chemotherapy: Potentiation of the antitumor activity of adriamycin, modulation of cytokine expression, and pharmacokinetics. *Int. J. Oncol.* **2007**, *30*, 947–953. [CrossRef]
8. Yennurajalingam, S.; Frisbee-Hume, S.; Palmer, J.L.; Delgado-Guay, M.O.; Bull, J.; Phan, A.T.; Tannir, N.M.; Litton, J.K.; Reddy, A.; Hui, D.; et al. Reduction of cancer-related fatigue with dexamethasone: A double-blind, randomized, placebo-controlled trial in patients with advanced cancer. *J. Clin. Oncol.* **2013**, *31*, 3076–3082. [CrossRef]
9. Wang, L.J.; Li, J.; Hao, F.R.; Yuan, Y.; Li, J.Y.; Lu, W.; Zhou, T.Y. Dexamethasone suppresses the growth of human non-small cell lung cancer via inducing estrogen sulfotransferase and inactivating estrogen. *Acta Pharmacol. Sin.* **2016**, *37*, 845–856. [CrossRef]
10. Lin, K.-T.; Sun, S.-P.; Wu, J.-I.; Wang, L.-H. Low-dose glucocorticoids suppresses ovarian tumor growth and metastasis in an immunocompetent syngeneic mouse model. *PLoS ONE* **2017**, *12*, e0178937. [CrossRef]
11. Gong, H.; Jarzynka, M.J.; Cole, T.J.; Lee, J.H.; Wada, T.; Zhang, B.; Gao, J.; Song, W.C.; DeFranco, D.B.; Cheng, S.Y.; et al. Glucocorticoids antagonize estrogens by glucocorticoid receptor-mediated activation of estrogen sulfotransferase. *Cancer Res.* **2008**, *68*, 7386–7393. [CrossRef] [PubMed]
12. Geng, Y.; Wang, J.; Jing, H.; Wang, H.W.; Bao, Y.X. Inhibitory effect of dexamethasone on lewis mice lung cancer cells. *Genet. Mol. Res.* **2014**, *13*, 6827–6836. [CrossRef] [PubMed]
13. Moon, E.Y.; Ryu, Y.K.; Lee, G.H. Dexamethasone inhibits in vivo tumor growth by the alteration of bone marrow cd11b(+) myeloid cells. *Int. Immunopharmacol.* **2014**, *21*, 494–500. [CrossRef] [PubMed]
14. Sau, S.; Banerjee, R. Cationic lipid-conjugated dexamethasone as a selective antitumor agent. *Eur. J. Med. Chem.* **2014**, *83*, 433–447. [CrossRef] [PubMed]
15. Komiya, A.; Shimbo, M.; Suzuki, H.; Imamoto, T.; Kato, T.; Fukasawa, S.; Kamiya, N.; Naya, Y.; Mori, I.; Ichikawa, T. Oral low-dose dexamethasone for androgen-independent prostate cancer patients. *Oncol. Lett.* **2010**, *1*, 73–79. [CrossRef] [PubMed]
16. Bray, F.; Ferlay, J.; Soerjomataram, I.; Siegel, R.L.; Torre, L.A.; Jemal, A. Global cancer statistics 2018: Globocan estimates of incidence and mortality worldwide for 36 cancers in 185 countries. *CA* **2018**, *68*, 394–424. [CrossRef]
17. Kim, J.; Gosnell, J.E.; Roman, S.A. Geographic influences in the global rise of thyroid cancer. *Nat. Rev. Endocrinol.* **2019**, *16*, 17–29. [CrossRef]
18. Pachmayr, E.; Treese, C.; Stein, U. Underlying mechanisms for distant metastasis—Molecular biology. *Visc. Med.* **2017**, *33*, 11–20. [CrossRef]
19. Yilmaz, M.; Christofori, G. Mechanisms of motility in metastasizing cells. *Mol. Cancer Res.* **2010**, *8*, 629–642. [CrossRef]
20. Paszek, M.J.; Zahir, N.; Johnson, K.R.; Lakins, J.N.; Rozenberg, G.I.; Gefen, A.; Reinhart-King, C.A.; Margulies, S.S.; Dembo, M.; Boettiger, D.; et al. Tensional homeostasis and the malignant phenotype. *Cancer Cell* **2005**, *8*, 241–254. [CrossRef]

21. Moore, S.W.; Roca-Cusachs, P.; Sheetz, M.P. Stretchy proteins on stretchy substrates: The important elements of integrin-mediated rigidity sensing. *Dev. Cell* **2010**, *19*, 194–206. [CrossRef] [PubMed]
22. Roussos, E.T.; Condeelis, J.S.; Patsialou, A. Chemotaxis in cancer. *Nat. Rev. Cancer* **2011**, *11*, 573–587. [CrossRef] [PubMed]
23. Brabletz, T.; Kalluri, R.; Nieto, M.A.; Weinberg, R.A. Emt in cancer. *Nat. Rev. Cancer* **2018**, *18*, 128–134. [CrossRef] [PubMed]
24. Yu, W.; Yang, L.; Li, T.; Zhang, Y. Cadherin signaling in cancer: Its functions and role as a therapeutic target. *Front. Oncol.* **2019**, *9*, 989. [CrossRef]
25. Taddei, M.L.; Giannoni, E.; Fiaschi, T.; Chiarugi, P. Anoikis: An emerging hallmark in health and diseases. *J. Pathol.* **2012**, *226*, 380–393. [CrossRef]
26. Paoli, P.; Giannoni, E.; Chiarugi, P. Anoikis molecular pathways and its role in cancer progression. *Biochim. Biophys. Acta* **2013**, *1833*, 3481–3498. [CrossRef]
27. Chang, T.T.; Hughes-Fulford, M. Molecular mechanisms underlying the enhanced functions of three-dimensional hepatocyte aggregates. *Biomaterials* **2014**, *35*, 2162–2171. [CrossRef]
28. Kopp, S.; Warnke, E.; Wehland, M.; Aleshcheva, G.; Magnusson, N.E.; Hemmersbach, R.; Corydon, T.J.; Bauer, J.; Infanger, M.; Grimm, D. Mechanisms of three-dimensional growth of thyroid cells during long-term simulated microgravity. *Sci. Rep.* **2015**, *5*, 16691. [CrossRef]
29. Kunz-Schughart, L.A. Multicellular tumor spheroids: Intermediates between monolayer culture and in vivo tumor. *Cell Biol. Int.* **1999**, *23*, 157–161. [CrossRef]
30. Martin, A.; Zhou, A.; Gordon, R.E.; Henderson, S.C.; Schwartz, A.E.; Schwartz, A.E.; Friedman, E.W.; Davies, T.F. Thyroid organoid formation in simulated microgravity: Influence of keratinocyte growth factor. *Thyroid* **2000**, *10*, 481–487. [CrossRef] [PubMed]
31. Bauer, J.; Grimm, D.; Gombocz, E. Semantic analysis of thyroid cancer cell proteins obtained from rare research opportunities. *J. Biomed. Inf.* **2017**, *76*, 138–153. [CrossRef] [PubMed]
32. Bauer, J.; Wehland, M.; Infanger, M.; Grimm, D.; Gombocz, E. Semantic analysis of posttranslational modification of proteins accumulated in thyroid cancer cells exposed to simulated microgravity. *Int. J. Mol. Sci.* **2018**, *19*, 2257. [CrossRef] [PubMed]
33. Krüger, M.; Melnik, D.; Kopp, S.; Buken, C.; Sahana, J.; Bauer, J.; Wehland, M.; Hemmersbach, R.; Corydon, T.J.; Infanger, M.; et al. Fighting thyroid cancer with microgravity research. *Int. J. Mol. Sci.* **2019**, *20*, 2553. [CrossRef] [PubMed]
34. Kopp, S.; Sahana, J.; Islam, T.; Petersen, A.G.; Bauer, J.; Corydon, T.J.; Schulz, H.; Saar, K.; Huebner, N.; Slumstrup, L.; et al. The role of nfkappab in spheroid formation of human breast cancer cells cultured on the random positioning machine. *Sci. Rep.* **2018**, *8*, 921. [CrossRef]
35. Corydon, T.J.; Mann, V.; Slumstrup, L.; Kopp, S.; Sahana, J.; Askou, A.L.; Magnusson, N.E.; Echegoyen, D.; Bek, T.; Sundaresan, A.; et al. Reduced expression of cytoskeletal and extracellular matrix genes in human adult retinal pigment epithelium cells exposed to simulated microgravity. *Cell. Physiol. Biochem.* **2016**, *40*, 1–17. [CrossRef]
36. Grosse, J.; Wehland, M.; Pietsch, J.; Ma, X.; Ulbrich, C.; Schulz, H.; Saar, K.; Hübner, N.; Hauslage, J.; Hemmersbach, R.; et al. Short-term weightlessness produced by parabolic flight maneuvers altered gene expression patterns in human endothelial cells. *Faseb J.* **2012**, *26*, 639–655. [CrossRef]
37. Ma, X.; Pietsch, J.; Wehland, M.; Schulz, H.; Saar, K.; Hübner, N.; Bauer, J.; Braun, M.; Schwarzwälder, A.; Segerer, J.; et al. Differential gene expression profile and altered cytokine secretion of thyroid cancer cells in space. *Faseb J.* **2014**, *28*, 813–835. [CrossRef]
38. Ma, X.; Wehland, M.; Schulz, H.; Saar, K.; Hubner, N.; Infanger, M.; Bauer, J.; Grimm, D. Genomic approach to identify factors that drive the formation of three-dimensional structures by ea.Hy926 endothelial cells. *PLoS ONE* **2013**, *8*, e64402. [CrossRef]
39. Ye, J.; Coulouris, G.; Zaretskaya, I.; Cutcutache, I.; Rozen, S.; Madden, T.L. Primer-blast: A tool to design target-specific primers for polymerase chain reaction. *BMC Bioinform.* **2012**, *13*, 134. [CrossRef]
40. Grosse, J.; Wehland, M.; Pietsch, J.; Schulz, H.; Saar, K.; Hübner, N.; Eilles, C.; Bauer, J.; Abou-El-Ardat, K.; Baatout, S.; et al. Gravity-sensitive signaling drives 3-dimensional formation of multicellular thyroid cancer spheroids. *Faseb J.* **2012**, *26*, 5124–5140. [CrossRef]
41. Pacifico, F.; Leonardi, A. Role of nf-kappab in thyroid cancer. *Mol. Cell. Endocrinol.* **2010**, *321*, 29–35. [CrossRef] [PubMed]

42. Giuliani, C.; Bucci, I.; Napolitano, G. The role of the transcription factor nuclear factor-kappa b in thyroid autoimmunity and cancer. *Front. Endocrinol.* **2018**, *9*, 471. [CrossRef] [PubMed]
43. Bauerle, K.T.; Schweppe, R.E.; Haugen, B.R. Inhibition of nuclear factor-kappa b differentially affects thyroid cancer cell growth, apoptosis, and invasion. *Mol. Cancer* **2010**, *9*, 117. [CrossRef] [PubMed]
44. Yamamoto, Y.; Gaynor, R.B. Therapeutic potential of inhibition of the nf-kappab pathway in the treatment of inflammation and cancer. *J. Clin. Investig.* **2001**, *107*, 135–142. [CrossRef]
45. Holbourn, K.P.; Acharya, K.R.; Perbal, B. The ccn family of proteins: Structure-function relationships. *Trends Biochem. Sci.* **2008**, *33*, 461–473. [CrossRef]
46. Chu, C.Y.; Chang, C.C.; Prakash, E.; Kuo, M.L. Connective tissue growth factor (ctgf) and cancer progression. *J. Biomed. Sci.* **2008**, *15*, 675–685. [CrossRef]
47. Asmis, L.M.; Gerber, H.; Kaempf, J.; Studer, H. Epidermal growth factor stimulates cell proliferation and inhibits iodide uptake of frtl-5 cells in vitro. *J. Endocrinol.* **1995**, *145*, 513–520. [CrossRef]
48. Colletta, G.; Cirafici, A.M.; Di Carlo, A. Dual effect of transforming growth factor beta on rat thyroid cells: Inhibition of thyrotropin-induced proliferation and reduction of thyroid-specific differentiation markers. *Cancer Res.* **1989**, *49*, 3457–3462.
49. Xu, J.; Lamouille, S.; Derynck, R. Tgf-β-induced epithelial to mesenchymal transition. *Cell Res.* **2009**, *19*, 156–172. [CrossRef]
50. Gugnoni, M.; Sancisi, V.; Manzotti, G.; Gandolfi, G.; Ciarrocchi, A. Autophagy and epithelial-mesenchymal transition: An intricate interplay in cancer. *Cell Death Dis.* **2016**, *7*, e2520. [CrossRef]
51. Bhatti, M.Z.; Pan, L.; Wang, T.; Shi, P.; Li, L. Reggamma potentiates tgf-beta/smad signal dependent epithelial-mesenchymal transition in thyroid cancer cells. *Cell Signal.* **2019**, *64*, 109412. [CrossRef]
52. Riwaldt, S.; Bauer, J.; Wehland, M.; Slumstrup, L.; Kopp, S.; Warnke, E.; Dittrich, A.; Magnusson, N.E.; Pietsch, J.; Corydon, T.J.; et al. Pathways regulating spheroid formation of human follicular thyroid cancer cells under simulated microgravity conditions: A genetic approach. *Int. J. Mol. Sci.* **2016**, *17*, 528. [CrossRef]
53. Chung, Y.J.; Lee, J.I.; Chong, S.; Seok, J.W.; Park, S.J.; Jang, H.W.; Kim, S.W.; Chung, J.H. Anti-proliferative effect and action mechanism of dexamethasone in human medullary thyroid cancer cell line. *Endocr. Res.* **2011**, *36*, 149–157. [CrossRef]
54. Scholzen, T.; Gerdes, J. The ki-67 protein: From the known and the unknown. *J. Cell. Physiol.* **2000**, *182*, 311–322. [CrossRef]
55. Chen, Z.Y.; Guo, S.; Li, B.B.; Jiang, N.; Li, A.; Yan, H.F.; Yang, H.M.; Zhou, J.L.; Li, C.L.; Cui, Y. Effect of weightlessness on the 3d structure formation and physiologic function of human cancer cells. *Biomed. Res. Int.* **2019**, *2019*, 4894083. [CrossRef]
56. Da, C.; Wu, K.; Yue, C.; Bai, P.; Wang, R.; Wang, G.; Zhao, M.; Lv, Y.; Hou, P. N-cadherin promotes thyroid tumorigenesis through modulating major signaling pathways. *Oncotarget* **2017**, *8*, 8131–8142. [CrossRef]
57. Vasko, V.; Espinosa, A.V.; Scouten, W.; He, H.; Auer, H.; Liyanarachchi, S.; Larin, A.; Savchenko, V.; Francis, G.L.; de la Chapelle, A.; et al. Gene expression and functional evidence of epithelial-to-mesenchymal transition in papillary thyroid carcinoma invasion. *Proc. Natl. Acad. Sci. USA* **2007**, *104*, 2803–2808. [CrossRef]
58. Su, H.; Bidere, N.; Zheng, L.; Cubre, A.; Sakai, K.; Dale, J.; Salmena, L.; Hakem, R.; Straus, S.; Lenardo, M. Requirement for caspase-8 in nf-kappab activation by antigen receptor. *Science* **2005**, *307*, 1465–1468. [CrossRef]
59. Schott, A.F.; Apel, I.J.; Nuñez, G.; Clarke, M.F. Bcl-xl protects cancer cells from p53-mediated apoptosis. *Oncogene* **1995**, *11*, 1389–1394.
60. Li, M.; Wang, D.; He, J.; Chen, L.; Li, H. Bcl-xl: A multifunctional anti-apoptotic protein. *Pharmacol. Res.* **2020**, *151*, 104547. [CrossRef]
61. Fiucci, G.; Ravid, D.; Reich, R.; Liscovitch, M. Caveolin-1 inhibits anchorage-independent growth, anoikis and invasiveness in mcf-7 human breast cancer cells. *Oncogene* **2002**, *21*, 2365–2375. [CrossRef] [PubMed]
62. Reginato, M.J.; Mills, K.R.; Paulus, J.K.; Lynch, D.K.; Sgroi, D.C.; Debnath, J.; Muthuswamy, S.K.; Brugge, J.S. Integrins and egfr coordinately regulate the pro-apoptotic protein bim to prevent anoikis. *Nat. Cell Biol.* **2003**, *5*, 733–740. [CrossRef] [PubMed]
63. Rohwer, N.; Welzel, M.; Daskalow, K.; Pfander, D.; Wiedenmann, B.; Detjen, K.; Cramer, T. Hypoxia-inducible factor 1alpha mediates anoikis resistance via suppression of alpha5 integrin. *Cancer Res.* **2008**, *68*, 10113–10120. [CrossRef] [PubMed]

64. Riwaldt, S.; Pietsch, J.; Sickmann, A.; Bauer, J.; Braun, M.; Segerer, J.; Schwarzwälder, A.; Aleshcheva, G.; Corydon, T.J.; Infanger, M.; et al. Identification of proteins involved in inhibition of spheroid formation under microgravity. *Proteomics* **2015**, *15*, 2945–2952. [CrossRef]
65. Warnke, E.; Pietsch, J.; Wehland, M.; Bauer, J.; Infanger, M.; Görög, M.; Hemmersbach, R.; Braun, M.; Ma, X.; Sahana, J.; et al. Spheroid formation of human thyroid cancer cells under simulated microgravity: A possible role of ctgf and cav1. *Cell Commun. Signal.* **2014**, *12*, 32. [CrossRef]
66. Abu-Absi, S.F.; Hu, W.-S.; Hansen, L.K. Dexamethasone effects on rat hepatocyte spheroid formation and function. *Tissue Eng.* **2005**, *11*, 415–426. [CrossRef]
67. Thiery, J.P. Epithelial–mesenchymal transitions in tumour progression. *Nat. Rev. Cancer* **2002**, *2*, 442–454. [CrossRef]
68. Zheng, Y.; Izumi, K.; Li, Y.; Ishiguro, H.; Miyamoto, H. Contrary regulation of bladder cancer cell proliferation and invasion by dexamethasone-mediated glucocorticoid receptor signals. *Mol. Cancer Ther.* **2012**, *11*, 2621–2632. [CrossRef]
69. Kim, J.H.; Hwang, Y.-J.; Han, S.H.; Lee, Y.E.; Kim, S.; Kim, Y.J.; Cho, J.H.; Kwon, K.A.; Kim, J.H.; Kim, S.-H. Dexamethasone inhibits hypoxia-induced epithelial-mesenchymal transition in colon cancer. *World J. Gastroenterol.* **2015**, *21*, 9887–9899. [CrossRef]
70. Jang, Y.H.; Shin, H.S.; Sun Choi, H.; Ryu, E.S.; Jin Kim, M.; Ki Min, S.; Lee, J.H.; Kook Lee, H.; Kim, K.H.; Kang, D.H. Effects of dexamethasone on the tgf-beta1-induced epithelial-to-mesenchymal transition in human peritoneal mesothelial cells. *Lab. Investig.* **2013**, *93*, 194–206. [CrossRef]
71. Parrelli, J.M.; Meisler, N.; Cutroneo, K.R. Identification of a glucocorticoid response element in the human transforming growth factor beta 1 gene promoter. *Int. J. Biochem. Cell Biol.* **1998**, *30*, 623–627. [CrossRef]
72. Huber, M.A.; Kraut, N.; Beug, H. Molecular requirements for epithelial-mesenchymal transition during tumor progression. *Curr. Opin. Cell Biol.* **2005**, *17*, 548–558. [CrossRef]
73. Ivanova, K.; Ananiev, J.; Aleksandrova, E.; Ignatova, M.M.; Gulubova, M. Expression of e-cadherin/beta-catenin in epithelial carcinomas of the thyroid gland. *Open Access Maced. J. Med. Sci.* **2017**, *5*, 155–159. [CrossRef]
74. Hinz, B. The extracellular matrix and transforming growth factor-β1: Tale of a strained relationship. *Matrix Biol.* **2015**, *47*, 54–65. [CrossRef]
75. Beheshti, A.; Ray, S.; Fogle, H.; Berrios, D.; Costes, S.V. A microrna signature and tgf-β1 response were identified as the key master regulators for spaceflight response. *PLoS ONE* **2018**, *13*, e0199621. [CrossRef]
76. Li, Z.; Chen, Y.; Cao, D.; Wang, Y.; Chen, G.; Zhang, S.; Lu, J. Glucocorticoid up-regulates transforming growth factor-β (tgf-β) type ii receptor and enhances tgf-β signaling in human prostate cancer pc-3 cells. *Endocrinology* **2006**, *147*, 5259–5267. [CrossRef]
77. Liu, L.; Aleksandrowicz, E.; Schonsiegel, F.; Groner, D.; Bauer, N.; Nwaeburu, C.C.; Zhao, Z.; Gladkich, J.; Hoppe-Tichy, T.; Yefenof, E.; et al. Dexamethasone mediates pancreatic cancer progression by glucocorticoid receptor, tgfbeta and jnk/ap-1. *Cell Death Dis.* **2017**, *8*, e3064. [CrossRef]
78. Ameri, W.A.; Ahmed, I.; Al-Dasim, F.M.; Mohamoud, Y.A.; AlAzwani, I.K.; Malek, J.A.; Karedath, T. Tgf-β mediated cell adhesion dynamics and epithelial to mesenchymal transition in 3d and 2d ovarian cancer models. *Biorxiv* **2018**, 465617. [CrossRef]
79. Sodek, K.L.; Ringuette, M.J.; Brown, T.J. Compact spheroid formation by ovarian cancer cells is associated with contractile behavior and an invasive phenotype. *Int. J. Cancer* **2009**, *124*, 2060–2070. [CrossRef]
80. Mitra, T.; Roy, S.S. Co-activation of tgfβ and wnt signalling pathways abrogates emt in ovarian cancer cells. *Cell. Physiol. Biochem.* **2017**, *41*, 1336–1345. [CrossRef]
81. Peinado, H.; Olmeda, D.; Cano, A. Snail, zeb and bhlh factors in tumour progression: An alliance against the epithelial phenotype? *Nat. Rev. Cancer* **2007**, *7*, 415–428. [CrossRef] [PubMed]
82. Yook, J.I.; Li, X.Y.; Ota, I.; Fearon, E.R.; Weiss, S.J. Wnt-dependent regulation of the e-cadherin repressor snail. *J. Biol. Chem.* **2005**, *280*, 11740–11748. [CrossRef]
83. Lin, R.Z.; Chou, L.F.; Chien, C.C.; Chang, H.Y. Dynamic analysis of hepatoma spheroid formation: Roles of e-cadherin and beta1-integrin. *Cell Tissue Res.* **2006**, *324*, 411–422. [CrossRef] [PubMed]
84. Smyrek, I.; Mathew, B.; Fischer, S.C.; Lissek, S.M.; Becker, S.; Stelzer, E.H.K. E-cadherin, actin, microtubules and fak dominate different spheroid formation phases and important elements of tissue integrity. *Biol. Open* **2019**, *8*, bio037051. [CrossRef]

85. Sahana, J.; Nassef, M.Z.; Wehland, M.; Kopp, S.; Krüger, M.; Corydon, T.J.; Infanger, M.; Bauer, J.; Grimm, D. Decreased e-cadherin in mcf7 human breast cancer cells forming multicellular spheroids exposed to simulated microgravity. *Proteomics* **2018**, *18*, e1800015. [CrossRef]
86. Pease, J.C.; Brewer, M.; Tirnauer, J.S. Spontaneous spheroid budding from monolayers: A potential contribution to ovarian cancer dissemination. *Biol. Open* **2012**, *1*, 622–628. [CrossRef]
87. Shimazui, T.; Schalken, J.A.; Kawai, K.; Kawamoto, R.; van Bockhoven, A.; Oosterwijk, E.; Akaza, H. Role of complex cadherins in cell-cell adhesion evaluated by spheroid formation in renal cell carcinoma cell lines. *Oncol. Rep.* **2004**, *11*, 357–360. [CrossRef]
88. Tsai, C.-W.; Wang, J.-H.; Young, T.-H. Core/shell multicellular spheroids on chitosan as in vitro 3d coculture tumor models. *Artif. Cells Nanomed. Biotechnol.* **2018**, *46*, S651–S660. [CrossRef]
89. Katsamba, P.; Carroll, K.; Ahlsen, G.; Bahna, F.; Vendome, J.; Posy, S.; Rajebhosale, M.; Price, S.; Jessell, T.M.; Ben-Shaul, A.; et al. Linking molecular affinity and cellular specificity in cadherin-mediated adhesion. *Proc. Natl. Acad. Sci. USA* **2009**, *106*, 11594–11599. [CrossRef]
90. Shannon, S.; Vaca, C.; Jia, D.; Entersz, I.; Schaer, A.; Carcione, J.; Weaver, M.; Avidar, Y.; Pettit, R.; Nair, M.; et al. Dexamethasone-mediated activation of fibronectin matrix assembly reduces dispersal of primary human glioblastoma cells. *PLoS ONE* **2015**, *10*, e0135951. [CrossRef]
91. Robinson, E.E.; Foty, R.A.; Corbett, S.A. Fibronectin matrix assembly regulates $\alpha5\beta1$-mediated cell cohesion. *Mol. Biol. Cell* **2004**, *15*, 973–981. [CrossRef]
92. Naves, M.A.; Pereira, R.M.; Comodo, A.N.; de Alvarenga, E.L.; Caparbo, V.F.; Teixeira, V.P. Effect of dexamethasone on human osteoblasts in culture: Involvement of beta1 integrin and integrin-linked kinase. *Cell Biol. Int.* **2011**, *35*, 1147–1151. [CrossRef]
93. Petrella, A.; Ercolino, S.F.; Festa, M.; Gentilella, A.; Tosco, A.; Conzen, S.D.; Parente, L. Dexamethasone inhibits trail-induced apoptosis of thyroid cancer cells via bcl-xl induction. *Eur. J. Cancer* **2006**, *42*, 3287–3293. [CrossRef]
94. Gazitt, Y.; Fey, V.; Thomas, C.; Alvarez, R. Bcl-2 overexpression is associated with resistance to dexamethasone, but not melphalan, in multiple myeloma cells. *Int. J. Oncol.* **1998**, *13*, 397–405. [CrossRef]
95. Lin, Y.; Fukuchi, J.; Hiipakka, R.A.; Kokontis, J.M.; Xiang, J. Up-regulation of bcl-2 is required for the progression of prostate cancer cells from an androgen-dependent to an androgen-independent growth stage. *Cell Res.* **2007**, *17*, 531–536. [CrossRef]
96. Toruner, M.; Fernandez-Zapico, M.; Sha, J.J.; Pham, L.; Urrutia, R.; Egan, L.J. Antianoikis effect of nuclear factor-kappab through up-regulated expression of osteoprotegerin, bcl-2, and iap-1. *J. Biol. Chem.* **2006**, *281*, 8686–8696. [CrossRef]
97. Bergin, E.; Levine, J.S.; Koh, J.S.; Lieberthal, W. Mouse proximal tubular cell-cell adhesion inhibits apoptosis by a cadherin-dependent mechanism. *Am. J. Physiol. Renal Physiol.* **2000**, *278*, F758–F768. [CrossRef]
98. Kantak, S.S.; Kramer, R.H. E-cadherin regulates anchorage-independent growth and survival in oral squamous cell carcinoma cells. *J. Biol. Chem.* **1998**, *273*, 16953–16961. [CrossRef]
99. Orford, K.; Orford, C.C.; Byers, S.W. Exogenous expression of beta-catenin regulates contact inhibition, anchorage-independent growth, anoikis, and radiation-induced cell cycle arrest. *J. Cell. Biol.* **1999**, *146*, 855–868. [CrossRef]
100. Riwaldt, S.; Bauer, J.; Pietsch, J.; Braun, M.; Segerer, J.; Schwarzwälder, A.; Corydon, T.J.; Infanger, M.; Grimm, D. The importance of caveolin-1 as key-regulator of three-dimensional growth in thyroid cancer cells cultured under real and simulated microgravity conditions. *Int. J. Mol. Sci.* **2015**, *16*, 28296–28310. [CrossRef]
101. Liu, W.R.; Jin, L.; Tian, M.X.; Jiang, X.F.; Yang, L.X.; Ding, Z.B.; Shen, Y.H.; Peng, Y.F.; Gao, D.M.; Zhou, J.; et al. Caveolin-1 promotes tumor growth and metastasis via autophagy inhibition in hepatocellular carcinoma. *Clin. Res. Hepatol. Gastroenterol.* **2016**, *40*, 169–178. [CrossRef] [PubMed]
102. Chatterjee, M.; Ben-Josef, E.; Thomas, D.G.; Morgan, M.A.; Zalupski, M.M.; Khan, G.; Andrew Robinson, C.; Griffith, K.A.; Chen, C.-S.; Ludwig, T.; et al. Caveolin-1 is associated with tumor progression and confers a multi-modality resistance phenotype in pancreatic cancer. *Sci. Rep.* **2015**, *5*, 10867. [CrossRef] [PubMed]
103. Sinha, B.; Köster, D.; Ruez, R.; Gonnord, P.; Bastiani, M.; Abankwa, D.; Stan, R.V.; Butler-Browne, G.; Vedie, B.; Johannes, L.; et al. Cells respond to mechanical stress by rapid disassembly of caveolae. *Cell* **2011**, *144*, 402–413. [CrossRef] [PubMed]
104. Moreno-Vicente, R.; Pavon, D.M.; Martin-Padura, I.; Catala-Montoro, M.; Diez-Sanchez, A.; Quilez-Alvarez, A.; Lopez, J.A.; Sanchez-Alvarez, M.; Vazquez, J.; Strippoli, R.; et al. Caveolin-1 modulates mechanotransduction

responses to substrate stiffness through actin-dependent control of yap. *Cell Rep.* **2018**, *25*, 1622–1635.e1626. [CrossRef] [PubMed]

105. Pietsch, J.; Ma, X.; Wehland, M.; Aleshcheva, G.; Schwarzwälder, A.; Segerer, J.; Birlem, M.; Horn, A.; Bauer, J.; Infanger, M.; et al. Spheroid formation of human thyroid cancer cells in an automated culturing system during the shenzhou-8 space mission. *Biomaterials* **2013**, *34*, 7694–7705. [CrossRef]
106. Cui, L.; Zhang, Q.; Mao, Z.; Chen, J.; Wang, X.; Qu, J.; Zhang, J.; Jin, D. Ctgf is overexpressed in papillary thyroid carcinoma and promotes the growth of papillary thyroid cancer cells. *Tumour Biol.* **2011**, *32*, 721–728. [CrossRef]
107. Dufau, I.; Frongia, C.; Sicard, F.; Dedieu, L.; Cordelier, P.; Ausseil, F.; Ducommun, B.; Valette, A. Multicellular tumor spheroid model to evaluate spatio-temporal dynamics effect of chemotherapeutics: Application to the gemcitabine/chk1 inhibitor combination in pancreatic cancer. *BMC Cancer* **2012**, *12*, 15. [CrossRef]
108. Engebraaten, O.; Bjerkvig, R.; Pedersen, P.H.; Laerum, O.D. Effects of egf, bfgf, ngf and pdgf(bb) on cell proliferative, migratory and invasive capacities of human brain-tumour biopsies in vitro. *Int. J. Cancer* **1993**, *53*, 209–214. [CrossRef]
109. Mueller-Klieser, W. Three-dimensional cell cultures: From molecular mechanisms to clinical applications. *Am. J. Physiol.* **1997**, *273*, C1109–C1123. [CrossRef]
110. Lichtenberger, B.M.; Tan, P.K.; Niederleithner, H.; Ferrara, N.; Petzelbauer, P.; Sibilia, M. Autocrine vegf signaling synergizes with egfr in tumor cells to promote epithelial cancer development. *Cell* **2010**, *140*, 268–279. [CrossRef]
111. Klein, M.; Vignaud, J.M.; Hennequin, V.; Toussaint, B.; Bresler, L.; Plenat, F.; Leclere, J.; Duprez, A.; Weryha, G. Increased expression of the vascular endothelial growth factor is a pejorative prognosis marker in papillary thyroid carcinoma. *J. Clin. Endocrinol. Metab.* **2001**, *86*, 656–658. [CrossRef] [PubMed]
112. Karaca, Z.; Tanriverdi, F.; Unluhizarci, K.; Ozturk, F.; Gokahmetoglu, S.; Elbuken, G.; Cakir, I.; Bayram, F.; Kelestimur, F. Vegfr1 expression is related to lymph node metastasis and serum vegf may be a marker of progression in the follow-up of patients with differentiated thyroid carcinoma. *Eur. J. Endocrinol.* **2011**, *164*, 277–284. [CrossRef] [PubMed]
113. Waleh, N.S.; Brody, M.D.; Knapp, M.A.; Mendonca, H.L.; Lord, E.M.; Koch, C.J.; Laderoute, K.R.; Sutherland, R.M. Mapping of the vascular endothelial growth factor-producing hypoxic cells in multicellular tumor spheroids using a hypoxia-specific marker. *Cancer Res.* **1995**, *55*, 6222–6226. [PubMed]
114. Vieira, J.M.; Santos, S.C.; Espadinha, C.; Correia, I.; Vag, T.; Casalou, C.; Cavaco, B.M.; Catarino, A.L.; Dias, S.; Leite, V. Expression of vascular endothelial growth factor (vegf) and its receptors in thyroid carcinomas of follicular origin: A potential autocrine loop. *Eur. J. Endocrinol.* **2005**, *153*, 701–709. [CrossRef] [PubMed]
115. Shim, S.H.; Hah, J.H.; Hwang, S.Y.; Heo, D.S.; Sung, M.W. Dexamethasone treatment inhibits vegf production via suppression of stat3 in a head and neck cancer cell line. *Oncol. Rep.* **2010**, *23*, 1139–1143. [CrossRef]
116. Grun, D.; Adhikary, G.; Eckert, R.L. Vegf-a acts via neuropilin-1 to enhance epidermal cancer stem cell survival and formation of aggressive and highly vascularized tumors. *Oncogene* **2016**, *35*, 4379–4387. [CrossRef]
117. Meng, X.G.; Yue, S.W. Dexamethasone disrupts cytoskeleton organization and migration of t47d human breast cancer cells by modulating the akt/mtor/rhoa pathway. *Asian Pac. J. Cancer Prev.* **2014**, *15*, 10245–10250. [CrossRef]
118. Srivastava, A.; Kumar, A.; Giangiobbe, S.; Bonora, E.; Hemminki, K.; Forsti, A.; Bandapalli, O.R. Whole genome sequencing of familial non-medullary thyroid cancer identifies germline alterations in mapk/erk and pi3k/akt signaling pathways. *Biomolecules* **2019**, *9*, 605. [CrossRef]

Permissions

All chapters in this book were first published by MDPI; hereby published with permission under the Creative Commons Attribution License or equivalent. Every chapter published in this book has been scrutinized by our experts. Their significance has been extensively debated. The topics covered herein carry significant findings which will fuel the growth of the discipline. They may even be implemented as practical applications or may be referred to as a beginning point for another development.

The contributors of this book come from diverse backgrounds, making this book a truly international effort. This book will bring forth new frontiers with its revolutionizing research information and detailed analysis of the nascent developments around the world.

We would like to thank all the contributing authors for lending their expertise to make the book truly unique. They have played a crucial role in the development of this book. Without their invaluable contributions this book wouldn't have been possible. They have made vital efforts to compile up to date information on the varied aspects of this subject to make this book a valuable addition to the collection of many professionals and students.

This book was conceptualized with the vision of imparting up-to-date information and advanced data in this field. To ensure the same, a matchless editorial board was set up. Every individual on the board went through rigorous rounds of assessment to prove their worth. After which they invested a large part of their time researching and compiling the most relevant data for our readers.

The editorial board has been involved in producing this book since its inception. They have spent rigorous hours researching and exploring the diverse topics which have resulted in the successful publishing of this book. They have passed on their knowledge of decades through this book. To expedite this challenging task, the publisher supported the team at every step. A small team of assistant editors was also appointed to further simplify the editing procedure and attain best results for the readers.

Apart from the editorial board, the designing team has also invested a significant amount of their time in understanding the subject and creating the most relevant covers. They scrutinized every image to scout for the most suitable representation of the subject and create an appropriate cover for the book.

The publishing team has been an ardent support to the editorial, designing and production team. Their endless efforts to recruit the best for this project, has resulted in the accomplishment of this book. They are a veteran in the field of academics and their pool of knowledge is as vast as their experience in printing. Their expertise and guidance has proved useful at every step. Their uncompromising quality standards have made this book an exceptional effort. Their encouragement from time to time has been an inspiration for everyone.

The publisher and the editorial board hope that this book will prove to be a valuable piece of knowledge for researchers, students, practitioners and scholars across the globe.

List of Contributors

Mehreen Ahmed, Nicholas Jinks, Hossein Kashfi and Abdolrahman S. Nateri
Cancer Genetics & Stem Cell Group, BioDiscovery Institute, Division of Cancer and Stem Cells, School of Medicine, University of Nottingham, Nottingham NG7 2UH, UK

Roya Babaei-Jadidi
Cancer Genetics & Stem Cell Group, BioDiscovery Institute, Division of Cancer and Stem Cells, School of Medicine, University of Nottingham, Nottingham NG7 2UH, UK
Respiratory Medicine, School of Medicine, University of Nottingham, Nottingham NG7 2UH, UK

Marcos Castellanos Uribe and Sean T. May
Nottingham Arabidopsis Stock Centre (NASC), Plant Science Building, School of Biosciences, University of Nottingham, Loughborough LE12 5RD, UK

Abhik Mukherjee
Department of Histopathology, Queen's Medical Centre, School of Medicine, University of Nottingham, Nottingham NG7 2UH, UK

Ruowen Ge and Chieh Kao
Department of Biological Sciences, National University of Singapore, Singapore 117558, Singapore

Dasom Kim, Jangsun Hwang, Yonghyun Choi, Yejin Kwon, Jaehee Jang, Semi Yoon and Jonghoon Choi
School of Integrative Engineering, Chung-Ang University, Seoul 06974, Korea

Elisabeth S. Gruber, Gerd Jomrich, Sebastian F. Schoppmann and Michael Gnant
Division of General Surgery, Department of Surgery, Comprehensive Cancer Center, Medical University of Vienna, 1090 Vienna, Austria

Georg Oberhuber
Institute of Pathology, Department of Experimental and Translational Pathology, Medical University of Vienna, 1090 Vienna, Austria
PIZ—Patho im Zentrum GmbH, 3100 St. Poelten, Lower Austria, Austria

Peter Birner and Michaela Schlederer
Institute of Pathology, Department of Experimental and Translational Pathology, Medical University of Vienna, 1090 Vienna, Austria

Michael Kenn and Wolfgang Schreiner
Section of Biosimulation and Bioinformatics, Center for Medical Statistics, Informatics and Intelligent Systems (CeMSIIS), Medical University of Vienna, 1090 Vienna, Austria

William Tse
James Graham Brown Cancer Center, University of Louisville School of Medicine, Louisville, KY 40202, USA
Division of Blood and Bone Marrow Transplantation, Department of Medicine, University of Louisville School of Medicine, Louisville, KY 40202, USA

Lukas Kenner
Institute of Pathology, Department of Experimental and Translational Pathology, Medical University of Vienna, 1090 Vienna, Austria
Christian Doppler Laboratory for Applied Metabolomics (CDL-AM), Medical University of Vienna, 1090 Vienna, Austria
Institute of Laboratory Animal Pathology, University of Veterinary Medicine Vienna, 1210 Vienna, Austria
CBmed Core Lab 2, Medical University of Vienna, 1090 Vienna, Austria

Hack Sun Choi
School of Biomaterials Sciences and Technology, College of Applied Life Science, Jeju National University, Jeju 63243, Korea
Subtropical/tropical Organism Gene Bank, Jeju National University, Jeju 63243, Korea

Ji-Hyang Kim
Interdisciplinary Graduate Program in Advanced Convergence Technology & Science, Jeju National University, Jeju 63243, Korea

Su-Lim Kim
School of Biomaterials Sciences and Technology, College of Applied Life Science, Jeju National University, Jeju 63243, Korea
Interdisciplinary Graduate Program in Advanced Convergence Technology & Science, Jeju National University, Jeju 63243, Korea

Nastaran Khazamipour, Nader Al-Nakouzi, Htoo Zarni Oo, Maj Ørum-Madsen and Mads Daugaard
Department of Urologic Sciences, University of British Columbia, Vancouver, BC V5Z 1M9, Canada
Vancouver Prostate Centre, Vancouver, BC V6H 3Z6, Canada

Dong-Sun Lee
School of Biomaterials Sciences and Technology, College of Applied Life Science, Jeju National University, Jeju 63243, Korea
Subtropical/tropical Organism Gene Bank, Jeju National University, Jeju 63243, Korea
Interdisciplinary Graduate Program in Advanced Convergence Technology & Science, Jeju National University, Jeju 63243, Korea

Dusana Majera, Zdenek Skrott, Katarina Chroma and Martin Mistrik
Laboratory of Genome Integrity, Institute of Molecular and Translational Medicine, Faculty of Medicine and Dentistry, Palacky University, 77 147 Olomouc, Czech Republic

Joanna Maria Merchut-Maya
Danish Cancer Society Research Center, 2100 Copenhagen, Denmark

Joen Svindt
Department of Biology, University of Copenhagen, 1353 Copenhagen, Denmark

Jiri Bartek
Laboratory of Genome Integrity, Institute of Molecular and Translational Medicine, Faculty of Medicine and Dentistry, Palacky University, 77 147 Olomouc, Czech Republic
Danish Cancer Society Research Center, 2100 Copenhagen, Denmark
Division of Genome Biology, Department of Medical Biochemistry and Biophysics, Science for Life Laboratory, Karolinska Institute, 171 77 Stockholm, Sweden

Ditte Marie Brix
Cell Death and Metabolism, Center for Autophagy, Recycling and Disease, Danish Cancer Society Research Center, 2100 Copenhagen, Denmark
Danish Medicines Council, Dampfærgevej 27-29, 2100 Copenhagen, Denmark

Knut Kristoffer Bundgaard Clemmensen
Cell Death and Metabolism, Center for Autophagy, Recycling and Disease, Danish Cancer Society Research Center, 2100 Copenhagen, Denmark

Tuula Kallunki
Cell Death and Metabolism, Center for Autophagy, Recycling and Disease, Danish Cancer Society Research Center, 2100 Copenhagen, Denmark
Department of Drug Design and Pharmacology, Faculty of Health Sciences, University of Copenhagen, 2200 Copenhagen, Denmark

Olivier Peulen, Gilles Rademaker, Sandy Anania, Akeila Bellahcène and Vincent Castronovo
Metastasis Research Laboratory, Giga Cancer, University of Liège, B4000 Liège, Belgium

Andrei Turtoi
Tumor Microenvironment Laboratory, Institut de Recherche en Cancérologie de Montpellier, INSERM U1194, 34000 Montpellier, France
Institut du Cancer de Montpeiller, 34000 Montpellier, France
Université de Montpellier, 34000 Montpellier, France

Sophie E. B. Ambjørner, Xamuel Loft Lund and Michael Gajhede
Department of Drug Design and Pharmacology, University of Copenhagen, 1353 Copenhagen, Denmark

Michael Wiese and Sebastian Christoph Köhler
Pharmaceutical Institute, University of Bonn, 53012 Bonn, Germany

Lasse Saaby and Birger Brodin
Department of Pharmacy, University of Copenhagen, 1353 Copenhagen, Denmark

Steffen Rump
SRConsulting, 31319 Sehnde, Germany

Henning Weigt
Division of Chemical Safety and Toxicity, Fraunhofer Institute of Toxicology and Experimental Medicine, 30625 Hannover, Germany

Nils Brünner and Jan Stenvang
Department of Drug Design and Pharmacology, University of Copenhagen, 1353 Copenhagen, Denmark
Scandion Oncology A/S, Symbion, 1353 Copenhagen, Denmark

Karina Smorodinsky-Atias and Nadine Soudah
Department of Biological Chemistry, The Institute of Life Science, The Hebrew University of Jerusalem, Jerusalem 91904, Israel

David Engelberg
Department of Biological Chemistry, The Institute of Life Science, The Hebrew University of Jerusalem, Jerusalem 91904, Israel
CREATE-NUS-HUJ, Molecular Mechanisms Underlying Inflammatory Diseases (MMID), National University of Singapore, 1 CREATEWAY, Innovation Wing, Singapore 138602, Singapore
Department of Microbiology, Yong Loo Lin School of Medicine, National University of Singapore, Singapore 117456, Singapore

Anne Steino
Vancouver Prostate Centre, Vancouver, BC V6H 3Z6, Canada
Department of Pathology and Laboratory Medicine, University of British Columbia, Vancouver, BC V5Z 1M9, Canada

Poul H Sorensen
Department of Pathology and Laboratory Medicine, University of British Columbia, Vancouver, BC V5Z 1M9, Canada
Department of Molecular Oncology, British Columbia Cancer Research Centre, Vancouver, BC V5Z1L3, Canada

Charles Robert Lichtenstern, Rachael Katie Ngu and Shabnam Shalapour
Department of Pharmacology, School of Medicine, University of California, San Diego, La Jolla, CA 92093, USA
Laboratory of Gene Regulation and Signal Transduction, Department of Pharmacology, School of Medicine, University of California, San Diego, La Jolla, CA 92093, USA

Michael Karin
Department of Pharmacology, School of Medicine, University of California, San Diego, La Jolla, CA 92093, USA
Laboratory of Gene Regulation and Signal Transduction, Department of Pharmacology, School of Medicine, University of California, San Diego, La Jolla, CA 92093, USA
Moores Cancer Center, University of California, San Diego, La Jolla, CA 92093, USA

Daniela Melnik and Mohamed Zakaria Nassef
Clinic for Plastic, Aesthetic and Hand Surgery, Otto von Guericke University, Leipziger Str. 44, 39120 Magdeburg, Germany

Jayashree Sahana
Department of Biomedicine, Aarhus University, Hoegh-Guldbergsgade 10, 8000 Aarhus C, Denmark

Thomas J. Corydon
Department of Biomedicine, Aarhus University, Hoegh-Guldbergsgade 10, 8000 Aarhus C, Denmark
Department of Ophthalmology, Aarhus University Hospital, Palle Juul-Jensens Boulevard 99, 8200 Aarhus N, Denmark

Sascha Kopp, Markus Wehland, Manfred Infanger and Marcus Krüger
Clinic for Plastic, Aesthetic and Hand Surgery, Otto von Guericke University, Leipziger Str. 44, 39120 Magdeburg, Germany
Research Group "Magdeburger Arbeitsgemeinschaft für Forschung unter Raumfahrt- und Schwerelosigkeitsbedingungen" (MARS), Otto von Guericke University, Universitätsplatz 2, 39106 Magdeburg, Germany

Daniela Grimm
Department of Biomedicine, Aarhus University, Hoegh-Guldbergsgade 10, 8000 Aarhus C, Denmark
Research Group "Magdeburger Arbeitsgemeinschaft für Forschung unter Raumfahrt- und Schwerelosigkeitsbedingungen" (MARS), Otto von Guericke University, Universitätsplatz 2, 39106 Magdeburg, Germany
Department of Microgravity and Translational Regenerative Medicine, Otto von Guericke University, Pfälzer Platz, 39106 Magdeburg, Germany

Index

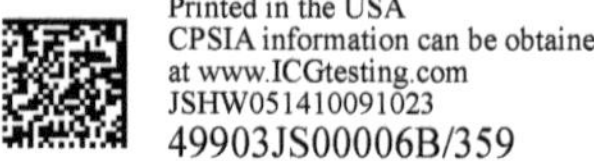

Printed in the USA
CPSIA information can be obtained
at www.ICGtesting.com
JSHW051410091023
49903JS00006B/359